T0289395

Managing Difficult Problems in Hand Surgery: Challenges, Complications, and Revisions

Editor

SONU A. JAIN

HAND CLINICS

www.hand.theclinics.com

Consulting Editor
KEVIN C. CHUNG

August 2023 • Volume 39 • Number 3

ELSEVIER

1600 John F. Kennedy Boulevard ● Suite 1800 ● Philadelphia, Pennsylvania, 19103-2899

http://www.theclinics.com

HAND CLINICS Volume 39, Number 3
August 2023 ISSN 0749-0712, ISBN-13: 978-0-323-94005-4

Editor: Megan Ashdown
Developmental Editor: Hannah Almira Lopez

Hand Clinics (ISSN 0749-0712) is published quarterly by Elsevier Inc., 360 Park Avenue South, New York, NY 10010-1710. Months of publication are February, May, August, and November. Business and Editorial Offices: 1600 John F. Kennedy Blvd., Ste. 1800, Philadelphia, PA 19103-2899. Customer Service Office: 3251 Riverport Lane, Maryland Heights, MO 63043. Periodicals postage paid at New York, NY and at additional mailing offices. Subscription price is $444.00 per year (domestic individuals), $878.00 per year (domestic institutions), $100.00 per year (domestic students/residents), $506.00 per year (Canadian individuals), $1023.00 per year (Canadian institutions), $568.00 per year (international individuals), $1023.00 per year (international institutions), $256.00 (international students/residents), and $100.00 (Canadian students/residents). Foreign air speed delivery is included in all *Clinics* subscription prices. All prices are subject to change without notice. **POSTMASTER:** Send address changes to *Hand Clinics*, Elsevier Health Sciences Division, Subscription Customer Service, 3251 Riverport Lane, Maryland Heights, MO 63043. Customer Service (orders, claims, online, change of address): Elsevier Health Sciences Division, Subscription **Customer Service, 3251 Riverport Lane, Maryland Heights, MO 63043. Tel: 1-800-654-2452 (U.S. and Canada); 314-447-8871 (outside U.S. and Canada). Fax: 314-447-8029. E-mail: journalscustomerservice-usa@elsevier.com (for print support); journalsonlinesupport-usa@elsevier.com (for online support).**

Reprints. For copies of 100 or more of articles in this publication, please contact the Commercial Reprints Department, Elsevier Inc., 360 Park Avenue South, New York, New York 10010-1710. Tel.: 212-633-3874; Fax: 212-633-3820; E-mail: reprints@elsevier.com.

Hand Clinics is covered in *MEDLINE/PubMed (Index Medicus), Current Contents/Clinical Medicine, EMBASE/Excerpta Medica,* and *ISI/BIOMED.*

Contributors

CONSULTING EDITOR

KEVIN C. CHUNG, MD, MS
Charles B.G. de Nancrede Professor of Surgery, Professor of Plastic Surgery and Orthopaedic Surgery, Chief of Hand Surgery, Department of Surgery, Section of Plastic Surgery, Michigan Medicine, Assistant Dean for Faculty Affairs, Associate Director of Global REACH, University of Michigan Medical School, Comprehensive Hand Center, University of Michigan, The University of Michigan Health System, Ann Arbor, Michigan, USA

EDITOR

SONU A. JAIN, MD
Professor of Plastic Surgery and Orthopaedics, Associate Program Director, Hand and Upper Extremity Surgery Fellowship, Associate Director, Hand and Upper Extremity Center, Chief, Division of Hand Surgery, Department of Plastic and Reconstructive Surgery, The Ohio State University Wexner Medical Center, Columbus, Ohio

AUTHORS

ANDREW D. ALLEN, MD
Resident Physician, Department of Orthopaedics, University of North Carolina School of Medicine, Chapel Hill, North Carolina, USA

HISHAM AWAN, MD
Director, OSU Hand and Upper Extremity Center, Professor of Orthopaedic Surgery, Program Director, Hand and Upper Extremity Fellowship, Chief, Orthopaedic Hand Surgery, Columbus, Ohio, USA

ABHIRAM R. BHASHYAM, MD, PhD
Hand and Upper Extremity Surgeon, Department of Orthopaedic Surgery, Massachusetts General Hospital, Assistant Professor of Orthopaedic Surgery, Harvard Medical School, Boston, Massachusetts, USA

REENA BHATT, MD
Associate Professor, Division of Plastic Surgery, The Warren Alpert Medical School of Brown University

DAVID J. BOZENTKA, MD
Professor of Orthopaedic Surgery, Chief, Hand Surgery, Hospital of the University of Pennsylvania, Philadelphia, Pennsylvania, USA

RONALD D. BROWN, MD
Assistant Professor, Department of Plastic and Reconstructive Surgery, The Ohio State University Hand and Upper Extremity Center, The Ohio State University, Columbus, Ohio, USA

NEAL C. CHEN, MD
Chief, Hand and Arm Center Department of Orthopaedic Surgery, Massachusetts General Hospital, Associate Professor, Harvard Medical School, Director, Hand Fellowship Program, Boston, Massachusetts, USA

KYLE J. CHEPLA, MD
Division of Plastic Surgery, MetroHealth Hospital, Columbus, Ohio, USA

KEVIN C. CHUNG, MD, MS
Charles B.G. de Nancrede Professor of
Surgery, Professor of Plastic Surgery and
Orthopaedic Surgery, Chief of Hand Surgery,
Department of Surgery, Section of Plastic
Surgery, Michigan Medicine, Assistant Dean
for Faculty Affairs, Associate Director of Global
REACH, University of Michigan Medical
School, Comprehensive Hand Center,
University of Michigan, The University of
Michigan Health System, Ann Arbor, Michigan,
USA

SZE RYN CHUNG, MBBCh, BAO, MRCS
Consultant, Department of Hand and
Reconstructive Microsurgery, Singapore
General Hospital, Singapore

R ADAMS COWLEY II, MD
Department of Orthopaedic Surgery, MedStar
Georgetown University Hospital, Georgetown
University School of Medicine, Washington,
DC, USA

NISHA CROUSER, MD
Department of Orthopaedics, The Ohio State
University Wexner Medical Center

REID W. DRAEGER, MD
Associate Professor, Department of
Orthopaedics, University of North Carolina
School of Medicine, Chapel Hill, North
Carolina, USA

CHRISTOPHER J. DY, MD, MPH
Department of Orthopaedic Surgery,
Washington University in St. Louis, St Louis,
Missouri, USA

KANU GOYAL, MD
Division of Hand Surgery, Department of
Orthopaedic Surgery, The Ohio State
University Wexner Medical Center, Columbus,
Ohio, USA

AMIT GUPTA, MD, FRCS
Clinical Professor, Department of Orthopedic
Surgery, University of Louisville, Director,
Louisville Arm & Hand, Louisville, Kentucky,
USA

WARREN C. HAMMERT, MD
Professor of Orthopaedic Surgery and Plastic
Surgery, Department of Orthopaedic Surgery,

Duke University Medical Center, Durham,
North Carolina, USA

CURTIS M. HENN, MD
Associate Professor of Orthopaedic Surgery,
Georgetown University School of Medicine,
Vice Chair, Quality and Safety, MedStar
Orthopaedic Institute, Washington Region,
Associate Residency Program Director,
MedStar Georgetown University Hospital,
Washington, DC, USA

SONU A. JAIN, MD, FACS
Professor of Plastic Surgery and Orthopaedics,
Associate Program Director, Hand and Upper
Extremity Surgery Fellowship, Associate
Director, Hand and Upper Extremity Center,
Chief, Division of Hand Surgery, Department of
Plastic and Reconstructive Surgery, The Ohio
State University Wexner Medical Center,
Columbus, Ohio

SALLY JO, MD
Department of Orthopaedic Surgery,
Washington University in St. Louis, St Louis,
Missouri, USA

STEPHEN A. KENNEDY, MD
Residency Program Director, Associate
Professor, Department of Orthopaedics and
Sports Medicine, University of Washington,
Harborview Medical Center, Seattle,
Washington, USA

JAEHON M. KIM, MD
Director, Hand and Upper Extremity
Fellowship, C.V. Starr Hand Center, Associate
Professor of Orthopedic Surgery, Icahn School
of Medicine at Mount Sinai, Department of
Orthopaedic Surgery, Mount Sinai Hospital,
New York, New York, USA

VICTOR KING, MD
Division of Plastic Surgery, The Warren Alpert
Medical School of Brown University

CHRISTOPHER S. KLIFTO, MD
Associate Professor, Department of
Orthopedic Surgery, Duke University Medical
Center, Durham, North Carolina, USA

ANTHONY LOGIUDICE, MD
Assistant Professor, Associate Program
Director, Hand & Upper Extremity Fellowship,

Department of Orthopaedic Surgery, Medical College of Wisconsin, Milwaukee, Wisconsin, USA

HANNAH C. LANGDELL, MD
Resident, Division of Plastic and Reconstructive Surgery, Duke University Medical Center, Durham, North Carolina, USA

JAMES S. LIN, MD
Resident, Department of Orthopaedics, The Ohio State University Wexner Medical Center, Columbus, Ohio, USA

BILAL MAHMOOD, MD
Assistant Professor, Department of Orthopaedic Surgery, University of Rochester, Rochester, New York, USA

SUHAIL K. MITHANI, MD
Associate Professor, Department of Orthopedic Surgery, Division of Plastic and Reconstructive Surgery, Duke University Medical Center, Durham, North Carolina, USA

ZINA MODEL, MD
Department of Orthopaedic Surgery, Massachusetts General Hospital, Boston, Massachusetts, USA

AMY M. MOORE, MD, FACS
Professor and Chair, Department of Plastic and Reconstructive Surgery, The Ohio State University, Columbus, Ohio, USA

STEVEN L. MORAN, MD
Professor of Plastic Surgery and Orthopedic Surgery, Mayo Clinic, Rochester, Minnesota, USA

CHAITANYA MUDGAL, MD, Ms(Orth), MCh (Orth)
Hand and Arm Orthopaedic Surgeon, Department of Orthopaedic Surgery, Massachusetts General Hospital, Associate Professor of Orthopaedic Surgery, Harvard Medical School, Boston, Massachusetts, USA

TYLER S. PIDGEON, MD
Associate Professor, Department of Orthopedic Surgery, Duke University Medical Center, Durham, North Carolina, USA

JILL PUTNAM, MD
The Hand and Upper Extremity Center, The Ohio State University, Columbus, Ohio, USA

MARCO RIZZO, MD
Professor of Orthopedic Surgery, Mayo Clinic, Rochester, Minnesota, USA

DAVID S. RUCH, MD
Professor, Division of Plastic and Reconstructive Surgery, Duke University Medical Center, Durham, North Carolina, USA

TIAM M. SAFFARI, MD, PhD, MSc
Department of Plastic and Reconstructive Surgery, The Ohio State University, Columbus, Ohio, USA

LUIS SCHEKER, MD
Associate Professor, Plastic and Reconstructive Surgery, University of Louisville School of Medicine, Glenview, Kentucky, USA

RYAN W. SCHMUCKER, MD
Assistant Professor, Department of Plastic and Reconstructive Surgery, The Ohio State University, Columbus, Ohio, USA

VIVIANA M. SERRA LOPEZ, MD, MS
Department of Orthopaedic Surgery, Hospital of the University of Pennsylvania, Philadelphia, Pennsylvania, USA

AMY SPEECKAERT, MD
Assistant Professor, Department of Orthopaedics, The Ohio State University Wexner Medical Center

BRIAN W. STARR, MD
Section of Plastic Surgery, Cincinnati Children's Hospital Medical Center, University of Cincinnati College of Medicine, Cincinnati, Ohio, USA

PATRICIA K. WELLBORN, MD
Resident Physician, Department of Orthopaedics, University of North Carolina School of Medicine, Chapel Hill, North Carolina, USA

CHIA H. WU, MD, MBA
Assistant Professor, Orthopedic Surgery, Hand and Upper Extremity Surgery, Baylor College of Medicine, Houston, Texas, USA

RYAN C. XIAO, MD
Department of Orthopaedic Surgery, Mount Sinai Hospital, New York, New York, USA

GLORIA X. ZHANG, BS
Department of Orthopedic Surgery, Duke University Medical Center, Durham, North Carolina, USA

Contents

Video content accompanies this article at http://www.hand.theclinics.com.

Small joint arthroplasty of the hand has been an established means of joint preservation and pain relief for over a half a century. Despite this, metacarpophalangeal (MCP) and proximal interphalangeal (PIP) joint arthroplasty has not achieved the long-term success seen with hip and knee arthroplasty. Problems following MCP, PIP, and carpometacarpal (CMC) joint arthroplasty can include intraoperative fracture, postoperative dislocation, recurrent pain, limitation of motion, and instability. The hand surgeon needs to be prepared for these problems and their management. This article addresses the management of the most common complications seen following MCP, PIP, and CMC arthroplasty.

Thumb carpometacarpal arthroplasty with complete trapeziectomy with or without suspensionplasty, ligament reconstruction, and/or tendon interposition is largely considered equivalent techniques in providing pain relief and improving function for patients with thumb carpometacarpal arthritis. In cases of continued pain, instability, and dysfunction following an index surgery, one must first identify the cause of failure. Any options for revision surgery depend on addressing the specific cause of persistent symptoms with awareness of available options. Most of the patients undergoing revision surgeries can achieve good to fair outcomes.

Traditional management of wrist arthritis consists of proximal row carpectomy, partial carpal fusions, or, in the event of pancarpal arthritis, total wrist fusion. Although proximal row carpectomy and partial wrist fusions preserve some motion at the wrist while relieving pain symptoms, the quality of results obtained from these procedures is not predictable or optimal in many instances. Management of hip, knee, ankle, and shoulder joints has evolved from arthrodesis to arthroplasty. The wrist joint is following the same pattern of evolution with the advent of reliable designs.

Compared with hip and knee arthroplasty, total elbow arthroplasty (TEA) has a higher complication rate and lower survivorship. Modern TEA implants most commonly require revision due to implant loosening, infection, and periprosthetic fracture. Concerns with revision TEA include handling of the soft tissues and possible necessity of flap coverage, triceps management, preservation of bone stock, and management of concurrent infection or fracture. In this review, we will discuss preoperative evaluation of the failed elbow arthroplasty, surgical approaches, techniques for revision, outcomes, and complications following revision total elbow arthroplasty.

augmented intraoperative decision-making, and an early postoperative mobilization therapy protocol.

HAND CLINICS

SERIES OF RELATED INTEREST:

Clinics in Plastic Surgery
www.plasticsurgery.theclinics.com

Orthopedic Clinics of North America
www.orthopedic.theclinics.com

Clinics in Sports Medicine
www.sportsmed.theclinics.com

THE CLINICS ARE AVAILABLE ONLINE!
Access your subscription at:
www.theclinics.com

Preface

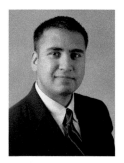

Sonu A. Jain, MD, FACS
Editor

We have all had the case that made us think, caused us to question, and forced us to try new techniques unexpectedly. We are able to navigate these situations based on our experiences and our adherence to principles. Given the ever-evolving state of hand surgery, we thought it would be important to have an issue of Hand Clinics devoted to challenging and complex conditions of the hand.

This issue of Hand Clinics truly highlights the diversity and complexity of hand and upper extremity surgery. In each chapter, experts share today's solutions on how to address the "tough" cases to help us provide the best possible care to our patients. From fractures to arthritis and from nerve to tendinopathies, treatment strategies are presented to maximize results and minimize complications for multiple hand conditions - all found in one book!

This issue was made possible by the contributing authors, the Elsevier staff and Dr. Chung. I am incredibly grateful for the opportunity and excited to share these 19 chapters with you. Lastly, I would like to thank my family for their incredible support.

Sonu A. Jain, MD, FACS
Hand and Upper Extremity Center
Division of Hand Surgery
Department of Plastic and Reconstructive Surgery
The Ohio State University Wexner Medical Center
Columbus, OH 43212, USA

E-mail address:
Sonu.Jain@osumc.edu

https://doi.org/10.1016/j.hcl.2023.05.013
0749-0712/23/© 2023 Published by Elsevier Inc.

hand.theclinics.com

Current Outcomes and Treatments of Complex Phalangeal and Metacarpal Fractures

Patricia K. Wellborn, MD, Andrew D. Allen, MD, Reid W. Draeger, MD*

KEYWORDS

• Metacarpal • Phalanx • Fracture • Complications • Stiffness • Malunion • Nonunion

KEY POINTS

- Complications after operative treatment of phalanx and metacarpal fractures occur in around 50% of patients, most often stiffness or malunion.
- Stiffness is the most common complication after phalangeal and metacarpal fractures, affecting up to 90% of patients after operative treatment.
- The guiding principle in the treatment of malunion is the functional impact and any potential, or already developed, functional limitations when determining operative or non-operative treatment.
- Nonunions in the hand are notoriously difficult to diagnose and are fortunately rare.

INTRODUCTION

There is little consensus in the management of most metacarpal and phalangeal fractures despite their prevalence and the high frequency of complications with current strategies. Fractures of the hand, wrist, and forearm account for 1.5% of all emergency department cases, with 41% of these injuries attributable to fractures of the metacarpals and phalanges.[1] Among collegiate athletes, hand and wrist injuries most commonly occur distal to the carpus and nearly 50% of these injuries either require surgical intervention or result in termination of play.[2] Often, the decision for operative or conservative treatment hinges on the presumed stability of the fracture.

The vast majority of metacarpal fractures can be treated non-operatively. Volar angulation is well tolerated, with even greater tolerance in the fourth and fifth metacarpals as compared to the second and third. Rotational forces are balanced by the strength of the intermetacarpal ligaments and do not play as large of a role as in phalangeal fractures.[3]

In contrast, phalangeal fractures are at high risk of rotational deformity.[3] The majority of phalangeal fractures occur in the proximal phalanx.[4] These fractures are often in the apex volar angulation due to the interossei flexing the proximal fragment and the central slip extending the distal fragment.[4–6] The rotational and angular nature of phalangeal fractures make them more susceptible to poor outcomes.

Functionally stable fractures, or those with a preserved range of motion and acceptable alignment, have demonstrated satisfactory outcomes with conservative management. Alternatively, unstable or open fractures have documented poor outcomes in over 50% of cases despite initial surgical management. Such poor outcomes translate to 30% of patients with difficulty after returning to work and 14% of patients transitioning occupations secondary to residual disability.[7] The subsequent management of complications in this group

Department of Orthopaedics, University of North Carolina School of Medicine, 130 Mason Farm Road, CB# 7055, Chapel Hill, NC 27599-7055, USA
* Corresponding author.
E-mail address: reid_draeger@med.unc.edu

Hand Clin 39 (2023) 251–263
https://doi.org/10.1016/j.hcl.2023.02.002
0749-0712/23/© 2023 Elsevier Inc. All rights reserved.

of fractures poses an additional challenge to the hand surgeon.

STIFFNESS
Background

Complications following operative treatment of metacarpal and phalangeal fractures are exceedingly common, the most frequently encountered being stiffness. Particularly among phalangeal fractures, stiffness may affect nearly 90% of patients following surgical treatment.[8] Hume and colleagues studied a group of healthy volunteers to determine both the normal and functional range of motion (ROM) of the joints of the hand. The normal ROM of the fingers was identified as 0° to 100°, 0° to 105°, and 0° to 85° at the metacarpophalangeal (MCP) joints, proximal interphalangeal (PIP) joints, and distal interphalangeal (DIP) joints, respectively. However, these normal values are not required to perform a variety of functional tasks. Functional ROM was documented as 33° to 73°, 36° to 86°, and 20° to 61° at the MCP joints, PIP joints, and DIP joints, respectively. In summing the ROM at each of these joints, the total active motion (TAM) is calculated and considered normal at 290°, and functional at 165°.[9] Other authors have set similar thresholds for acceptable finger ROM with poor ROM considered as TAM of less than 180° or TAM less than 50% of the contralateral.[7,8,10,11]

In the setting of fracture, early active motion is considered a key tenant of successful recovery. When unstable, fracture fixation is often performed for allowing the initiation of early motion. Early motion decreases edema, joint effusions, and improves tendon gliding.[12] However, despite diligent implementation of early motion, stiffness remains a complex multifactorial complication based on the location of the fracture, type of fixation, intraoperative soft tissue dissection, initial degree of soft tissue injury, and patient-specific factors such as age.[10,12–14] Furthermore, overzealous dissection in an effort to provide more stable fixation may counterproductively induce stiffness. To decrease the risk of stiffness, surgeons should minimize dissection, avoid stripping the periosteum, and if possible, attempt closed reduction.[12]

In a study of 105 metacarpal or phalangeal fractures treated with plate fixation, Page and Stern found an exceedingly high rate of post-operative stiffness, with only 11% of phalangeal fractures and 76% of metacarpal fractures demonstrating good or excellent ROM. In addition to phalangeal fracture, other factors associated with stiffness included open fractures and the use of minicondylar as opposed to straight plates.[8] In an effort

to assess newer, low-profile mini-frag plates, Brei-Thoma and colleagues assessed ROM following plate fixation in fractures without extensive soft tissue injury. Despite newer designs, 67% of patients suffered an extension lag and 25% of patients had <180° of TAM. Over 21% of patients required secondary surgery for reduced mobility.[15]

Differing evidence exists regarding the impact of plate positioning on post-operative ROM. Robinson and colleagues[16] compared lateral versus dorsal plating and found that final TAM did not differ between groups. On the other hand, Onishi and colleagues documented 3.0 times increased risk with dorsal positioning when compared to lateral. Screws alone were optimal, reducing the risk of stiffness by 5.9 times.[14] Among lateral plating for phalangeal fractures, Katayama identified the importance of plate edge distance from the joint line, where a closer distance between the plate edge and the joint line was associated with increased stiffness.[17] When certain fracture patterns are not amenable to screw fixation or when involving the periarticular region of the metacarpal or phalanx, the need for additional surgical intervention for stiffness has been reported at nearly 40%.[11]

Management
The treatment of the stiff finger should be guided by the underlying pathology, as determined by a physical examination. Kaplan described a classification system of the stiff finger, which includes eight finger types, each of which exhibits a different combination of limits in active flexion, passive flexion, active extension, or passive extension.[18] Limitations in extension are addressed by releasing volar structures and limitations in flexion are addressed with dorsal releases. In general, passive motion deficits involve the capsuloligamentous structures whereas active motion deficits are more likely associated with tendon adhesions.

Aggressive therapy is the mainstay of preoperative and post-operative management. In the case of passive flexion deficits, initial measures include taping, dynamic and static splinting, or joint slings. For extension deficits, spring finger extension splints, safety pin splinting, and static or dynamic splinting may be utilized.[18] Dynamic splinting has demonstrated a mean improvement of 18° by 4 months for PIP joint contractures initially measured as <45°.[19] Gains in passive motion should be prioritized before addressing limitations in active motion. When soft tissue equilibrium is achieved and improvements in ROM reach a plateau, further surgical intervention is indicated.[18] Patients who fail to regain significant motion by

3 months should be considered for operative intervention.[20]

Surgical options to address passive motion deficits include percutaneous collateral ligament release, external fixation, and open capsuloligamentous releases. Percutaneous collateral ligament release, while appealing as a minimally invasive technique, has demonstrated poor long-term outcomes with 70% contracture recurrence and nearly 30% rate of extensor lag by 10 months.[21] Regarding external fixation, encouraging data suggest an average gain of nearly 40° maintained at 21 months for PIP joint flexion contractures treated in extension external fixators.[22] As opposed to extension external fixators in which the volar structures are lengthened, gradual distraction external fixation allows for the lengthening of all periarticular structures. Houshian and colleagues[23] documented a mean active extension gain of 47° and a total active ROM gain of 63° with 16 days of distraction at a follow-up of 34 months.

Open releases are often performed to simultaneously address both passive and active motion deficits. Deficits in passive flexion are addressed with dorsal capsulectomy, which may include releases of the transverse retinacular ligament, dorsal capsule, intra-articular adhesions, and, if persistently stiff, the dorsal fibers of the proper collateral ligament. When addressing limited passive extension, volar capsulectomy should include the volar plate, checkrein ligaments, accessory collateral, ligaments, and proper collateral ligaments.[18] When active motion is also compromised, flexor tenolysis through a mid-lateral incision or extensor tenolysis through a dorsal incision is warranted. Post-operatively, the surgeon should employ aggressive therapy to maximize gains. When both volar and dorsal disease exists, procedures should be staged to avoid extensive surgical insult leading to counterproductive swelling, pain, and marginal wound necrosis.[18,20]

In a study of long-term outcomes following open surgical management of PIP joint contractures, Ghidella and colleagues identified an average gain in the arc of motion of 7.5° at an average of 35 months.[24] Further analysis revealed significant differences based on contracture etiology, where simple diagnoses such as laceration, fracture, or dislocation experienced significantly increased gains (17°) compared with complex injuries including crush or revascularization (0.5°). Overall, 29% of patients lost motion following open release. Factors correlating with a worse prognosis include increased age, increased number of prior procedures, and increased pre-operative arc of motion. Among patients with post-traumatic stiffness, Lutsky and colleagues[25] documented a 41-

degree improvement in TAM following open release, with 21% of patients experiencing a net decrease. Risk factors included delay in postoperative therapy >7 days and involvement of worker's compensation. These studies suggest that candidates for open surgical release should include a selective population, ideally younger patients with a more limited pre-operative ROM, and ability to comply with post-operative therapy.

MALUNION
Background

Malunion, or healing in a non-anatomic position, of metacarpal and phalangeal fractures, is the second most common complication after stiffness.[26] Malunion can occur in the form of shortening, rotational, angular, or a combination of these deformities.[26] The degree of deformity plays a significant role in the degree of functional impact. The functional impact of malunion can range from no impact on hand function to substantial limitations. Substantial limitations occur due to tendon imbalance and associated contractures from the altered position of the metacarpal/phalanx.[27]

Metacarpal
Metacarpal malunions most often occur due to sagittal plane deformity, with apex dorsal angulation being the most common.[5] Sagittal plane deformity is typically the most well-tolerated of the deformities.[26,28] Balaram and colleagues[26] describe various ranges of acceptable dorsal angular deformity: 10° for the index and long fingers, 20° for the ring finger, and 30° for the small finger. There is an increasing tolerance for deformity in the fourth and fifth carpometacarpal (CMC) joints due to the degree of mobility in these joints. The second and third CMC joints are more rigid, and therefore, less tolerant to angular deformity.[5,28]

The next best-tolerated deformity is shortening of the metacarpal. Shortening is typically limited to less than 3 to 4 mm due to the strength of the intermetacarpal ligaments, which hold fractures out to length, except in cases where multiple metacarpals are fractured.[5] The greatest concern with metacarpal shortening is the creation of an extensor lag at the MCP joint. For every 2 mm of metacarpal shortening, a 7-degree extensor lag is created at the MCP joint.[5,26,27] The MCP joints have a natural ability to hyperextend on average around 20°. Therefore, the MCP joint can adequately compensate for an extensor lag of up to 20° or metacarpal shortening of around 6 mm.[26]

Rotational deformities of the metacarpals are the most poorly tolerated.[5] Fortunately, rotational deformities are also the least common of the deformities in metacarpals due to the strength of the intermetacarpal ligaments. The border digits (first and fifth metacarpals) are most likely to incur rotational deformity given only one intermetacarpal ligament is present.[5] The degree of rotation at the metacarpal has amplified effects in the malrotation of the digit. Several authors have attempted to elucidate the degree of impact metacarpal rotational malunion has on the digits. Freeland and colleagues[5] report that for each degree of metacarpal malrotation, 5° of malrotation is created at the fingertips. They also state that around 10° of metacarpal rotational deformity results in 2 cm of fingertip overlap. Similarly, Balaram and colleagues[26] report that 5° of metacarpal malrotation can cause 1.5 cm of fingertip overlap. Thus, even minor metacarpal malrotation can cause dramatic functional limitations at the fingertips.

Phalanx

Phalangeal malunions are more common than metacarpal malunions. Phalangeal malunions are typically sagittal plane or rotational deformities. Rotational malalignment is common with these fractures as the proximal phalanx lacks the stabilization of the intermetacarpal ligaments. Any rotational malalignment can cause substantial functional repercussions. Thus, consideration to correcting malrotated phalangeal malunions should be considered to curb functional limitations due to malrotation. Concerning sagittal plane deformities, in the proximal phalanx, malunions are typically in the apex volar angulation.[4,5,26] Functional limitations in motion begin with around 25° of angulation.[5] As angulation increases, the phalanx is essentially shortened. This creates a functional extensor lag at the proximal interphalangeal joint.[5] Held reports that for every 1 mm of functional phalangeal shortening, a 12-degree extensor lag is created at the PIP.[4] To compensate for the PIP extensor lag, the distal interphalangeal joint hyperextends. This leads to extensor tendon adherence and functional shortening which may remain present despite malunion surgical correction.[5]

In the middle and distal phalanx, malunions are typically a combination of rotational and sagittal plane deformities given the paucity of soft tissue attachments. The middle phalanx may be either apex volar or dorsal depending on the location of the fracture. If the fracture occurs proximal to the flexor digitorum superficialis (FDS) insertion, the fracture will angulate dorsally. If distal to FDS insertion, the fracture will be in volar angulation.[5] Rotational malunion is determined by examining

for overlapping, or "scissoring", of digits as the patient makes a complete fist.

Management

The treatment of metacarpal and phalangeal malunions is dictated by a combination of the timing of malunion presentation, radiographic parameters of the malunion, and, most importantly, the degree of functional limitation caused by the malunion.

Timing of malunion presentation

Malunion presentation is typically divided into three periods: acute, subacute, and chronic. Acute presentation occurs within the first 7 to 10 days in children and within the first 2 to 2½ weeks in adults after injury. If a patient presents within the acute period, there is still ample time to intervene as no significant healing has yet occurred. Options for management include non-operative in the form of reduction or, more commonly, operative intervention in the form of closed reduction/percutaneous pinning (CRPP), open reduction/percutaneous pinning (ORPP), or open reduction internal fixation (ORIF).

The subacute period is defined as between 2 and around 4 weeks. Early healing and bone formation have occurred but the fracture is not yet fully healed/united. Lester and colleagues define this period as "no man's land." Some surgeons advocate for watchful waiting with aggressive therapy to work toward the best possible functional outcome. Others advocate for more aggressive ORIF or primary arthrodesis.

The final phase of the presentation is the chronic malunion that is already fully healed. This occurs around 4 to 8 weeks post-injury. Treatment at this phase requires osteotomy, arthrodesis, bone resection, or arthroplasty.[29]

Radiographic parameters of the malunion

Although functional limitations are the guiding principle, some have suggested general radiographic guidelines to guide management. Freeland and colleagues propose that malunions be revised if angulation is greater than 15° in the proximal or middle phalanx and greater than 30° in the metacarpal in the sagittal plane. They also suggest revision for malrotation greater than 10° in either the metacarpal or phalanx that is symptomatic or functionally limiting.[5] Although radiographic parameters provide an important framework for guiding malunion treatment, radiographic appearance should not be considered in isolation as a functional digit with an abnormal radiographic appearance is far superior to a digit with limited function and a normal radiographic appearance.

Functional limitations due to the malunion

Arguably the most important indication for malunion treatment is the degree of functional limitation. If a patient is asymptomatic or functioning at a high level, non-operative treatment remains the preferred option. This is especially pertinent in individuals presenting in the chronic/healed period or if a bridging callus is already seen on radiographs.[5] It is crucial to consider the functional impact and any potential, or already developed, functional limitations when determining operative or non-operative treatment.

In the patient with substantial functional limitations and who is relatively early in the recovery period, operative revision of the malunion is recommended as soon as possible. Operative treatment includes removal of immature/maturing callus, anatomic reduction, and stabilization at the fracture site. The goal of the immediate operative revision is to intervene before the full maturation of adhesions and scar tissue and before development of contractures.[5]

In a patient with functional limitations and a fully healed malunion, surgery is not performed immediately. In this patient, the goal shifts toward achieving maximal function in the digit. It is recommended that surgery not be considered until at least 3 months after injury. Aggressive therapy should be pursued with the goal of maximal ROM and function. In a portion of these patients, adequate function will be regained obviating surgery altogether.[5] Additionally, a patient's compliance with therapy pre-operatively likely correlates with compliance post-operatively should surgical treatment be entertained. As the success of any operative treatment is largely dependent on formal or self-guided therapy in the post-operative period, a trial of pre-operative therapy can help the surgeon in counseling a patient regarding treatment options and prognosticating the likelihood of success of surgical management.

Operative treatment of malunions

In mild deformities, simply removing the protruding bony deformity may be enough to allow for adequate tendon gliding and remove any joint impingement. This can be especially helpful in managing pediatric phalangeal neck malunions with restricted pre-operative flexion due to bony impingement.[30]

In more severe deformities, osteotomy either at the original fracture site or in a different location is required. Either a closing or opening wedge osteotomy may be used. Although a closing wedge osteotomy is technically easier, an opening wedge osteotomy has the advantage of preserving the original length of the bone. Maintaining adequate length is crucial to maintaining the tendon balance and preventing the development of extensor lag and stiffness.[29]

Appropriate pre-operative planning must be utilized for osteotomies to make appropriate multiplanar corrections. Though multiplanar opening or closing wedge osteotomies may be required for some phalangeal malunions, those with severe deformities who have not undergone extensive bony remodeling may be managed successfully with osteotomy at the fracture site and fixation (**Fig. 1**). Internal fixation with plate and/or screw fixation is nearly always used as an extensive open approach is already being utilized for the osteotomy portion of the procedure. Plate and/or screw fixation offers substantial rigid stability to the osteotomy site and can allow for early aggressive therapy.

In a study by Buchler and colleagues,[31] phalangeal malunion revision with rigid internal fixation was performed on 59 patients. A concomitant tenolysis was performed in 50% of the subjects. For malunions with pure dorsal angulation or coronal deformities, a transverse incomplete opening wedge osteotomy was performed. For pure volar angulation, a transverse incomplete opening wedge osteotomy was utilized. For pure malrotation deformities, a complete transverse osteotomy was performed at the fracture site. More commonly, malunions in several planes were treated with complete transverse osteotomies. Rigid internal fixation was performed in all patients. Union was achieved in all patients. Improvements in active ROM were present in 89% of patients and there was satisfactory correction in 76% of patients. They achieved "excellent" or "good" results as determined by an author-developed grading system in 96% of patients treated for pure malunion. However, only 64% of those with injuries to other soft tissue structures achieved these results. Injuries to soft tissue structures in addition to bone are critical to consider as these concomitant injuries may have substantial implications on the prognosis of treatment. Patients with combined injuries must be appropriately counseled about their guarded prognosis before revision.[26,31]

In a similar study, Trumble, and colleagues performed in situ osteotomy of the proximal phalanx malunion site and performed internal fixation with a dorsal plate. Patients with pure rotational deformities were treated with an in situ complete osteotomy and fixed so that the finger was parallel to the other digits with the PIP joint in 90° of flexion. Patients with both rotational and angular deformities were treated with a wedge resection

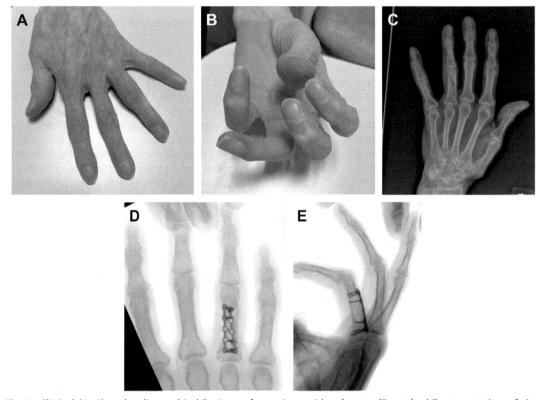

Fig. 1. Clinical (*A, B*) and radiographic (*C*) views of a patient with subacute (5-week-old) presentation of ring finger proximal phalanx malunion demonstrating substantial malrotation. Rigid fixation (*D, E*) re-established anatomic alignment and allowed for early post-operative ROM work with hand therapy.

osteotomy. All patients were allowed immediate active and passive ROM. All patients had correction of digit overlap and achieved union within 7 weeks. On average, patients had improved flexion of 15° at the PIP and 10° at DIP.[32]

Metacarpal malunions can be treated with either in situ osteotomy or derotational osteotomy at the base of the metacarpal. In situ osteotomy allows for direct correction at the malunion site. Metacarpal base osteotomy has the advantage of better bone healing at the meta-diaphyseal junction and avoids an approach through scar tissue.[5,26,29] This approach works well for rotational malunions but does not have the ability to correct for angular deformities. A proximal metaphyseal osteotomy has the powerful ability to correct up to 18 to 20° of malrotation.[28]

If the metacarpal malunion is both angulated and rotated, an in situ osteotomy will need to be performed with either an opening or closing wedge.[28] Karthik and colleagues describe a corrective osteotomy technique for these fractures. A dorsal approach is taken to the metacarpal at the level of the malunion site. A Kirschner wires (K-wire) is driven through the metacarpal head and proximal to the level of the malunion. A closing or opening wedge osteotomy is then performed. The K-wire is then used in a joystick-type fashion and driven proximally into the proximal metacarpal after performing derotation. The osteotomy site is then secured with a dorsal plate and the K-wire is removed. All patients are allowed immediate ROM. All patients had complete correction and union. Both functional and patient-reported scores improved after revision.[33] Although symptomatic and functionally-limiting metacarpal malunions are rare, both types of osteotomies can be successful when used in the correct manner.

NONUNION
Background

Nonunion of metacarpal and phalangeal fractures is rare, seen in fewer than 1% of phalangeal fractures and 7% of metacarpal fractures. Among those nonunions, those patients with functional or clinical impacts are even fewer.[28,34] Diagnosing nonunions in the hand is much more difficult than in the remainder of the body. Radiographic healing is not seen until around 5 months post-injury and fracture lines may be present on radiographs for up to a year in hand fractures that ultimately heal uneventfully. Clinically diagnosed union is typically seen in around one-fourth of the time needed to have radiographic union.[27] Clinical signs and symptoms are far more reliable than radiographic findings when diagnosing nonunion. These predictors include instability, gross deformity, implant failure, and persistent pain[27] (**Fig. 2**). Varying definitions of nonunion in the hand exist but several authors agree upon a definition of no clinical or radiographic evidence of healing at 4 months or if a radiographic fracture line remains present at 14 months post-injury.[26–28]

The vast majority of nonunions in the hand are atrophic, with no significant bone formation present.[26–28] This is typically a result of soft tissue trauma involving bone loss or loss of blood supply, including open fracture, nerve injury, or infection[26,28] (**Fig. 3**). In atrophic nonunions, surgical management includes debridement, bone grafting, and fixation. Although rare, hypertrophic nonunions of the hand do occur. This is typically a result of soft tissue interposition at the fracture site and requires open debridement and rigid fixation.[28]

Although phalangeal nonunions are extremely rare, when they do occur, it is typically a sequelae of either significant soft tissue trauma as described above or by problems with surgical fixation. Wray and colleagues performed a case series on phalangeal nonunions and found that they occur in fewer than 1% of all fractures. The most common cause of nonunion was fractures fixed in

distraction with K-wire in either CRPP or ORPP. All nonunions in the series were treated with revision reduction and K-wire fixation with bone graft in a subset of patients. All were allowed aggressive ROM within 3 weeks and all went on to eventual union.[34]

Metacarpal nonunions occur more frequently than in the phalanges but are still overall rare. They occur most frequently in transverse fractures that are displaced. Kollitz and colleagues report that nonunion occurs in 30% of transverse pattern fractures that are treated non-operatively, although a portion of these may ultimately be asymptomatic. Therefore, pure transverse metacarpal shaft fractures should be more aggressively treated surgically.[28]

Management

Management of phalangeal and metacarpal nonunions is focused on optimizing functional outcomes of the finger and hand. A mainstay of all treatment options involves aggressive hand therapy both pre-operatively and post-operatively to regain ROM and strength. If the finger is already stiff, it is unlikely that the finger will regain greater motion even if the nonunion can heal.[27] This is a critical point to explain to patients, especially if the primary complaint is stiffness rather than pain.

Nonunions in the setting of significant soft tissue trauma, segmental bone loss, and/or nerve injury are difficult to manage. These individuals have poor biology in the form of disrupted soft tissue

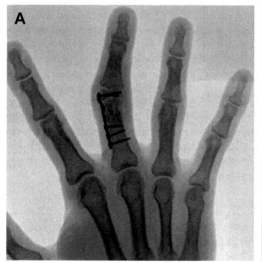
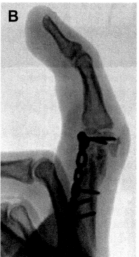
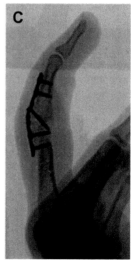

Fig. 2. A highly comminuted proximal phalanx fracture. Nonunion diagnosed with progressive ulnar deviating deformity (*A*) and screw pullout (*B*). PIP arthrodesis performed as salvage procedure (*C*). (*From* Ring D. Malunion and Nonunion of the Metacarpals and Phalanges. Journal of Bone and Joint Surgery. 2005;87(6):1380-1388; with permission.)

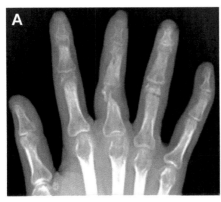
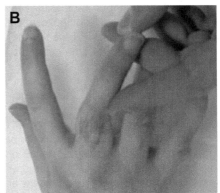

Fig. 3. A case of phalangeal nonunion after severe soft tissue injury. (*A*) Radiograph (*B*) Clinical examination demonstrating gross motion at the fracture site. (*From* Balaram AK & Bednar MS. Complications after the fractures of metacarpal and phalanges. Hand Clinics. 2010;26(2):169–177; with permission.)

or blood supply. If there is a severe soft tissue injury, a nonunion revision is not indicated as the outcome is likely to be the same and functional outcomes are poor.[26] Similarly, if the finger is insensate, there is no indication for revision as that finger will have a poor functional outcome and pain is not present.[26]

Atrophic nonunions should be treated with debridement and correction of the underlying biology problem. Soft tissues should be allowed to heal fully before nonunion revision and all infections should be eradicated. After this, bone grafting and fixation, either internal or external, may be utilized.[28] Bone grafting may take the form of non-vascularized cortico-cancellous or cancellous bone or vascularized bone grafting, which has been described as harvested from multiple sites including the medial femoral condyle and scapula.[35] Hypertrophic nonunions should be treated with open debridement, to ensure no interposed tissue and revision fixation. Importantly, all nonunions should be counseled on early aggressive ROM. These patients are at high risk for stiffness and fixation needs to be stable enough to allow for early passive and active ROM.[28]

In cases with severe soft tissue injury, nerve injury, and nonunion, the prognosis of treatment can be poor. In consideration of the patient's functional status and functional goals, amputation may be a feasible and expeditious treatment option (**Fig. 4**). Amputation may alleviate stiffness in the surrounding digits as well as the affected digit and may allow patients to return to activity and work more rapidly. In these patients, amputation should be presented as a viable option alongside digit salvage, which may ultimately require fewer procedures and less post-operative therapy to give satisfactory functional results.

ARTICULAR DEFECTS
Background

Intra-articular metacarpal and phalangeal fractures pose a particularly increased risk of loss of function secondary to stiffness and early post-traumatic arthritis.[36] Given the complexity surrounding articular fractures and fracture dislocations, optimal treatment remains controversial. Most commonly, fractures involving the PIP joints are treated with open reduction and internal fixation (65%), followed by percutaneous pinning (11%).[36] However, depending on the nature of the injury, management may include external fixation, volar plate arthroplasty, extension block pinning, hemi-hamate arthroplasty, silicone arthroplasty, and primary arthrodesis.[36,37] Oflazoglu and colleagues[36] observed a 16% reoperation rate among PIP joint fractures, with a significantly increased risk among open fractures (26%) and crush injuries (64%). Most commonly, reoperation is performed to address stiffness and/or persistent joint subluxation. Varying rates of recurrent pain and post-traumatic arthritis are documented in the literature, though post-traumatic arthritis has been documented as high as 46% with extension block pinning.[38] Revision surgery most often involves silicone arthroplasty or arthrodesis, though joint-preserving operations are often utilized in younger patient populations.

Management

Goals of management for articular fractures of the hand include providing sufficient stability for early motion, restoration of gliding joint motion, and restoration of articular surface congruity.[37] Treatment should be guided by the severity of the injury and integrity of the soft tissues. The most widely used classification system for PIP joint fracture/

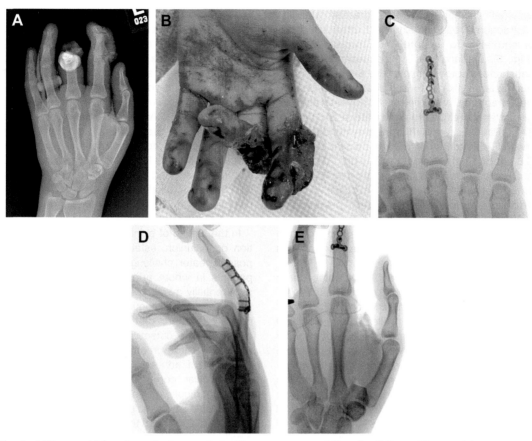

Fig. 4. A 20-year-old female patient presented with severe osseous (*A*) and soft tissue (*B*) wounds/near amputation after having her hand pinned out of a car window during an accident. The original high degree of comminution and poor status of the soft tissues led to long finger PIP arthrodesis to increase function (*C, D*). Though the patient did well with the index finger initially despite its instability and deformity, she eventually elected for index ray amputation (*E*) a year after injury as she continued to struggle with stiffness and pain in the hand.

dislocations is based on fracture stability, where a stable fracture involves less than 30% of the articular surface, a tenuous fracture involves 30% to 50%, and unstable fractures involve greater than 50%.[38]

Minicondylar plates have been widely used with the reported benefit of providing sufficient stability for early ROM.[39,40] Although open reduction and fixation with minicondylar plates has demonstrated acceptable results in allowing early motion with low rates of nonunion and malunion, the benefits are countered by high rates of hardware failure or symptomatic hardware, stiffness, and infeasibility in the setting of soft-tissue compromise. Overall complication rates are documented as greater than 50%.[40] Hardware is removed in 45% of cases and 20% of patients require additional secondary procedures, most commonly for extensor lag or contracture.[39,40] Small condylar fractures not amenable to mini-fragment plating have been treated successfully with interfragmentary screw

fixation. As opposed to K-wire fixation, mini screws allow for compression of the fracture and can be advanced beneath the chondral surface. Among 11 condylar fractures, Tan and colleagues documented a 100% union rate and near full preservation of motion, though did report one complication of screw subsidence.

CRPP and volar plate arthroplasty have demonstrated the greatest post-operative PIP joint ROM and lowest reoperation rates, however, these patients typically present with less severe injury and smaller articular defects.[38] Volar plate arthroplasty is a technique in which the volar plate is advanced into the joint to resurface small volar lip defects at the base of the middle phalanx. Advancement of the volar plate can re-establish stability in cases of dorsal subluxation and increase articular congruity when a small volar lip fragment is unable to be reconstructed.[37]

Among larger articular defects or pilon-type fractures, hemi-hamate arthroplasty (HHA) or external fixation provides greater stability. Distraction through an external fixator utilizes ligamentotaxis to restore the articular surface (**Fig. 5**). Dailiana and colleagues documented satisfactory outcomes with the 6-week use of a mini-external fixator for metacarpal and phalangeal fractures, with nearly 80% restoration of grip strength relative to contralateral and 210° of TAM. Patients reported limited dysfunction with mean DASH scores of 7.9 and satisfaction rated 8.8 out of 10 at 29-month follow-up.[41] Houshian and colleagues additionally reported the mini-external fixator to be useful in cases of intra-articular fracture with delayed presentation (>20 days). Though results are limited to a 6-month follow-up, this cohort regained grip strength of 93% relative to the contralateral hand and 100% satisfaction.[42]

HHA is a well-established treatment of large articular defects at the volar lip of the middle phalanx and has demonstrated acceptable functional outcomes. Calfee and colleagues performed HHA in both acute and chronic defects of the volar lip involving >50% of the articular surface and found that PIP joint arc of motion was satisfactory in both acute and chronic cases, averaging approximately 70° at a 4.5-year follow-up. Grip strength was documented at 95% of contralateral and patient reported outcomes revealed minimal pain and dysfunction despite average flexion

contracture of 19°.[43] Though typically for volar defects, Dai and colleagues utilized hamate osteochondral autograft to address central and dorsal defects of the base of the middle phalanx. Union wa0s achieved in all cases and PIP joint ROM improved 60° for volar lip reconstruction, 25° for dorsal lip reconstruction, and 90° for central defect reconstruction.[44] As an alternative to hamate donor site, rib costal cartilage autograft has also been described for treatment of phalangeal articular defects.[45] However, Hasegawa and colleagues[45] reported chondrolysis and ankylosis in 2/7 cases, likely secondary to inadequate harvest of the osseous portion of the costo-osteochondral graft.

In the setting of significantly delayed presentation or malunion, established articular deformity poses greater challenge, particularly in younger patients in whom arthrodesis or arthroplasty is preferentially avoided. In a series of five patients, Harness, and colleagues treated malunited unicondylar fracture of the proximal phalanx with extra-articular osteotomy. Management via an extra-articular approach seeks to avoid the complications of adhesions and stiffness related to intra-articular correction. The authors describe an extra-articular closing wedge osteotomy opposite the side of the malunited condyle followed by combined K-wire and tension band fixation. In this small cohort, union was achieved in all cases,

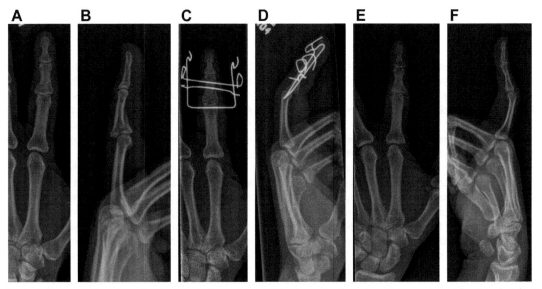

Fig. 5. A 47-year-old male patient presented in a delayed fashion after jamming his finger playing cricket. AP (*A*) and lateral (*B*) radiographs revealed a highly comminuted, non-united pilon-type fracture of the base of the middle phalanx with dorsal dislocation of the PIP joint as evidenced by the "V-sign" on lateral radiographs. A dynamic external fixator (*C, D*) in the style of Suzuki, and colleagues[49] was placed to treat the pilon fracture as the degree of comminution precluded ORIF. Upon removal, the PIP joint was congruently reduced (*E, F*) and the patient regained substantial, but not full, PIP ROM.

average angular deformity improved from 25 to 1 degree, ROM improved a mean of 50°, and no patient reported pain at a minimum 12-month follow-up.[46]

Management of metacarpal head defects, though less common, poses a unique challenge among younger patients in whom arthroplasty does not provide a durable solution. Kitay and colleagues describe a case report of osteochondral autograft transplantation surgery from the non-weightbearing portion of the knee to fill a focal metacarpal head defect. In the single case, authors demonstrate feasibility and describe excellent, painless ROM without donor site morbidity. However, long-term outcomes and larger studies are lacking to further validate this procedure.[47]

As a final salvage operation prior to arthroplasty or arthrodesis, free vascularized joint transfer has been described, though not without significant donor site morbidity and limited ROM.[45] Kuzu and colleagues describe the technique for free vascularized toe to hand PIP joint transfer with improved, though limited outcomes. PIP joint ROM improved from 3.6° to 24.1° postoperatively and DASH scores decreased by a mean of 11 points from 41 to 30. The procedure is overall limited by the technical difficulty and severity of potential complications, including one case requiring early post-operative exploration due to arterial compression.[48]

SUMMARY

Although the majority of metacarpal and phalangeal fractures can be treated non-operatively with little to no complication of treatment, a subset of these fractures remains difficult to treat and fraught with complications. The stability of the fracture continues to guide the management and determination of operative or non-operative treatment. Stiffness remains the most common complication and often the most difficult complication to treat. The primary principle should remain the prevention of stiffness from occurring in the first place. This is guided by maximizing the stability of the fracture with the least immobilization possible. Surgical treatment should provide enough stability to allow for early motion and the importance of post-operative therapy cannot be underemphasized. Malunion and nonunion revision should be guided by the function of the finger and the inherent functional limitations of the malunion rather than radiographic findings. It is crucial to evaluate the entire extent of the initial injury including soft tissue and nerve damage.

CLINICS CARE POINTS

- Fractures of the hand, wrist, and forearm account for 1.5% of all emergency department cases, with 41% of these injuries attributable to fractures of the metacarpals and phalanges.[1]

- Functionally stable fractures, or those with preserved ROM and acceptable alignment, have demonstrated satisfactory outcomes with conservative management.

- Unstable or open fractures have documented poor outcomes in over 50% of cases despite initial surgical management.

- Among phalangeal fractures, stiffness may affect nearly 90% of patients following surgical treatment.[8]

- To decrease the risk of stiffness, surgeons should minimize dissection, avoid stripping the periosteum, and if possible, attempt closed reduction.[12]

- Aggressive therapy is the mainstay of preoperative and post-operative management of stiffness.

- Functional impact of malunion can range from no impact on hand function to substantial limitations.

- Treatment of metacarpal and phalangeal malunions is dictated by a combination of the timing of malunion presentation, radiographic parameters of the malunion, and, most importantly, the degree of functional limitation caused by the malunion.

- Malunion revision surgery may involve in situ or remote osteotomy. Phalangeal malunions are typically treated in situ whereas metacarpal malunions may be treated either in situ or with a derotational osteotomy at the base of the metacarpal.

- Nonunion of metacarpal and phalangeal fractures is rare, seen in fewer than 1% of phalangeal fractures and 7% of metacarpal fractures. Among those nonunions, those patients with functional or clinical impacts are even fewer.[28,34]

- Varying definitions of nonunion in the hand exist but several authors agree upon a definition of no clinical or radiographic evidence of healing at 4 months or if a radiographic fracture line remains present at 14 months post-injury.[26–28]

- In cases with severe soft tissue injury, nerve injury, and nonunion, the prognosis of treatment can be poor. Amputation often provides the best functional outcome.

- Intra-articular metacarpal and phalangeal fractures pose a particularly increased risk of loss of function secondary to stiffness and early post-traumatic arthritis.[36]
- Goals of management for articular fractures of the hand include providing sufficient stability for early motion, restoration of gliding joint motion, and restoration of articular surface congruity.[37]

DISCLOSURE

The authors have no pertinent conflicts of interest to disclose for this work.

REFERENCES

1. Chung KC, Spilson S. The frequency and epidemiology of hand and forearm fractures in the United States. J Hand Surg 2001;26(5):908–15.
2. Chan JJ, Xiao RC, Hasija R, et al. Epidemiology of Hand and Wrist Injuries in Collegiate-Level Athletes in the United States. J Hand Surg 2021. https://doi.org/10.1016/j.jhsa.2021.10.011.
3. Boeckstyns MEH. Current methods, outcomes and challenges for the treatment of hand fractures. J Hand Surg: European 2020;45(6):547–59.
4. Held M, Jordaan P, Laubscher M, et al. Conservative treatment of fractures of the proximal phalanx: an option even for unstable fracture patterns. Hand Surg 2013;18(2):229–34.
5. Freeland AE, Lindley SG. Malunions of the finger metacarpals and phalanges. Hand Clin 2006;22(3): 341–55.
6. Lögters TT, Lee HH, Gehrmann S, et al. Proximal phalanx fracture management. Hand (N Y) 2018; 13(4):376–83.
7. Pun WK, Chow SP, So YC, et al. A prospective study on 284 digital fractures of the hand. J Hand Surg 1989;14(3):474–81.
8. Page SM, Stern PJ. Complications and range of motion following plate fixation of metacarpal and phalangeal fractures. J Hand Surg Am 1998;23(5): 827–32.
9. Hume MC, Gellman H, McKellop H, et al. Functional range of motion of the joints of the hand. J Hand Surg Am 1990;15(2):240–3.
10. Duncan RW, Freeland AE, Jabaley ME, et al. Open hand fractures: an analysis of the recovery of active motion and of complications. J Hand Surg Am 1993; 18(3):387–94.
11. Omokawa S, Fujitani R, Dohi Y, et al. Prospective outcomes of comminuted periarticular metacarpal and phalangeal fractures treated using a titanium plate system. J Hand Surg 2008;33(6):857–63.
12. Neumeister MW, Winters JN, Maduakolum E. Phalangeal and metacarpal fractures of the hand: preventing stiffness. Plast Reconstr Surg 2021; 9(10):e3871.
13. Shimizu T, Omokawa S, Akahane M, et al. Predictors of the postoperative range of finger motion for comminuted periarticular metacarpal and phalangeal fractures treated with a titanium plate. Injury 2012;43(6):940–5.
14. Onishi T, Omokawa S, Shimizu T, et al. Predictors of postoperative finger stiffness in unstable proximal phalangeal fractures. Plast Reconstr Surg 2015;3(6). https://doi.org/10.1097/GOX.0000000000000396.
15. Brei-Thoma P, Vögelin E, Franz T. Plate fixation of extra-articular fractures of the proximal phalanx: do new implants cause less problems? Arch Orthop Trauma Surg 2015;135(3):439–45.
16. Robinson LP, Gaspar MP, Strohl AB, et al. Dorsal versus lateral plate fixation of finger proximal phalangeal fractures: a retrospective study. Arch Orthop Trauma Surg 2017;137(4):567–72.
17. Katayama T, Furuta K, Ono H, et al. Clinical outcomes of unstable metacarpal and phalangeal fractures treated with a locking plate system: a prospective study. J Hand Surg: European 2020;45(6):582–7.
18. Kaplan FTD. The stiff finger. Hand Clin 2010;26(2): 191–204.
19. Prosser R. Splinting in the management of proximal interphalangeal joint flexion contracture. J Hand Ther 1996;9(4):378–86.
20. Houshian S, Jing SS, Chikkamuniyappa C, et al. Management of posttraumatic proximal interphalangeal joint contracture. J Hand Surg 2013;38(8):1651–8.
21. Stanley JK, Jones WA, Lynch MC. Percutaneous accessory collateral ligament release in the treatment of proximal interphalangeal joint flexion contracture. J Hand Surg Br 1986;11(3):360–3.
22. Houshian S, Gynning B, Schrøder HA. Chronic flexion contracture of proximal interphalangeal joint treated with the compass hinge external fixator. A consecutive series of 27 cases. J Hand Surg Br 2002;27(4):356–8.
23. Houshian S, Chikkamuniyappa C, Schroeder H. Gradual joint distraction of post-traumatic flexion contracture of the proximal interphalangeal joint by a mini-external fixator. J Bone Joint Surg Br 2007; 89(2):206–9.
24. Ghidella SD, Segalman KA, Murphey MS. Long-term results of surgical management of proximal interphalangeal joint contracture. J Hand Surg 2002; 27(5):799–805.
25. Lutsky KF, Matzon JL, Dwyer J, et al. Results of operative intervention for finger stiffness after fractures of the hand. Hand 2016;11(3):341–6.
26. Balaram AK, Bednar MS. Complications after the fractures of metacarpal and phalanges. Hand Clin 2010;26(2):169–77.

27. Ring D. Malunion and nonunion of the metacarpals and phalanges. J Bone Joint Surg 2005;87(6): 1380–8.
28. Kollitz KM, Hammert WC, Vedder NB, et al. Metacarpal fractures: treatment and complications. Hand 2014;9(1):16–23.
29. Lester B, Mallik A. Impending malunions of the hand treatment of subacute, malaligned fractures. Clin Orthop Relat Res 1996;327:55–62.
30. Kaoru T, Kazuo I, Katsuro T. Malunion of fractures of the proximal phalangeal neck in children. Journal of Plastic Surgery and Hand Surgery 2010;44(1): 69–71.
31. Buchler U, Gupta A, Rut S. Corrective osteotomy for post-traumatic malunion of the phalanges in the hand. J Hand Surg 1996;21(1):33–42.
32. Trumble T, Gilbert M. In situ osteotomy for extra-articular malunion of the proximal phalanx. J Hand Surg 1998;23A(5):821–7.
33. Karthik K, Tahmassebi R, Khakha RS, et al. Corrective osteotomy for malunited metacarpal fractures: long-term results of a novel technique. J Hand Surg 2015;40E(8):840–5.
34. Wray RC, Glunk R. Treatment of delayed union, nonunion, and malunion of the phalanges of the hand. Ann Plast Surg 1989;22(1):14–8.
35. Christen T, Krahenbuhl SM, Muller CT, et al. Periosteal medial femoral condyle free flap for metacarpal nonunion. Microsurgery 2022;42(3):226–30.
36. Oflazoglu K, Wilkens SC, Rakhorst H, et al. Reoperation after operative fixation of proximal interphalangeal joint fractures. Hand 2021;16(3):338–47.
37. Haase SC, Chung KC. Current concepts in treatment of fracture-dislocations of the proximal interphalangeal joint. Plast Reconstr Surg 2014;134(6): 1246–57.
38. Gianakos A, Yingling J, Athens CM, et al. Treatment for acute proximal interphalangeal joint fractures and fracture-dislocations: a systematic review of the literature. Journal of Hand and Microsurgery 2020;12(S 01):S9–15. https://doi.org/10.1055/s-0040-1713323.
39. Büchler U, Fischer T. Use of a minicondylar plate for metacarpal and phalangeal periarticular injuries. Clin Orthop Relat Res 1987;214:53–8.
40. Oullette EA, Freeland AE. Use of the minicondylar plate in metacarpal and phalangeal fractures. Clin Orthop Relat Res 1996;327:38–46.
41. Dailiana Z, Agorastakis D, Varitimidis S, et al. Use of a mini-external fixator for the treatment of hand fractures. J Hand Surg 2009;34(4):630–6.
42. Houshian S, Jing SS. A new technique for closed management of displaced intra-articular fractures of metacarpal and phalangeal head delayed on presentation: Report of eight cases. J Hand Surg: European Volume 2014;39(3):232–6.
43. Calfee RP, Kiefhaber TR, Sommerkamp TG, et al. Hemi-hamate arthroplasty provides functional reconstruction of acute and chronic proximal interphalangeal fracture-dislocations. J Hand Surg 2009;34(7):1232–41.
44. Dai J, Zheng Y, Yang C, et al. Osteochondral autograft from the hamate for treating partial defect of the proximal interphalangeal joint. J Hand Surg 2022. https://doi.org/10.1016/j.jhsa.2021.11.007.
45. Hasegawa T, Yamano Y. Arthoplasty of the proximal interphalangeal joint using costal cartilage grafts. J Hand Surg: European Volume 1992;17(5):583–5.
46. Harness NG, Chen A, Jupiter JB. Extra-articular osteotomy for malunited unicondylar fractures of the proximal phalanx. J Hand Surg 2005;30(3):566–72.
47. Kitay A, Waters PM, Bae DS. Osteochondral autograft transplantation surgery for metacarpal head defects. J Hand Surg 2016;41(3):457–63.
48. Kuzu IM, Kayan RB, Öztürk K, et al. Functional improvement with free vascularized toe-to-hand proximal interphalangeal (PIP) joint transfer. Plast Reconstr Surg 2018;6(7). https://doi.org/10.1097/GOX.0000000000001775.
49. Suzuki Y, Matsunaga T, Sato S, et al. The pins and rubbers traction system for treatment of comminuted intraarticular fractures and fracture-dislocations in the hand. J Hand Surg Br 1994;19(1):98–107.

Scaphoid and Carpal Bone Fracture
The Difficult Cases and Approach to Management

Abhiram R. Bhashyam, MD, PhD*, Chaitanya Mudgal, MD, MS(Orth), MCh(Orth)

KEYWORDS

- Scaphoid fracture • Scaphoid nonunion • Carpal fracture • Wrist fracture • Wrist instability

KEY POINTS

- Fractures of the carpal bones, except the scaphoid, are quite rare.
- Any fracture involving the carpal bones should heighten suspicion for wrist instability.
- Systematic preoperative imaging is critical to identify fractures that may require stabilization. Special views and/or cross-sectional imaging are often required for diagnosis and surgical planning.
- Nondisplaced fractures can be treated nonoperatively but may require prolonged immobilization for bones with tenuous blood supply, such as the scaphoid, lunate, and capitate. Scaphoid fractures, especially fractures of the proximal pole are predisposed to nonunion or avascular necrosis because the scaphoid is almost completely covered with hyaline cartilage creating an environment with limited periosteum and vascular supply.
- Displaced carpal bone fractures, and those associated with carpal instability, require open reduction internal fixation.

INTRODUCTION

Fractures of the carpus can have a significant impact on functional activity of patients and their quality of life. Wrist and hand motion depends on the normal alignment of the carpal bones, whose synchronized movement allow for flexion, extension, radial deviation, and ulnar deviation of the wrist. Disruption to normal carpal alignment can have significant effects on wrist motion and the likelihood of posttraumatic arthritis—especially if the injury is not identified promptly and treated appropriately. Additionally, displaced carpal fractures may be predisposed to nonunion and posttraumatic arthritis given the potential for vascular disruption and joint incongruency due to their intra-articular location.

Definition: Challenging Scaphoid and Carpal Bone Fractures

In this article, we will focus on our approach to managing challenging scaphoid and carpal bone fractures. Challenging scaphoid fractures can be categorized into 3 groups: acute fractures (proximal pole and waist), previously operated fractures (partial union or nonunion, proximal pole fragmentation), and nonunions.[1] In the treatment of nonunions, we will review fixation and bone graft options including nonvascularized grafts (distal radius, iliac crest, cancellous graft, proximal hamate), vascularized pedicled grafts (volar carpal artery, 1,2-Intercompartmental Supraretinacular Artery [ICSRA], dorsal capsular), and free vascularized grafts (medial femoral condyle/trochlea,

Department of Orthopaedic Surgery, Hand & Arm Center, Massachusetts General Hospital, Boston, MA, USA
* Corresponding author. Department of Orthopaedics, Hand & Arm Center, Massachusetts General Hospital, 55 Fruit Street, Boston, MA 02114.
E-mail address: abhashyam@partners.org

Hand Clin 39 (2023) 265–277
https://doi.org/10.1016/j.hcl.2023.02.003
0749-0712/23/© 2023 Elsevier Inc. All rights reserved.

rib). Finally, we will review the management for carpal bones other than the scaphoid.

Epidemiology and Pathophysiology

Scaphoid fractures account for approximately 80% of all carpal fractures.[2] The overall incidence of scaphoid fractures is ~43 per 100,000.[3] The triquetrum is the second most commonly injured bone. Fractures of the remaining carpal bones are quite rare and together account for only 2% of all carpal fractures.[4] Carpal fractures occur most commonly after falls in young, highly active individuals.[5] Typically, the fall onto an outstretched hand produces an extension moment on the carpus, inducing tensile stress on the volar aspect and compression or shear stress on the dorsal aspect. In higher energy hyperextension injuries, this tensile stress on the volar side of the wrist may result in a perilunate dislocation if the volar wrist ligaments are disrupted. A scaphocapitate perilunate dislocation is a specific fracture pattern whereby both the scaphoid and capitate fracture in a hyperextension injury, and the subsequent shortening of the carpus prevents the reduction of the proximal capitate, and instead causes it to rotate 180°. Scaphocapitate syndrome has been classified by Vance and Gelberman into 6 different types and a further type was added by Mudgal and Lovell.[6] Compression stress on the dorsal aspect typically results in dorsal cortical comminution (eg, triquetral avulsion fracture).

Applied Anatomy and Classification

The 8 carpal bones are divided into the following: (1) the proximal row—scaphoid, lunate, triquetrum, and pisiform and (2) the distal row—trapezium, trapezoid, capitate, and hamate. Their relationships are maintained by radiocarpal, ulnocarpal, and intercarpal ligaments. From radial to ulnar, the volar extrinsic ligaments are the radioscaphocapitate, radioscapholunate, long radiolunate, and short radiolunate. Individual carpal bones are also connected through the interosseous intracarpal ligaments (**Fig. 1A–C**).

The scaphoid is almost completely covered with hyaline cartilage, creating an environment with limited periosteum and vascular supply that is predisposed to nonunion and dysvascularity, which in turn can lead to avascular necrosis. Scaphoid fractures are commonly classified using the Herbert classification, which distinguishes between acute fractures (stable/unstable) and nonunions (**Table 1**).[7] Similarly, more than 80% of the lunate is covered in cartilage, with only 2 areas of vascular supply on the volar and dorsal surface. Lunate fractures are classified based on their vascular anatomy using the Teisen and Kjarbeck classification,[8] which splits lunate fractures into 5 groups (**Table 2**). Trapezium fractures can be divided into body fractures and palmar ridge fractures. Trapezial body fractures can be classified according to the Walker classification, which divides fractures into 5 groups (**Table 3**).[9] Triquetral fractures are classified simply as dorsal avulsion fractures, volar avulsion fractures, and body fractures. Hamate fractures are classified as hook fractures and body fractures. There is no specific useful classification system for capitate, pisiform, or trapezoid fractures. In general, intraobserver and interobserver reliability in carpal fracture classification schemes is poor due to difficulty of interpreting carpal fractures on plain radiographs.[10]

DISCUSSION
Clinical Assessment

Ecchymosis, swelling, and deformity are common physical examination findings in patients with carpal fractures. Palpation of bony landmarks can also raise suspicion for these injuries, especially when there is tenderness over the distal radius, volar scaphoid tubercle, anatomic snuffbox, pisiform, or hook of hamate. For example, in young men with a clear history of sports injury and anatomic snuffbox tenderness on ulnar deviation and tenderness of the scaphoid tubercle, the risk of a scaphoid waist fracture is 91% when all 4 of the aforementioned factors are present.[11] In patients with triquetrum fractures, a simple test to make a clinical diagnosis is done as follows. With the wrist resting at neutral, the examiner places an index finger on the pisiform and applies a dorsally directed force. This makes the triquetrum prominent dorsally, allowing for ease of palpation, eliciting focal tenderness, and diagnosing a triquetral fracture. Similarly, hamate fractures may be diagnosed by local tenderness dorsally as well as volarly over the hook of the hamate. Wright and colleagues described a specific test for hook of hamate fractures. The hand is held in ulnar deviation because the patient flexes the interphalangeal joints of the ulnar 2 digits, using the flexor digitorum profundi against resistance applied by the examiner. The flexor tendons act as a deforming force on the fracture site, and the maneuver elicits pain.[12]

Neurologic examination is important in patients with suspected fracture of the carpus because some types of carpal bone injuries can be associated with acute carpal tunnel syndrome (perilunate fracture dislocations, concomitant fractures of the distal radius and carpus) and others are associated with ulnar nerve injury (hook of hamate

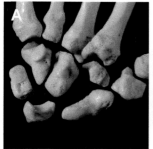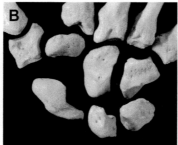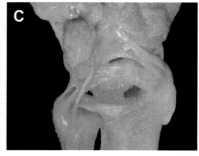

Fig. 1. (*A*) Volar appearance of the carpus. (*B*) Dorsal appearance of the carpus. (*C*) Volar carpal ligaments. (*Courtesy of* Amit Gupta, MD, FRCS, Louisville, KY.)

fractures and fracture dislocations). Objective measures such as static 2-point discrimination should be used to test sensation because light touch sensation is unreliable after acute trauma. Should the examiner wish to test light touch, it is imperative that this testing be done before installation of any local anesthetic in any reduction maneuvers. In motor testing, it is important to distinguish true deficit from weakness secondary to pain. Motor testing may provide a spurious response because the patient may not be able to demonstrate appropriate function due to pain inhibition.

Radiologic Evaluation

Radiographic evaluation begins with posteroanterior (PA), lateral, and oblique views of the hand and wrist. In most circumstances when there is concern for altered carpal relationships which may suggest ligament injury, it is prudent to obtain radiographs of the uninjured side for comparison. On the standard PA view, Gilula's lines should be examined for any discontinuities,[13] which would indicate fracture or dislocation (**Fig. 2**). A "cortical ring" sign can be caused by excessive scaphoid flexion, which can be a sign of scaphoid fracture

or scapholunate dissociation. The lunate should appear to be trapezoid in shape,[14] and a triangular shape can be an indication of perilunate dislocation (**Fig. 3**). The absence of a cortical ring over the hamate on the PA view can be a clue indicating a hook of hamate fracture. Displaced fractures of the scaphoid, body of the trapezium and of the capitate can also typically be readily seen on the PA view.

On the lateral view, the radius, lunate, capitate, and third metacarpal should be collinear when the wrist is at neutral rotation. The absence of the lunate would indicate perilunate dislocation (**Fig. 4**). Dorsal cortical fractures of the triquetrum, which are the most common triquetral fractures, can also be readily seen on the lateral view. However, the absence of radiographic evidence of a dorsal triquetral avulsion fracture on the lateral radiograph does not always imply that there is no fracture. Due to the curvature of the carpus, some dorsal avulsion fractures of the triquetrum may not be adequately visualized on standard radiographs.

Specialized views are helpful for visualizing certain carpal fractures. A scaphoid view is a PA view with the wrist in ulnar deviation, which better

Table 1		
Herbert classification of scaphoid fractures		
Type A	A1	Tubercle fractures
	A2	Nondisplaced waist fractures
Type B	B1	Oblique fracture of distal third
	B2	Displaced or mobile waist fractures
	B3	Proximal pole fractures
	B4	Fracture dislocation of carpus
	B5	Comminuted fractures
Type C	C	Delayed union
Type D	D1	Fibrous nonunion
	D1	Sclerotic nonunion

Table 2	
Teisen and Hjarbeck classification of lunate fractures	
Group 1	Fracture of volar pole possibly affecting nutrient vessel
Group 2	Chip fracture not affecting nutrient vessel
Group 3	Fracture of dorsal pole possibly affecting nutrient vessel
Group 4	Sagittal fracture through body
Group 5	Tranverse fracture through wrist

Table 3
Walker classification of trapezial body fractures

1	Horizontal fractures
2A	Radial tuberosity fractures through the carpometacarpal (CMC) joint
2B	Radial tuberosity fractures through the ST joint
3	Ulnar tuberosity fractures
4	Fractures of the CMC joint
5	Fractures of the ST joint

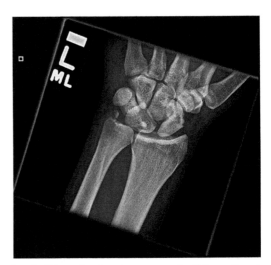

Fig. 3. Triangular lunate as seen in this perilunate fracture dislocation.

visualizes the scaphoid along its entire extended length. However, up to 40% of scaphoid waist fractures may not be seen on any of these views. Radial deviation views can be helpful to see palmar cortical fractures of the triquetrum. A semipronated PA view can better visualize the trapezium and the Scaphotrapeziotrapezoidal (STT) joint. Semisupinated views (45° PA) and carpal tunnel views may be helpful for identifying pisiform and hook of hamate fractures, respectively (**Fig. 5**). A clenched fist PA view is most sensitive for identifying scapholunate diastasis.[5,13,14]

Advanced imaging is often required to accurately identify carpal fractures due to the significant bony overlap between carpal bones on plain radiographs. For example, the sensitivity for detecting scaphoid fracture on plain radiographs alone is only 75%.[15] In the acute setting, computed tomography (CT) scans and MRI can be helpful in identifying radiographically occult carpal fractures in instances of clinical suspicion and inconclusive radiographs. Currently available data suggest that an MRI is more sensitive and specific than a CT scan in the diagnosis of occult scaphoid fractures.[16] CT and MRI scans can be very helpful for delineating fracture geometry, displacement, and comminution. This makes them especially helpful for fracture assessment, planning surgical tactics, and placement of any hardware. Evaluation of healing with advanced imaging (CT) is frequently performed during the treatment of acute scaphoid fractures and nonunions; however, reliability may not always be improved compared with conventional radiographs.[10,17]

Treatment Principles

Treatment of nondisplaced carpal fractures is commonly nonoperative with splinting. Treatment of displaced fractures can be variable, ranging from open reduction internal fixation (ORIF) to surgical excision to splinting. Typical surgical approaches to the treatment of carpal bone fractures will be reviewed, followed by the principles of management for each carpal bone.

tThe workhorse approaches for the management of most carpal fractures are the modified volar Henry, extended carpal tunnel, and midline dorsal. The modified volar Henry follows the line of the flexor carpi radialis (FCR) tendon, which can be easily palpated in most patients. Once the floor of the

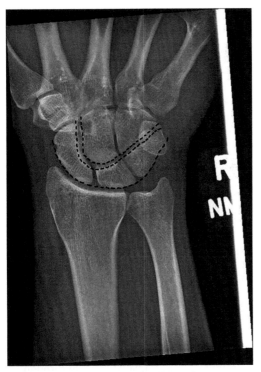

Fig. 2. Gilula's lines. Disruption of these lines suggests a carpal injury.

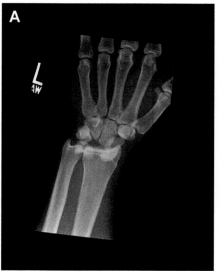
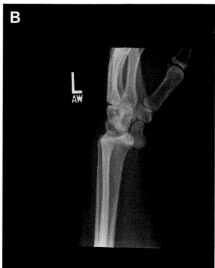

Fig. 4. Perilunate dislocation. (*A*) AP view, (*B*) Lateral view.

FCR sheath is incised to open Parona space and thenar muscles split, the volar radiocarpal ligaments and wrist capsule are quickly exposed. A longitudinal or anatomic capsulotomy then provides access to the scaphoid and STT joint. Contemporary data has not revealed the superiority of one capsulotomy over the other, and it seems that the choice of capsulotomy is largely dependent on surgeon. In the extended carpal tunnel approach, the carpal tunnel contents are retracted radially and the ulnar neurovascular bundle ulnarly, to open Parona space. This approach provides excellent access to the intermediate column of the radius, the lunate, and the hook of hamate. In addition, this approach allows easy access to the space of Poirier, especially in cases of volar lunate dislocation when lunate reduction is performed through the volar capsular rent in the space of Poirier. A technical tip to aid exposure in this approach, consists of flexing the wrist and supporting it in the

flexed position with a large bolster placed along the dorsal surface of the hand. This wrist flexion allows gentle retraction of the flexor tendons and median nerve in a radial direction, reduces tension on the volar ligaments and allows easy reduction of a dislocated lunate. In the dorsal midline approach, a longitudinal incision with radial and ulnar full-thickness flaps is used to visualize the extensor tendon compartments. Once the EPL is transposed and the second and fourth compartments raised subperiosteally, the dorsal wrist capsule is easily exposed. A longitudinal or ligament-sparing capsulotomy then reveals the dorsal aspect of the carpal bones.

Pisiform and some hamate injuries require an flexor carpi ulnaris (FCU) approach to visualize and protect the ulnar neurovascular bundle. A Guyon canal release should be performed when exposing the hamate hook volarly. This is because at the level of the carpus, the ulnar nerve arborizes, and the deep motor branch turns nearly 90° around the base of the hook of hamate (**Fig. 6**). Hook of hamate fractures may also be approached through a more traditional carpal tunnel release approach as previously described. The hamate hook may be exposed circumferentially by subperiosteal dissection to protect the ulnar neurovascular bundle allowing safe excision of the hamate hook.

Scaphoid Fractures

Challenging scaphoid fractures can be categorized into 3 groups: acute fractures (proximal pole and waist), previously operated fractures (partial union or nonunion, proximal pole fragmentation), and nonunions.[1] In previously operated fractures, the surgical approach is typically more

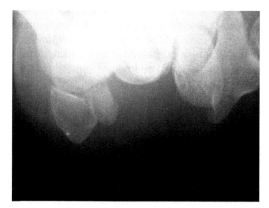

Fig. 5. Carpal tunnel view.

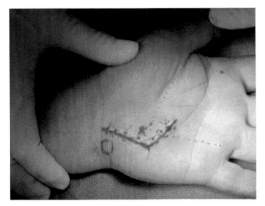

Fig. 6. Incision for hook of hamate fracture.

extensile but the treatment principles are similar to the treatment of a scaphoid nonunion. For this reason, we recommend classifying scaphoid fractures as acute fractures or nonunions when planning treatment.

Current best evidence suggests that nondisplaced, acute waist (<4 weeks from injury), and/or distal pole/third fractures can be treated nonsurgically with adequate immobilization for 6 to 12 weeks using a thumb spica or regular short-arm cast.[18,19] Displacement is typically defined as more than 1 mm of translation, more than 10° angular displacement, radiolunate angle greater than 15°, scapholunate angle greater than 60°, or intrascaphoid angle greater than 35°. Scaphoid waist fractures with less than 2 mm of displacement may be initially treated with cast immobilization but these injuries should be followed closely with immediate conversion to surgical fixation when suspected development of a nonunion is confirmed.[19] In general, fracture displacement is best assessed on a CT scan, which must be done along the long axis of the scaphoid. Displacement is best noted in the coronal plane as a cortical mismatch at the scapho-capitate articulation, or as a dorsal opening of the fracture line when viewed along the long axis, which causes an increase in the intrascaphoid angle. Fracture displacement can also occur as a result of protonation of the distal fragment in up to 36% patients, which can be challenging to diagnose even on a CT scan and often needs 3-dimensional reconstruction ot the scaphoid to make the diagnosis.[20] In contrast, displaced fractures are prone to nonunion and are best treated surgically. Displaced fractures have been shown to have a doubled risk of nonunion for each 0.5 mm of translation.[21] Factors associated with the development of nonunion include delayed diagnosis or treatment, inadequate immobilization, proximal pole fracture, initial and progressive fracture

displacement, comminution, and presence of associated carpal injuries (eg, perilunate injuries).[14]

The primary goal of surgical treatment is the attainment of an anatomic reduction with stable fixation, except in cases of distal pole or tuberosity nonunion, where excision of the distal pole nonunion fragment may allow for the patient to have a painless, stable functional wrist. Acute scaphoid fractures can be managed through a percutaneous or open approach. Previously operated fractures and scaphoid nonunions are managed via an open approach. Indications for percutaneous fixation include nondisplaced scaphoid waist fractures, displaced scaphoid waist fractures that can be closed reduced, and nondisplaced proximal pole fractures. Operative treatment is recommended for all displaced scaphoid fractures because increasing displacement is correlated with increasing risk of nonunion and avascular necrosis, particularly in proximal pole fractures. Volar and/or dorsal open approaches can be used to facilitate fracture reduction and fixation based on fracture characteristics and surgeon preference. It is the senior authors' preference to approach all proximal pole fractures and scaphoid waist fractures dorsally because this approach allows predictable, consistent, and replicable placement of the screw fixation within the central portion of the scaphoid, a factor related to improving the chances of obtaining union after fixation.[22] When fixing acute fractures, it is prudent to use a smaller screw size. If the volar approach is chosen to fix either a distal third or a waist fracture, it is imperative that the trapezial ridge be generously rongeured out, so as to allow central screw placement. An alternate method to ensure central screw placement is to place the screw through the transtrapezial approach.[23]

Common fixation strategies to obtain stable rigid fixation for the treatment of acute scaphoid fractures and scaphoid nonunions are K-wires, headless compression screws, and plates. Headless compression screws may be inserted along the central axis of the scaphoid or perpendicular to the fracture plane within the middle third of the scaphoid based on fracture anatomy and surgeon preference.[24] Although screw placement perpendicular to the fracture plane would make intuitive sense, finite element analysis of screw relation to fracture plane has not shown the superiority of screw placement perpendicular to the fracture site. The power of K-wires in difficult situations should not be underestimated: a recent retrospective cohort study comparing clinical and radiographic outcomes between K-wire and cannulated compression screw fixation in the treatment of scaphoid nonunions found no difference in bony healing or functional outcomes at the time of final follow-up.[24,25] Indeed, this study replicated the findings of Fernandez as well as Nagle.[26,27] Plate fixation of scaphoid fractures is relatively more recent and typically indicated in settings of significant comminution or segmental bone loss that is treated with bone grafting.[28]

Bone graft is typically used in the treatment of scaphoid nonunions. Bone grafts can be divided based on 2 characteristics: (1) structural versus nonstructural and (2) vascularized versus nonvascularized. Structural bone graft is typically used in the correction of humpback deformity or segmental defects within the scaphoid but there is significantly more debate regarding the need for vascularized versus nonvascularized bone graft. A recent national database study comparing rates of revision surgery after the treatment of scaphoid nonunions using vascularized versus nonvascularized bone grafts found similar rates of reoperation, suggesting that nonvascularized bone grafting may be a reasonable first option.[29] Common sources for nonvascularized graft include the distal radius and iliac crest. Vascularized bone grafts are either pedicled (eg, volar carpal artery, 1,2-intercompartmental supraretinacular artery) or free (eg, medial femoral condyle/medial femoral trochlea [MFT]).[30,31] Proximal pole reconstruction after scaphoid nonunion has historically been a challenging problem to treat. It is important to remember the role of adequate fracture surface preparation, and cancellous bone grafting with screw fixation even in these challenging situations. Two recent studies have shown a high rate of union using this treatment methodology.[32,33] Recent literature has also highlighted the utility of 2 new bone grafts: the proximal hamate nonvascularized bone graft and the MFT osteochondral free flap.[34–36] Long-term follow-up results in larger cohorts of patients are needed for these options.

AUTHOR'S APPROACH TO MANAGEMENT OF SCAPHOID FRACTURES

We prefer volar percutaneous fixation in fractures that are in the distal third or in the distal portion of the waist. The volar scaphoid tubercle is palpated and marked. A small incision is made over the tubercle, just large enough to accommodate the drill guide as well as to rongeur the volar lip of the trapezium. A blunt instrument is used to spread down to the bone. The guidewire is then placed onto the tubercle in line with the thumb aiming about 45° both ulnarly and dorsally. Once the starting point and trajectory is satisfactory, the guidewire is advanced. A screw that is 4 mm shorter than the measured length of the guidewire is typically chosen. A cannulated drill is then used to drill across the fracture, and the screw is inserted over the guidewire and compressed.

For displaced waist fractures, we prefer an open volar approach. Once the fracture is exposed, 0.045 or 0.062 inch K-wires are placed into the proximal and distal fragments to use as joysticks to facilitate reduction. A pointed reduction clamp is applied to hold the reduction, and the surgeon then places the screw as above. For mid-waist and proximal pole fractures, we prefer a dorsal approach and use a similar K-wire technique followed by rigid fixation. For predictable central screw placement, it is vital to start the guidewire just radial to the attachment of the scapholunate interosseous ligament and the trajectory of the guidewire should aim along the axis of the thumb metacarpal.

In the setting of scaphoid nonunion, we prefer nonvascularized bone grafting with rigid fixation, even in the setting of proximal pole nonunions. Vascularized bone grafting is used if nonvascularized bone grafting fails. For complete proximal pole necrosis or avascular necrosis (AVN), we prefer the MFT osteochondral free flap versus expectant management.

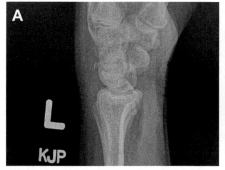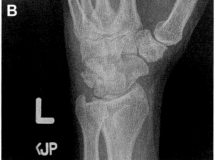

Fig. 7. Triquetral body and dorsal avulsion fractures. (*A*) AP view, (*B*) Lateral view.

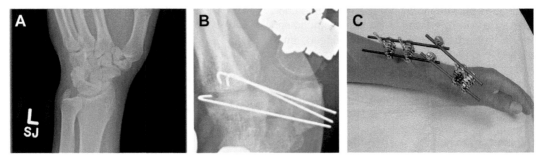

Fig. 8. (A) Trapezium fracture, (B) Treated with open reduction internal fixation with (C) adjuvant external fixation.

Triquetrum Fractures

Dorsal cortical fractures can be treated with immobilization for 4 to 6 weeks. The immobilization is primarily to treat the underlying soft tissue injury. In rare circumstances, a painful nonunion of the displaced fragment is treated with surgical excision. Most triquetral body fractures may also be treated nonoperatively but ORIF has been described for displaced triquetral body fractures.[37] Surgical management should be considered in cases of suspected carpal instability (**Fig. 7**).

Trapezium Fractures

Nondisplaced trapezial body fractures and palmar trapezial ridge fractures can be treated in a short-arm thumb spica cast for 4 to 6 weeks. Painful nonunited palmar ridge fractures can be treated with excision. Displaced body fractures should be treated with closed versus open reduction and

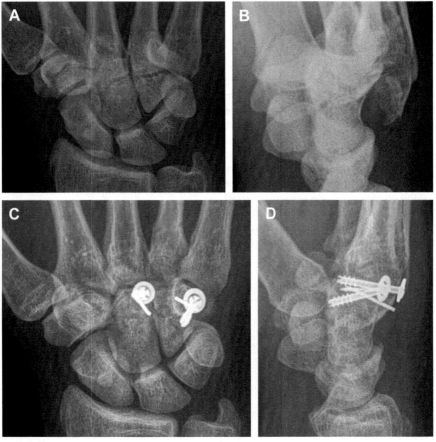

Fig. 9. Hamate and capitate fractures. (A) AP view, (B) Lateral view, (C,D) AP and lateral view after open reduction internal fixation.

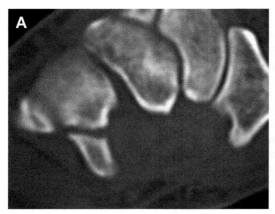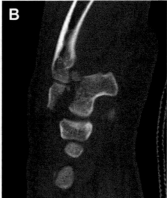

Fig. 10. (*A*) CT of hook of hamate fracture. (*B*) CT of hamate body fracture.

internal fixation. Fractures can be exposed through the Wagner approach using headless compression screws, K-wires or a combination of both. Displaced fractures can be treated with ORIF plus additional external fixation if needed. The first metacarpal can be pinned to the second metacarpal to provide traction on the trapezium in cases of comminuted fractures. Trapezial fractures are often associated with base of first metacarpal fractures, which should also be addressed (**Fig. 8**).

Capitate Fractures

Isolated nondisplaced capitate fractures can be treated with a thumb spica cast, typically for 6 to 8 weeks or more. As the head of the capitate is completely covered in cartilage, the proximal capitate is supplied by retrograde blood flow and is subject to the same difficulties of vascularity as the proximal pole of the scaphoid. Displaced capitate fractures and those associated with transscaphoid or transcapitate perilunate dislocations are managed operatively through a dorsal approach (**Fig. 9**).

Hamate Fractures

Nondisplaced hook of hamate fractures can be treated nonoperatively. A short-arm cast is applied for 6 weeks and union is confirmed with a CT scan. Displaced or chronic hook of hamate fractures (**Fig. 10**A) is typically treated with excision because an untreated fracture can lead to rupture of the long flexors of the ring and small fingers.[38] However, because the hook of hamate acts as a pully for the ulnar digital flexors, some have advocated for ORIF to prevent decreased small finger function.[39] It is worth noting that this suggestion has not been replicated. Nondisplaced hamate body fractures can also be treated nonoperatively with casting. Displaced fractures that involve the carpometacarpal joint should be managed with ORIF (**Fig. 10**B).

Pisiform Fractures

Nondisplaced pisiform fractures can be treated with casting. Displaced and comminuted fractures and symptomatic nonunions should be treated with excision. The pisiform can be accessed volarly. As with the hamate, particular attention must be paid to identify and isolate the ulnar neurovascular bundle.

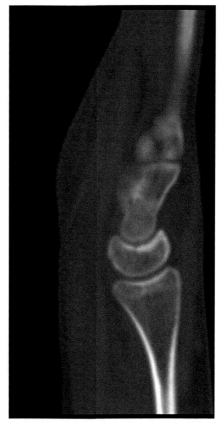

Fig. 11. Lunate fracture.

Trapezoid Fractures

Due to its protected location, isolated trapezoid fractures are extremely rare and fewer than 20 cases have been reported in the literature.[5] Displaced isolated fractures should be treated with ORIF.

Lunate Fractures

The lunate is also in a relatively protected location. Isolated lunate fractures are rare. Nondisplaced fractures without associated instability can be treated with immobilization (**Fig. 11**). Displaced fractures and those associated with carpal instability must be treated surgically, either with closed reduction and pinning or ORIF. Avulsions of the scapholunate interosseous ligament may be repaired with suture anchors, and the carpus reduced and pinned.

If open reduction is required, lunate body fractures can be approached via a volar or dorsal approach (**Fig. 12**A–C). The fragments can be fixed with either headless compression screws or Kirschner wires. Scaphocapitate pinning has

been advocated by some authors because it may take some load off the healing lunate. In instances of a nonreconstructable lunate, either proximal row carpectomy or scaphocapitate fusion with lunate excision is indicated.

Complications/Prognosis

The scaphoid, lunate, and head of the capitate are covered in large part by cartilage, and both the proximal scaphoid and capitate head are supplied by retrograde blood flow. These factors increase the likelihood of nonunion due to limited perfusion after trauma. Therefore, it is common to obtain a CT scan at 3 to 4 months after treatment to confirm healing. We recommend operative treatment of nondisplaced scaphoid fractures treated nonoperatively if there is no evidence of healing on CT at 3 to 4 months. For operatively treated scaphoid fractures, revision ORIF may be necessary.

Given the tenuous blood supply, the proximal pole of the scaphoid and the head of the capitate are prone to dysvascularity. This may be due to the amount of displacement in the initial injury.

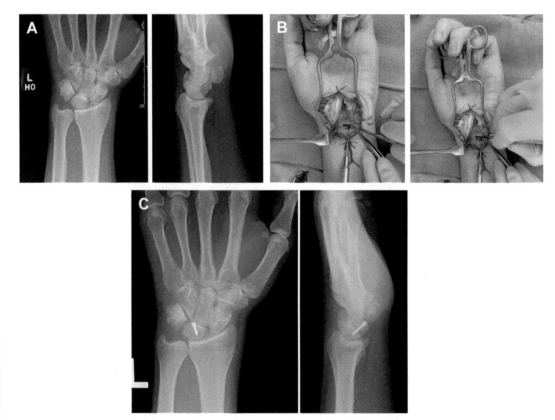

Fig. 12. Volar approach for displaced lunate fracture. (*A*) AP and lateral radiographs demonstrating displaced lunate fracture, (*B*) Clinical photos demonstrating displaced volar lunate fracture (*forceps*), (*C*) AP and lateral radiographs after open reduction internal fixation. (*Courtesy of* Jeffrey Friedrich, MD, FACS, Seattle, WA.)

Dysvascularity can also be iatrogenic, from violating the blood supply during surgical dissection. Contrast-enhanced MRI may be used to assess for vascularity, although its use is controversial. Proximal pole avascular necrosis of the scaphoid can be treated with pedicled or free vascularized bone graft. Capitate AVN is rare and there are no series with long-term results of revascularization.[32]

Osteoarthritis is one other complication of carpal injury. Scaphoid nonunion advanced collapse (SNAC) is a well-known progression of degenerative changes. It begins with cystic changes of the scaphoid, followed by radioscaphoid arthritis, and is concluded by pan-carpal arthritis. Operative treatment of scaphoid injuries may also predispose patients to degenerative changes through iatrogenic injury to the cartilage at the scaphotrapezial joint at the time of screw insertion. However, although this phenomenon has been documented radiographically, it seems that it is of minimal clinical relevance. Treatment of SNAC wrist is typically with proximal row carpectomy, scaphoid excision with 4-corner fusion, or total wrist arthrodesis depending on the extent of arthritis. Wrist denervation can also be considered.

SUMMARY

Carpal fractures are rare, with the scaphoid being the most commonly affected bone and accounting for about 80% of all carpal fractures. They most commonly present in young, male patients because of sports related or other low mechanism injury. Higher energy injuries such as falls from height and motor vehicle accidents can also cause carpal fractures with the possibility for carpal instability.

Carpal fractures can easily be missed on conventional radiographs, and special views or advanced cross-sectional imaging is often necessary for diagnosis. Early and accurate diagnosis is crucial because displaced carpal fractures can have significant impact to long-term hand and wrist function. Nondisplaced fractures can often be treated effectively with casting but displaced carpal fractures almost always require fixation. Some of the carpal bones—the scaphoid, lunate, and capitate—are covered almost entirely with cartilage and thus have limited blood supply. Thus, avascular necrosis, delayed union, and nonunion are potential complications following nonoperative or operative treatment of fractures. Finally, displaced carpal fractures can lead to posttraumatic arthritis. Treatment of these complications include revision ORIF, proximal row carpectomy, limited intercarpal fusion, and total wrist arthrodesis.

CLINICS CARE POINTS

- Fractures of the carpal bones, except the scaphoid, are quite rare
- Any fracture involving the carpal bones should heighten suspicion for wrist instability
- Systematic preoperative imaging is critical to identify fractures that may require stabilization. Special views and/or cross-sectional imaging are often required for diagnosis and surgical planning.
- Nondisplaced fractures can be treated nonoperatively but may require prolonged immobilization for bones with tenuous blood supply, such as the scaphoid, lunate and capitate. Scaphoid fractures are predisposed to nonunion because the scaphoid is almost completely covered with hyaline cartilage creating an environment with limited periosteum and vascular supply
- Displaced carpal bone fractures, and those associated with carpal instability require open reduction internal fixation.

DECLARATION OF INTERESTS

No potential conflicts of interest exist with respect to the research, authorship, and/or publication of this article. This article was funded in part by the Jesse B. Jupiter/Wyss Medical Foundation Fund.

REFERENCES

1. Cooney WP, Dobyns JH, Linscheid RL. Fractures of the scaphoid: a rational approach to management. Clin Orthop Relat Res 1980;149:90–7.
2. Van Tassel DC, Owens BD, Wolf JM. Incidence estimates and demographics of scaphoid fracture in the U.S. population. J Hand Surg Am 2010;35(8): 1242–5.
3. Adler JB, Shaftan GW. Fractures of the capitate. J Bone Joint Surg Am 1962;44-A:1537–47.
4. Wolf JM, Dawson L, Mountcastle SB, et al. The incidence of scaphoid fracture in a military population. Injury 2009;40(12):1316–9.
5. Vigler M, Aviles A, Lee SK. Carpal fractures excluding the scaphoid. Hand Clin 2006;22(4): 501–16.
6. Mudgal C, Lovell M. Scapho-capitate syndrome: distant fragment migration. Acta Orthop Belg 1995; 61(1):62–5.

7. Herbert TJ, Fisher WE. Management of the fractured scaphoid using a new bone screw. J Bone Joint Surg Br 1984;66(1):114–23.

8. Teisen H, Hjarbaek J. Classification of fresh fractures of the lunate. J Hand Surg Br 1988;13(4):458–62.

9. Walker JL, Greene TL, Lunseth PA. Fractures of the body of the trapezium. J Orthop Trauma 1988;2(1):22–8.

10. Drijkoningen T, ten Berg PWL, Guitton TG, et al. Reliability of Diagnosis of Partial Union of Scaphoid Waist Fractures on Computed Tomography. J Hand Microsurg 2018;10(3):130–3.

11. Duckworth AD, Buijze GA, Moran M, et al. Predictors of fracture following suspected injury to the scaphoid. J Bone Joint Surg Br 2012;94(7):961–8.

12. Wright TW, Moser MW, Sahajpal DT. Hook of hamate pull test. J Hand Surg Am 2010;35(11):1887–9.

13. Gilula LA. Carpal injuries: analytic approach and case exercises. AJR Am J Roentgenol 1979;133(3):503–17.

14. Leslie IJ, Dickson RA. The fractured carpal scaphoid. Natural history and factors influencing outcome. J Bone Joint Surg Br 1981;63-B(2):225–30.

15. Lozano-Calderón S, Blazar P, Zurakowski D, et al. Diagnosis of scaphoid fracture displacement with radiography and computed tomography. J Bone Joint Surg Am 2006;88(12):2695–703.

16. Rua T, Malhotra B, Vijayanathan S, et al. Clinical and cost implications of using immediate MRI in the management of patients with a suspected scaphoid fracture and negative radiographs results from the SMaRT trial. Bone Joint Lett J 2019;101-B(8):984–94.

17. Matzon JL, Lutsky KF, Tulipan JE, et al. Reliability of Radiographs and Computed Tomography in Diagnosing Scaphoid Union After Internal Fixation. J Hand Surg 2021;46(7):539–43.

18. Buijze GA, Doornberg JN, Ham JS, et al. Surgical compared with conservative treatment for acute nondisplaced or minimally displaced scaphoid fractures: a systematic review and meta-analysis of randomized controlled trials. J Bone Joint Surg Am 2010;92(6):1534–44.

19. Dias JJ, Brealey SD, Fairhurst C, et al. Surgery versus cast immobilisation for adults with a bicortical fracture of the scaphoid waist (SWIFFT): a pragmatic, multicentre, open-label, randomised superiority trial. Lancet 2020;396(10248):390–401.

20. Nakamura R, Imaeda T, Horii E, et al. Analysis of scaphoid fracture displacement by three-dimensional computed tomography. J Hand Surg Am 1991;16(3):485–92.

21. Grewal R, Suh N, Macdermid JC. Use of computed tomography to predict union and time to union in acute scaphoid fractures treated nonoperatively. J Hand Surg Am 2013;38(5):872–7.

22. Trumble TE, Gilbert M, Murray LW, et al. Displaced Scaphoid Fractures Treated with Open Reductio and Internal Fixation with a Cannulated Screw. JBJS 2000;82(5):633.

23. Verstreken F, Meermans G. Transtrapezial Approach for Fixation of Acute Scaphoid Fractures. JBJS Essent Surg Tech 2015;5(4):e29.

24. Engel H, Xiong L, Heffinger C, et al. Comparative outcome analysis of internal screw fixation and Kirschner wire fixation in the treatment of scaphoid nonunion. J Plast Reconstr Aesthet Surg 2020;73(9):1675–82.

25. Mahmoud M, Hegazy M, Khaled SA, et al. Radiographic Parameters to Predict Union after Volar Percutaneous Fixation of Herbert Type B1 and B2 Scaphoid Fractures. J Hand Surg Am 2016;41(2):203–7.

26. Nagle DJ. Scaphoid nonunion. Treatment with cancellous bone graft and Kirschner-wire fixation. Hand Clin 2001;17(4):625–9.

27. Fernandez DL, Eggli S. Non-union of the scaphoid. Revascularization of the proximal pole with implantation of a vascular bundle and bone-grafting. J Bone Joint Surg Am 1995;77(6):883–93.

28. Schormans PMJ, Kooijman MA, Ten Bosch JA, et al. Mid-term outcome of volar plate fixation for scaphoid nonunion. Bone Joint Lett J 2020;102-B(12):1697–702.

29. Ross PR, Lan WC, Chen JS, et al. Revision surgery after vascularized or non-vascularized scaphoid nonunion repair: A national population study. Injury 2020;51(3):656–62.

30. Aibinder WR, Wagner ER, Bishop AT, et al. Bone Grafting for Scaphoid Nonunions: Is Free Vascularized Bone Grafting Superior for Scaphoid Nonunion? Hand (N Y) 2019;14(2):217–22.

31. Rancy SK, Swanstrom MM, DiCarlo EF, et al. Success of scaphoid nonunion surgery is independent of proximal pole vascularity. J Hand Surg Eur 2018;43(1):32–40.

32. Shoji KE, Simeone FJ, Ozkan S, et al. Outcomes of Local Bone Graft and Fixation of Proximal Pole Scaphoid Nascent Nonunions and Nonunions. J Wrist Surg 2020;9(3):203–8.

33. Luchetti TJ, Rao AJ, Fernandez JJ, et al. Fixation of proximal pole scaphoid nonunion with non-vascularized cancellous autograft. J Hand Surg Eur 2018;43(1):66–72.

34. Chan AHW, Elhassan BT, Suh N. The Use of the Proximal Hamate as an Autograft for Proximal Pole Scaphoid Fractures: Clinical Outcomes and Biomechanical Implications. Hand Clin 2019;35(3):287–94.

35. Kakar S, Greene RM, Elhassan BT, et al. Topographical Analysis of the Hamate for Proximal Pole Scaphoid Nonunion Reconstruction. J Hand Surg Am 2020;45(1):69.e1–7.

36. Pet MA, Assi PE, Yousaf IS, et al. Outcomes of the Medial Femoral Trochlea Osteochondral Free Flap for Proximal Scaphoid Reconstruction. J Hand Surg Am 2020;45(4):317–26.e3.

37. Porter ML, Seehra K. Fracture-dislocation of the triquetrum treated with a Herbert screw. J Bone Joint Surg Br 1991;73(2):347–8.

38. Klausmeyer MA, Mudgal CS. Hook of hamate fractures. J Hand Surg Am 2013;38(12):2457–60. quiz 2460.

39. Watson HK, Rogers WD. Nonunion of the hook of the hamate: an argument for bone grafting the nonunion. J Hand Surg Am 1989;14(3):486–90.

Recognizing and Treating Unique Distal Radius Fracture Patterns that are Prone to Displacement

Sze Ryn Chung, MBBCh BAO, MRCS[a], Kevin C. Chung, MD, MS[b],*

KEYWORDS

- Distal radius fracture • Unstable • Volar plate • Dorsal plate • Fragment-specific fixation
- Dorsal spanning plate

KEY POINTS

- Distal radius fracture is considered unstable when the fracture cannot resist displacement after initial closed reduction.
- Treatment options depend on radiographic parameters of instability (eg, absence of volar cortical hook, dorsal comminution) and patient factors (eg, age, functional demand, preference).
- Although most distal radius fractures can be managed with volar plates, some fracture patterns are more amenable to fragment-specific fixation.
- Die-punch fractures may require an additional dorsal plate or a dorsal spanning plate.
- Intra-articular fracture with a step-off or gap of more than 2 mm would benefit from arthroscopic-assisted fixation.

INTRODUCTION

The initial management of patients with distal radius fractures (DRFs) consists of closed reduction and plaster immobilization.[1–3] However, despite acceptable postreduction radiographs, up to 64% of patients have repeat displacement following closed reduction.[4] Most surgeons would agree that the inability of a fracture to resist displacement after initial closed reduction is considered an unstable fracture. The question is, what parameters should be used to determine that a fracture is unstable?

The use of volar locking plates (VLPs) has revolutionized the treatment of DRFs. With the innovations in variable-angled plating design, locking construct, and technique, the VLP affords stable anatomical fixation allowing earlier mobilization and return to function.[5] However, not all DRFs can be treated with VLPs. Some fracture patterns may do well simply with reduction and immobilization. In addition, severely comminuted DRFs may benefit from fragment- or column-specific fixation.

Therefore, understanding the distal radius' 3-dimensional anatomy is crucial in recognizing subtle differences among fracture patterns.[6] Secondary displacement of fractures can occur if specific fracture patterns are not appreciated and addressed surgically. This article focuses on recognizing unstable DRF patterns, assessing them through radiographic imaging, and managing these unstable fractures.

FACTORS OF INSTABILITY

Several factors of instability have been proposed in the literature to identify DRFs that are prone to displacement.[7] Although no consensus exists regarding which parameters to use, the authors

[a] Department of Hand and Reconstructive Microsurgery, Singapore General Hospital, 20, College Road, 169856 Singapore; [b] Section of Plastic Surgery, Department of Surgery, University of Michigan Medical School, Ann Arbor, MI, USA
* Corresponding author. Section of Plastic Surgery, The University of Michigan Health System, 1500 East Medical Center Drive, 2130 Taubman Center, SPC 5340, Ann Arbor, MI 48109-5340.
E-mail address: kecchung@med.umich.edu

Hand Clin 39 (2023) 279–293
https://doi.org/10.1016/j.hcl.2023.02.004

adopt some criteria to decide which fractures benefit from surgery.

The authors consider Lafontaine factors of instability when assessing the initial radiographs of a patient with DRF: dorsal angulation greater than 20°, dorsal comminution, intra-articular fracture extension, associated ulnar fracture, and age over 60 years.[8] The presence of 3 or more factors is considered unstable. According to Walenkamp and colleagues,[7] the most significant predictors of fracture instability were age over 60, female sex, and fractures with dorsal comminution. Despite the high risk of fracture instability, geriatric patients tend to cope well with malunited DRF.[9,10]

Another criterion that the authors adopt is the presence of volar cortical integrity (volar hook)[11] (**Fig. 1**). The volar hook is the strongest predictor in preventing dorsal angulation and final carpal alignment during healing. Therefore, restoring the volar hook during manipulation and reduction of a DRF with a translated volar cortex will ensure fracture stability.

The classical rule of 11 helps one appreciate the acceptable radiographic parameters in patients with DRF.[12] The rule of 11 entails re-establishing the distal radius height of 11 mm, ulnar variance of 1 mm, radial inclination of 22°, and volar tilt of 11°. The fracture reduction is considered acceptable once these radiographic parameters are established. If the postreduction radiographs showed repeat displacement outside acceptable parameters, most surgeons would agree that dorsal angulation greater than 10 to 15°, greater than 2 to 5 mm of ulnar shortening, less than 15° of radial inclination, or intra-articular step-off greater than 2 mm would benefit from surgical fixation.[13,14]

Currently, there are no standard criteria for assessing the stability of DRFs. The described

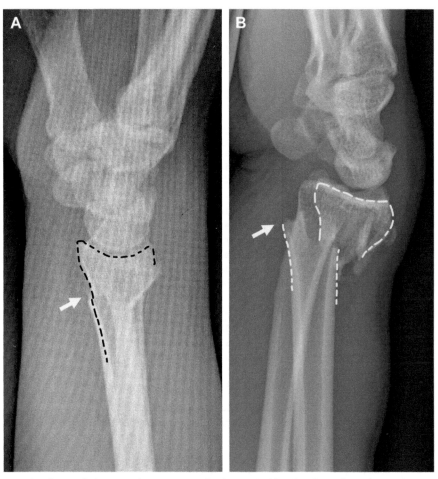

Fig. 1. (*A*) Lateral radiograph showing the presence of volar cortical hook, where the volar cortices are in contact with one another, as shown by the (*black dotted lines*). (*Yellow arrow*) indicates the fracture site. (*B*) Translated volar cortex (*yellow dotted line*) is a strong predictor of instability.[12]

criterion mainly serves as a guide to identify unstable DRF and facilitate shared decision making between patients and surgeons. Therefore, the treatment of DRF should be individualized based on fracture patterns and patient factors.

RADIOGRAPHIC EVALUATION

Accurate interpretation of radiographs is essential for the effective management of DRFs. Subtle changes in radiographic landmarks can provide a great deal of information regarding a fracture pattern and the extent of the injury.

Radiographs

Radiographic evaluation of DRF requires the standard wrist posteroanterior (PA) and lateral projection views.[6] In comminuted fractures, oblique views may provide a different perspective of the fracture pattern than the standard views. Traction views help identify small fracture fragments that would otherwise be missed in standard views. A 10° tilt PA, 45° pronated oblique, and 20° inclined lateral might help assess the presence of joint penetration following implant fixation.[15] Widening the distal radioulnar joint (DRUJ) on PA view or dorsal subluxation of the ulna in relation to the radius on lateral view may represent DRUJ instability from unstable sigmoid notch fracture or triangular fibrocartilage complex (TFCC) injury.

The volar rim of the lunate facet (teardrop) is best appreciated through the 10° lateral view. The teardrop angle is measured from the central axis of the teardrop (parallel to the subchondral bone) to the axis of the radial shaft, which is typically 70° (see **Fig. 7**). An increase in anterior-posterior (AP) distance on the lateral view indicates a die-punch fracture, usually from an axial injury (**Fig. 2**). Articular separation with gaps on PA and lateral views indicates incomplete apposition of the intra-articular fragments.[6]

The intra-articular fracture patterns tend to be predictable because of the strong extrinsic ligaments attached to the fragments.[16]

Computed Tomography

A computed tomography (CT) scan is valuable for patients with complex intraarticular DRF. It allows one to study the articular fracture patterns more closely and provide important information for preoperative evaluation, planning, and intraoperative navigation.[17] By reconstructing data from conventional 2-dimensional CT scan images, one can produce 3D images of the articular surface (see **Fig. 15**).

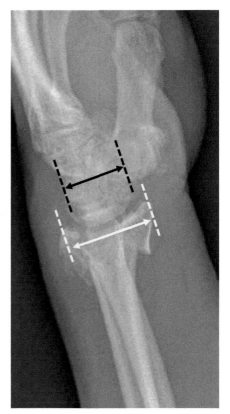

Fig. 2. Lateral radiograph showing increased AP distance of the die-punch fracture (*yellow*) compared with the AP distance of the lunate (*black*). Black dotted lines: Anterior and posterior border of the lunate bone; Yellow dotted lines: Anterior and posterior rims of the distal radius. AP: Anterior posterior.

TREATMENT BASED ON FIXATION TECHNIQUES
Volar Plate Fixation

Intraarticular distal radius fracture

Recent designs of variable angled VLPs have enabled surgeons to place the plates close to the watershed line. In addition, these plates are more anatomical, allowing a more distal plate placement and thus better purchase in smaller articular fractures that are difficult to capture with the traditional T-plates. Such plates should be seated distal to the fracture line to provide a buttress and prevent the volar rim fragments from displacing forward (**Fig. 3**).

Fig. 4 is an example of an unstable DRF with significant radial shortening, dorsal angulation, and a translated volar cortex. Following initial reduction and temporary immobilization, the radiographs showed inadequate restoration of the volar cortical hook with persistent displacement of the volar fragments. The authors prefer an extended flexor carpi radialis (FCR) approach for most of their intra-

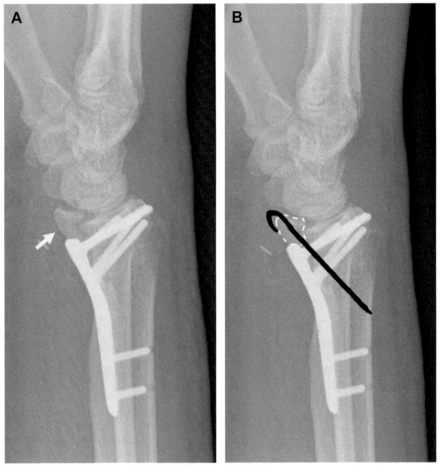

Fig. 3. (*A*) Lateral radiographs revealed an unstable volar rim fracture (*yellow arrow*) not adequately addressed with a VLP. (*B*) A fragment-specific implant such as a K-wire (*black*) may be used to stabilize the fragment. (*Yellow dotted*) lines show the outline of the unstable fracture fragment. VLP, Volar locking plate.

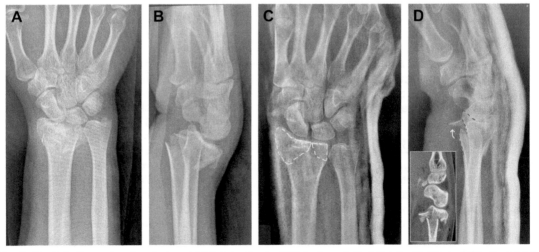

Fig. 4. (*A, B*) Radiographs of a displaced (*C*) intra-articular DRF (*yellow dotted lines*) with the inability to restore the (*D*) volar cortical hook (*red dotted lines*). The (*yellow arrow*) indicates the comminuted volar cortical fragment.

articular DRFs. The brachioradialis tendon was released to facilitate the correction of the radial shortening, translation, and restoration of articular congruity.[18,19] The pronator quadratus was raised subperiosteally, and the intermediate column was exposed to reduce the intermediate fragments accurately, particularly the sigmoid notch.

An Orbay approach was employed by pronating the proximal fragment with lobster claw forceps to access the dorsal aspect of the fracture site.[20] This approach facilitates debridement of the fracture callus and organized hematoma. The fracture was reduced by matching the volar cortices like a jigsaw using maneuvers such as longitudinal traction. In addition, an osteotome was used to lever the distal fragment through the fracture site, correcting the dorsal angulation and dorsal translation. A rolled green towel was then placed behind the dorsum of the hand with the wrist flexed to facilitate the correction of dorsal angulation. The distal fragment was temporarily stabilized with an interfocal 1.4 mm K-wire from the styloid tip to the proximal radius (**Fig. 5**A – black wire).

To stabilize the intermediate column, one may place a second oblique wire from the proximal radius to the intermediate column distally (see **Fig. 5**A–blue wire). In cases with a sagittal split with a significant gap between the radial and the intermediate column, the authors use bone tenaculum forceps (**Fig. 5**B) to assist with the reduction. A transverse K-wire may be placed to stabilize the fragments (see **Fig. 5**A – red wire) Radial height can be achieved by ulnar deviation and intrafocal K-wires to lever the radial column fragments radially.

The authors employ the lift technique to correct the dorsal angulation.[21,22] **Fig. 6** depicts the steps for performing the lift technique. A simple tip to determine the distal screw direction is to place a hypodermic needle into the radiocarpal joint. The drill should be oriented in a direction parallel to the joint surface. In fractures with a coronal split, manual pressure or reduction of the fragments in an AP direction using bone tenaculum forceps may be helpful.

Before closure, the DRUJ is routinely balloted for stability. Although there is a high prevalence of concomitant ligamentous injury associated with intra-articular DRFs, there is no strong evidence to suggest the benefits of repairing them.[23,24] The authors prefer to fix concomitant ulnar styloid fractures if the DRUJ is unstable.

Volar shearing fractures volar Barton

Volar shearing fractures are frequently associated with subluxation or dislocation of the carpus because of the loss of palmar support of the carpus. The fracture may be simple or comminuted.[25] The lateral radiograph may show an abnormal teardrop angle, indicating a displaced volar lunate facet (**Fig. 7**). This creates functional

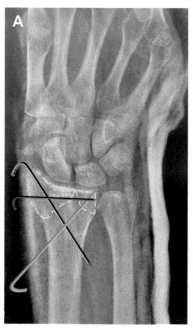
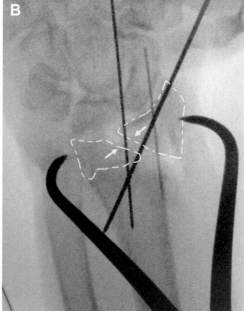

Fig. 5. (A) Multiple K-wire configurations that one can adopt to stabilize the radial and intermediate columns temporarily. (B) A bone tenaculum clamp is 1 trick to reduce the radial and intermediate column. The (yellow dotted lines) show the outline of the radial and intermediate column fragments; (*Yellow arrow*) indicates the reduction of the fragments using a bone tenaculum clamp.

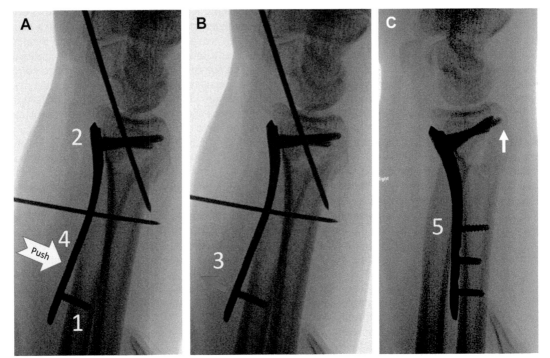

Fig. 6. (*A–C*) Lateral radiographs depict the steps of performing a lift technique to correct dorsal angulation of DRF. First, a locking screw is placed into the proximal hole without entering the bone (lift screw). Next, distal locking screws are inserted parallel to the joint line, distal to fracture site. The proximal lift screw is removed (*red arrow*). The plate is approximated to the radial shaft by inserting a cortical screw along the shaft of the plate. This effectively lifts the distal fragment, correcting the volar tilt (*white arrow*). Finally, locking screws are placed to secure the plate further.

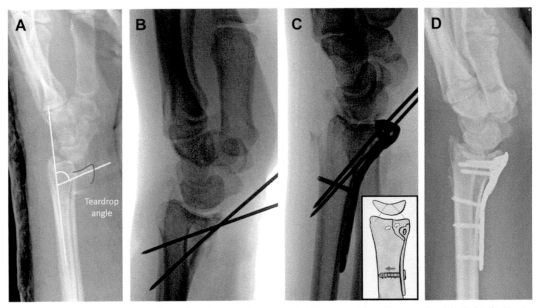

Fig. 7. (*A*) Lateral radiographs of a volar shearing fracture with increased teardrop angle. (*B*) Multiple K-wires were inserted to stabilize the fragments, and (*C*) a volar buttress plate was placed to compress the fragment (*yellow arrow*) to the stable dorsal cortex with a cortical shaft screw (*red arrow*). (*D*) Placement of locking screws to stabilize the fracture. (*Courtesy of* A/Prof Teoh Lam Chuan, Tan Tock Seng, Singapore.)

incompetence of the short radiolunate ligament, leading to radiocarpal instability.

Surgery aims to realign the articular surface to less than 2 mm step-off. The authors prefer fixing these fractures with a volar buttress plate via an extended FCR approach. Once the fracture site is exposed, a rolled green towel is placed under the dorsum of the wrist with the shoulder abducted at a 90° angle and the forearm in supination. The wrist is hyperextended to aid the reduction of the volar fragment.

Multiple K-wires were placed to reduce the teardrop fragment, followed by a volar buttress plate to stabilize the fracture. The authors initiate early motion exercises within 1 week postoperatively if the fracture is stable.

Dorsal Plate Fixation

Dorsal shearing fractures dorsal Barton

The goal in managing distal radius shearing fractures is to restore joint congruency within 2 mm of the articular step-off. Closed reduction and cast immobilization may not be sufficient to stabilize this fracture pattern.

The authors prefer dorsal buttress plates in such injuries, especially in cases with dorsal wall comminution. This is achieved through a dorsal longitudinal approach between the third and fourth extensor compartments (EC). The extensor pollicis longus (EPL) is released, exteriorized, and transposed radially. Subperiosteal elevation of the second and fourth EC is then made, exposing the fracture site. To ease reduction, one may choose to leave the periosteum attached to the comminuted fragments.

Fig. 8 shows a dorsal Barton fracture fixed with 2.4 mm dorsal buttress plates. The authors used bone grafts to fill the bone defects from the comminution. One helpful tip is to bend the distal end of the plate (see **Fig. 8**–yellow arrow) to create a better buttress effect. In addition, a transverse dorsal capsulotomy was performed to facilitate visualization and reduction of the articular joint surface.

After fixation, the periosteum was repaired over the implant to prevent extensor tendon irritation. Secondary plate removal is advised because of the risk of tendon irritation.

Dorsal rim fractures

Dorsal wall fragments provide a footprint for the origin of the dorsal radiocarpal ligament. Failure to address the dorsal rim fragment will lead to the displacement of the fragments and dorsal carpal subluxation (**Fig. 9**). Because of dorsal bending or axial loading forces in DRFs, the fragments of the dorsal wall can be comminuted or impacted into the metaphysis.[19]

Fig. 10 depicts an intra-articular DRF with comminuted dorsal rim fragments and dorsal angulation. There was also an unstable dorsal ulnar corner fragment, as shown on the CT scan (yellow asterisk) (see **Fig. 10**B). Dorsal plating was indicated in this case, as the volar fracture line was distal to the watershed line (see **Fig. 10**B – yellow arrow).

The fracture was fixed with 2.4 mm dorsal buttress plates, similar to the case in **Fig. 8**. Osteotomes were used to lever and correct the dorsal angulation intraoperatively, followed by bone graft placement.

Sandwich Plate Fixation

Sandwich plating or combined volar/dorsal plating is an effective technique for achieving near-anatomic reconstruction of intra-articular DRF with volar and dorsal comminution. A possible alternative to this treatment would be a dorsal

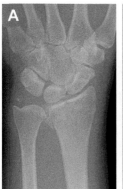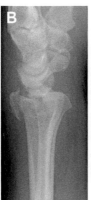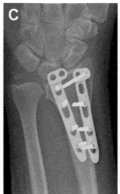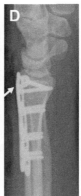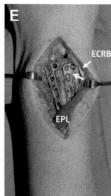

Fig. 8. (A, B) Radiographs showing a dorsal shearing fracture treated with dorsal buttress plates (C–E). The plate has been bent (*yellow arrow*) to create a better buttress effect, and the screws were directed proximally. (*Courtesy of* A/Prof Teoh Lam Chuan, Tan Tock Seng, Singapore.)

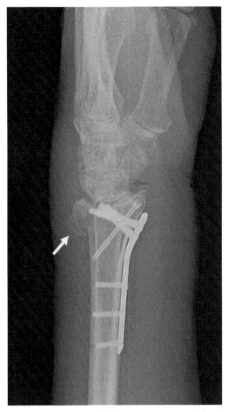

Fig. 9. Lateral radiograph showing an unstable dorsal wall fragment (*yellow arrow*) following a VLP with carpus subluxation (*red arrow*).

spanning plate (DSP) in patients with severe die-punch fractures.[26]

Fig. 11 shows a die-punch intra-articular DRF in a 70-year-old functionally active woman. The lateral radiograph showed an increase in AP distance of the distal radius. An osteotome was used to recreate the fracture site through the volar

incision. A VLP was placed with the wrist in axial traction and ulnar deviation. The authors then proceeded with the dorsal incision, exposing the dorsal comminuted fragments. The dorsal wall was reconstituted with bone allografts and was stabilized with a dorsal buttress plate (**Fig. 12**). The patient was placed on a cast postoperatively for 1 month and was subsequently started on gentle wrist mobilization.

In the authors' experience, osteoporotic bone with extensive comminution often requires VLP with bone augmentation, such as bone graft or bone substitute to fill the metaphyseal defect. However, complications as high as 26% have been reported in the literature from extensor tendon rupture, median neuropathy, wound infections, and wrist collapse.[27]

Fragment-Specific Implant Fixation

DRFs that are distal to or close to the watershed line are indicated for FSF. One of the aims of FSF is to restore the distal radius geometry by applying low-profile implants on specific fracture components. The placement of multiplanar fragment-specific implants creates a rigid load-sharing construct, and such fixation relies on strong ipsilateral bone proximally.[28] Four main categories of FSF implants have been described:[29]

- Pin plates
- Hook plates
- Wire-forms and clamps
- Volar buttress plates

Fig. 13 shows a teardrop avulsion fracture with volar carpus subluxation. Through the extended FCR approach, the teardrop fragment was exposed, reduced, and stabilized with a 1.0 mm K-wire followed by hook plate fixation.

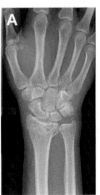
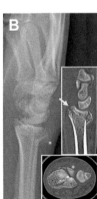
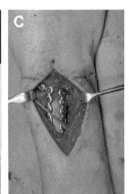
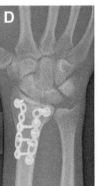
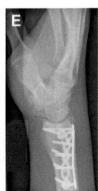

Fig. 10. (*A, B*) Radiographs and CT images of intraarticular DRF fixed with (*C–E*) dorsal buttress plates with correction of dorsal angulation and stabilization of the dorsal wall fragments. The (*yellow arrow*) indicates the volar fracture line located at or distal to the watershed line, and the (*yellow asterisks*) show the unstable dorsal ulnar corner fragment.

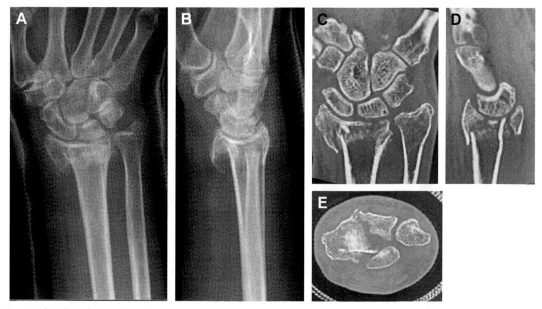

Fig. 11. (*A–E*) Radiographs and CT images show a comminuted intraarticular DRF with die-punch fragments.

Hand fixation plates can also be fabricated and cut into hook or buttress plates (**Fig. 14**). A volar ulnar approach may also be employed. However, the authors find that the extended FCR approach is sufficient to expose the intermediate column.

Arthroscopic-Assisted Distal Radius Fixation

Distal radius fractures with an intra-articular step or gap larger than 2 mm may benefit from an arthroscopic-associated distal radius fixation (AADRF) because of the risk of developing radiographic arthritis.[30,31] Although the degree of radiographic arthritis and its correlation with functional outcome remain controversial, many surgeons have had positive results with arthroscopic reduction.[31,32] In addition to evaluating the congruency of the articular surfaces, arthroscopy can detect any concomitant soft tissue injuries that may require repair.

Ideally, DRFs that require arthroscopic-assisted reduction should be fixed within 1 week to

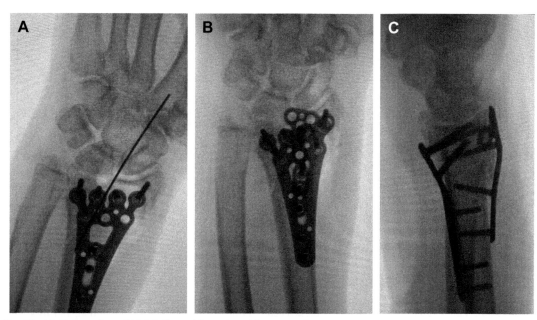

Fig. 12. (*A–C*) Insertion of VLP followed by a dorsal buttress plate.

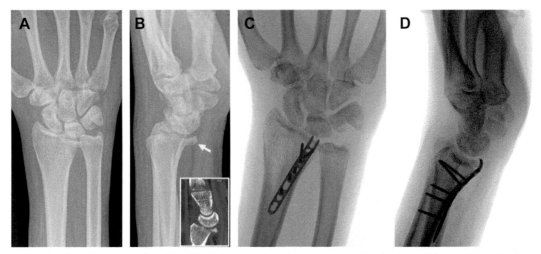

Fig. 13. (*A, B*) Radiographs of a DRF with displaced volar ulna corner stabilized using a 2.0 mm distal ulna hook plate (*C, D*). (*Courtesy of* A/Prof Teoh Lam Chuan, Tan Tock Seng, Singapore.)

facilitate easy mobilization of fracture fragments. The authors prefer to place the arthroscope to fine-tune the intra-articular reduction after provisional fixation of the DRF. Either a 30° or 0° arthroscope can be used. The authors prefer to use a 1.9 mm scope with a 6-R portal as a viewing portal and a 3-4 portal as a working portal.

Figs. 15 and 16 show a DRF with intra-articular step-off and a gap of 2 mm. Reduction and provisional fixation were performed with multiple K-wires and a VLP through the standard volar approach (**Fig 17**A). A cortical screw is placed in the oblong hole of the plate, allowing the plate to be adjusted during the fixation if necessary.[33]

The arthroscope is then introduced through the standard wrist arthroscopy setup with the wrist in vertical traction. The authors' preference is to use the dry wrist arthroscopy technique described by Del Pinal to assess the articular surfaces.[34] An arthroscopic shaver with intermittent irrigation is used to remove blood and debris.

The authors prefer first to stabilize the larger fragments and then match the smaller fragments to them. This provides a stable template to gauge the reduction of other fragments. The authors often use K-wires of 1.0 mm or 1.2 mm diameter to joystick the fracture fragments under arthroscopic visualization before screw insertion. The

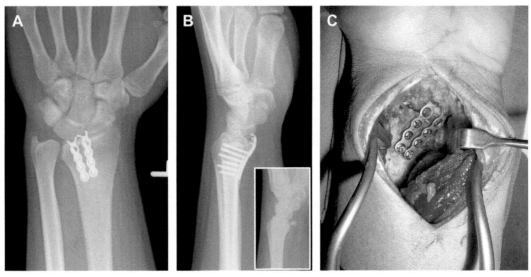

Fig. 14. (*A, B*) This is a similar case of ateardrop fracture pattern treated with hook plates fabricated from (*C*) hand fixation plates. Anatomical reduction was achieved. (*Courtesy of* A/Prof Teoh Lam Chuan, Tan Tock Seng, Singapore.)

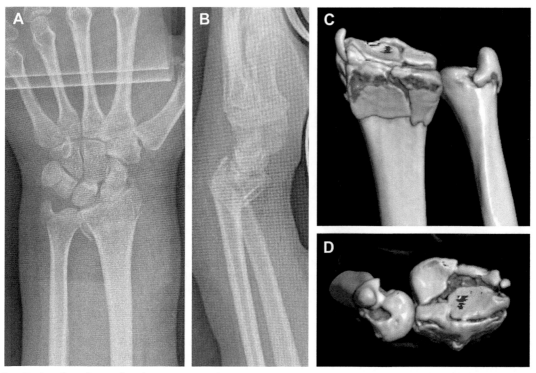

Fig. 15. (*A, B*) Radiographs of a comminuted intraarticular DRF, with (*C, D*) 3-dimensional CT images showing intra-articular step and gap.

wires were placed distal to the plate in the subchondral bone to lever the fracture fragments (**Fig. 17**B). A Freer elevator and probe also aid the reduction process. Once the reduction is acceptable, locking screws are placed to secure the fixation (**Fig. 17**C, D).

Dorsal Spanning Plate Fixation

Dorsal spanning plates (DSP) are indicated in high-energy, severely comminuted DRFs that are not amenable to conventional plate fixation. They can serve either as a temporary or a

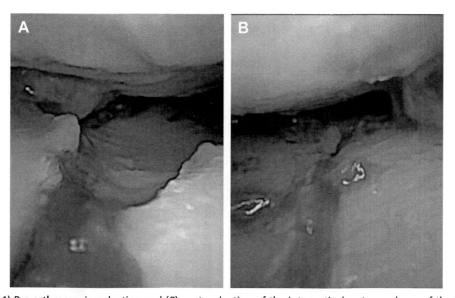

Fig. 16. (*A*) Pre-arthroscopic reduction and (*B*) post-reduction of the intra-articular step and gap of the intermediate column–from the 6-R portal.

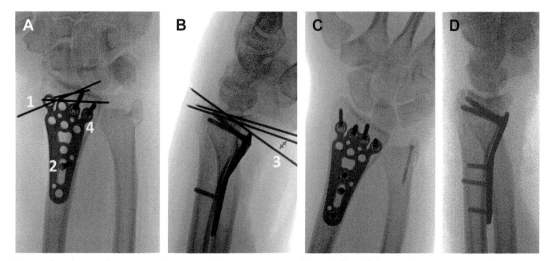

Fig. 17. (*A, B*) A preliminary reduction with K-wires was performed first, followed by placement of a VLP, and secured with a cortical screw in the oblong hole. An arthroscope was then placed, and the distal K-wires were used as a joystick to fine-tune the reduction under arthroscopic visualization. (*C, D*) Once the reduction was satisfactory, locking screws were placed to secure the fixation.

definitive fixation device. Indications are similar to those for bridging external fixators (BEF). However, DSPs are generally preferred implants, because they do not carry the risk of pin site infections associated with BEFs.[35] The DSP uses ligamentotaxis for fracture reduction and provides a dorsal buttress preventing dorsal angulation and subsidence.

Dorsal spanning plates could be centered over the second or third metacarpal. Centering over the third metacarpal provides greater implant rigidity compared with the second metacarpal.[36]

The authors make two 4 cm incisions, one over the third metacarpal shaft and the other along the radius diaphysis. Dissection is made down to the bone, and soft tissue dissection is made with a freer elevator from distal to proximal. The authors prefer to place the plate from distal to proximal beneath the fourth extensor compartment. One must avoid extensor tendon entrapment from the plate, particularly the EPL tendon.[37] Centering the plate over the second metacarpal allows the plate to be positioned beneath the second extensor compartment.

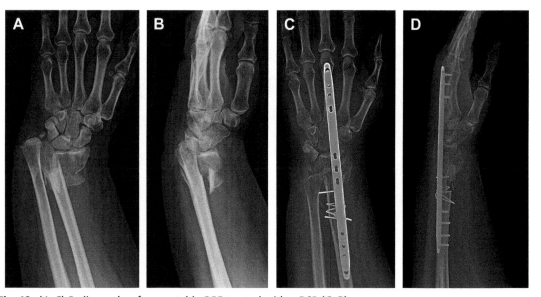

Fig. 18. (*A, B*) Radiographs of an unstable DRF treated with a DSP (*C, D*).

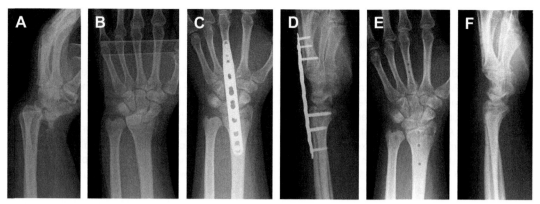

Fig. 19. (*A–F*) Another example of an unstable fracture treated with a DSP. (*Courtesy of* A/Prof Teoh Lam Chuan, Tan Tock Seng, Singapore.)

Fig. 18 shows an unstable DRF with a segmental fracture of the metaphysis that was fixed with a DSP. Cerclage and K-wires were further applied to stabilize the fragments. One of the concerns of DSP is stiffness from prolonged immobilization of the carpus. Therefore, the plate was removed 4 months after the bone had healed, and the patient was immediately started on wrist mobilization therapy. **Fig. 19** is another case of a volar radiocarpal fracture-dislocation treated using a wrist fusion plate as a dorsal spanning plate.

SUMMARY

Managing DRFs is challenging, especially when extensive comminution, bone loss, or multiple critical fracture fragments are present. Every fracture presents differently. Therefore, understanding the fracture mechanism and the functional anatomy of the distal radius is crucial to managing such a complex injury. Distal radius fractures do not always require surgical fixation, and many elderly patients are able to function well despite malunion. Treatment options should be tailored to the patient and the injury. Therefore, it is essential to be versatile with all surgical techniques and understand the importance of restoring critical fragments to prevent repeat displacement and complications.

CLINICS CARE POINTS

- Distal radius fracture is considered unstable when the fracture cannot resist displacement after initial closed reduction.
- Treatment option depends on radiographic parameters of instability (eg, absence of volar

cortical hook, dorsal and comminution) and patient factors (eg, age, functional demand, and preference).

- Although most distal radius fractures can be managed with volar plates, some fracture patterns are more amenable to fragment-specific fixation.
- Die-punch fractures may require an additional dorsal plate or a dorsal spanning plate.
- Intra-articular fracture with a step-off or gap of more than 2 mm would benefit from arthroscopic-assisted fixation.

FINANCIAL DISCLOSURE

Dr K.C. Chung receives funding from the National Institutes of Health, United States and book royalties from Wolters Kluwer and Elsevier. He also receives funding from a research grant from Sonex to study carpal tunnel outcomes.

ACKNOWLEDGMENTS

The authors thank A/Prof Teoh Lam Chuan from Tan Tock Seng Hospital, Singapore, for his contribution to this article.

REFERENCES

1. Arora R, Lutz M, Deml C, et al. A prospective randomized trial comparing nonoperative treatment with volar locking plate fixation for displaced and unstable distal radial fractures in patients sixty-five years of age and older. J Bone Joint Surg Am 2011;93(23):2146–53.
2. Earnshaw SA, Aladin A, Surendran S, et al. Closed reduction of Colles fractures: comparison of manual manipulation and finger-trap traction: a prospective,

　　randomized study. J Bone Joint Surg Am 2002; 84(3):354–8.

3. Mackenney PJ, McQueen MM, Elton R. Prediction of instability in distal radial fractures. J Bone Joint Surg Am 2006;88(9):1944–51.

4. Makhni EC, Ewald TJ, Kelly S, et al. Effect of patient age on the radiographic outcomes of distal radius fractures subject to nonoperative treatment. J Hand Surg Am 2008;33(8):1301–8.

5. Orbay JL, Fernandez DL. Volar fixed-angle plate fixation for unstable distal radius fractures in the elderly patient. J Hand Surg Am 2004;29(1):96–102.

6. Medoff RJ. Essential radiographic evaluation for distal radius fractures. Hand Clin 2005;21(3):279–88.

7. Walenkamp MM, Aydin S, Mulders MA, et al. Predictors of unstable distal radius fractures: a systematic review and meta-analysis. J Hand Surg Eur 2016; 41(5):501–15.

8. Lafontaine M, Hardy D, Delince P. Stability assessment of distal radius fractures. Injury 1989;20(4): 208–10.

9. Chung KC, Kim HM, Malay S, et al, WRIST Group. Comparison of 24-month outcomes after treatment for distal radius fracture: the WRIST randomized clinical trial. JAMA Netw Open 2021;4(6):e2112710.

10. Nelson GN, Stepan JG, Osei DA, et al. The impact of patient activity level on wrist disability after distal radius malunion in older adults. J Orthop Trauma 2015;29(4):195–200.

11. LaMartina J, Jawa A, Stucken C, et al. Predicting alignment after closed reduction and casting of distal radius fractures. J Hand Surg Am 2015; 40(5):934–9.

12. Gupta A. Why and how I fix distal radius fractures— a personal perspective. 10th FESSH Meeting, 15-18 Jun 2005, Goteborg, Sweden.

13. American Association of Orthopaedic Surgeons, Management of distal radius fractures evidence-based clinical practice guide. AAOS, Available at: https://www.Aaos.org/globalassets/quality-and-practice-resources/distal-radius/drfcpg.pdf. Accessed April 2, 2022.

14. Del Piñal F, Jupiter JB, Rozental TD, et al. Distal radius fractures. J Hand Surg Eur 2022;47(1):12–23.

15. Smith DW, Henry MH. The 45 degrees pronated oblique view for volar fixed-angle plating of distal radius fractures. J Hand Surg Am 2004;29(4):703–6.

16. Melone CP. Articular fractures of the distal radius. Orthop Clin North Am 1984;15(2):217–36.

17. Kong L, Zhang Z, Lu J, et al. Clinical utility of 3-dimensional reconstruction images to predict conservative treatment outcomes of intra-articular distal radius fractures. Med Sci Monit 2020;26:e926894.

18. Koh S, Andersen CR, Buford WL Jr, et al. Anatomy of the distal brachioradialis and its potential relationship to distal radius fracture. J Hand Surg Am 2006;31(1):2–8.

19. Rhee PC, Medoff RJ, Shin AY. Complex distal radius fractures: an anatomic algorithm for surgical management. J Am Acad Orthop Surg 2017;25(2): 77–88.

20. Orbay JL, Badia A, Indriago IR, et al. The extended flexor carpi radialis approach: a new perspective for the distal radius fracture. Tech Hand Up Extrem Surg 2001;5(4):204–11.

21. Sreedharan S, Mohd Fadil MF, Lim WS. Intraoperative correction of volar tilt of distal radius fractures using volar locking plate as reduction tool: review of 24 cases. Hand Surg 2014;19(3): 363–8.

22. Sechachalam S, Satku M, Wong JH, et al. Trigonometry-integrated 'lift' technique (TILT) for restoring volar tilt in distal radius fractures: description of technique and preliminary results. J Hand Surg Asian Pac 2017;22(1):53–8.

23. Lindau T, Arner M, Hagberg L. Intraarticular lesions in distal fractures of the radius in young adults. A descriptive arthroscopic study in 50 patients. J Hand Surg Br 1997;22:638–643..

24. Swart E, Tang P. The effect of ligament injuries on outcomes of operatively treated distal radius fractures. Am J Orthop (Belle Mead NJ) 2017;46(1): E41–6.

25. Mehara AK, Rastogi S, Bhan S, et al. Classification and treatment of volar Barton fractures. Injury 1993;24(1):55–9.

26. Ruch DS, Ginn TA, Yang CC, et al. Use of a distraction plate for distal radial fractures with metaphyseal and diaphyseal comminution. J Bone Joint Surg Am 2005;87(5):945–54.

27. Day CS, Kamath AF, Makhni E, et al. "Sandwich" plating for intra-articular distal radius fractures with volar and dorsal metaphyseal comminution. Hand (N Y) 2008;3(1):47–54.

28. Medoff RJ, Kopylov P. Immediate internal fixation and motion of comminuted distal radius fractures using a new fragment specific fixation system. Orthop Trans 1998;22:165.

29. Benson LS, Medoff RJ. Fragment-specific fixation of distal radius fractures. In: Slutsky DJ, Osterman AL, editors. Fractures and injuries of the distal radius and carpus, Chapter 12. Philadelphia: W.B. Saunders; 2009.

30. Knirk JL, Jupiter JB. Intra-articular fractures of the distal end of the radius in young adults. J Bone Joint Surg Am 1986;68(5):647–59.

31. Yao J, Fogel N. Arthroscopy in distal radius fractures: indications and when to do it. Hand Clin 2021;37(2):279–91.

32. Saab M, Wunenburger PE, Guerre E, et al. Does arthroscopic assistance improve reduction in distal articular radius fracture? A retrospective comparative study using a blind CT assessment. Eur J Orthop Surg Traumatol 2019;29(2):405–11.

33. Abe Y, Fujii K. Arthroscopic-assisted reduction of intra-articular distal radius fracture. Hand Clin 2017;33(4):659–68.
34. Del Piñal F. Technical tips for (dry) arthroscopic reduction and internal fixation of distal radius fractures. J Hand Surg Am 2011;36(10):1694–705.
35. Fares AB, Childs BR, Polmear MM, et al. Dorsal bridge plate for distal radius fractures: a systematic review. J Hand Surg Am 2021;46(7):627.e1–8.
36. Alluri RK, Bougioukli S, Stevanovic M, et al. A biomechanical comparison of distal fixation for bridge plating in a distal radius fracture model. J Hand Surg Am 2017;42(9):748.e1–8.
37. Lewis S, Mostofi A, Stevanovic M, et al. Risk of tendon entrapment under a dorsal bridge plate in a distal radius fracture model. J Hand Surg Am 2015;40(3):500–4.

Complications and Revision Surgery of Forearm Fractures

Viviana M. Serra Lopez, MD, MS[a,*], Chia H. Wu, MD, MBA[b],
David J. Bozentka, MD[a]

KEYWORDS

- Nonunion • Malunion • Both bone forearm fractures • Compression plating
- Heterotopic ossification

KEY POINTS

- Complications following forearm fractures include nonunion, malunion, infection, and refracture.
- Malalignment of forearm anatomy is poorly tolerated, and correction of anatomic alignment should also restore rotational stability.
- In the case of nonunion, workup should include evaluation for infection, nutritional status, and/or endocrine workup to resolve any underlying causes before pursuing revision fixation.

INTRODUCTION

Forearm fractures may lead to dysfunction from restricted range of motion or persistent pain. Possible complications include malunion, in which the fracture heals but fails to restore anatomic alignment, and nonunion, in which the fracture does not heal or refracture. Soft tissue complications, such as ectopic bone growth and stiffness, may also occur.

The configuration of the forearm is frequently described as a ring; the radius and the ulna articulate through the proximal radioulnar joint (PRUJ) and the distal radioulnar joint (DRUJ). The interosseous membrane (IOM) maintains the relationship between the radius and the ulna, provides forearm stability, and transmits loads from the elbow to the wrist. The forearm is also unique in that it allows the radius to rotate around a fixed ulna, resulting in pronation and supination. For this reason, restoration of the radial bow in cases of fracture is essential to restoring forearm motion. This includes restoration of both the maximum radial bow in length, as well as its location in the radial shaft by comparing it to a normal contralateral radiograph (**Fig. 1**).

The mainstay of operative treatment of forearm fractures is restoring anatomic alignment through open reduction and internal fixation (ORIF). Plate and screw fixation can achieve union in 96% to 97% of cases.[1–3] Functional outcomes have a positive association with restoration of the radial bow, both in terms of range of motion of the forearm and recovery of grip strength.[4] Residual angulation of 20° or more in midshaft fractures may limit motion due to impingement of the radius and ulna or by excessive tension on the IOM.[5] Functional outcomes have been found to correlate negatively with decreased range of motion of the wrist and forearm after fixation of both bone fractures.[6]

BACKGROUND

Nonunions

A nonunion is a fracture that will not heal without additional intervention. There is currently no consensus on the timeline required to diagnose a forearm nonunion; however, failure to demonstrate

[a] Department of Orthopaedic Surgery, Hospital of the University of Pennsylvania, 3737 Market Street, 6th Floor, Philadelphia, PA 19104, USA; [b] Baylor College of Medicine, 7200 Cambridge Street, 10th Floor, Houston, TX 77030, USA
* Corresponding author.
E-mail address: serra.viviana@gmail.com

Hand Clin 39 (2023) 295–306
https://doi.org/10.1016/j.hcl.2023.02.005

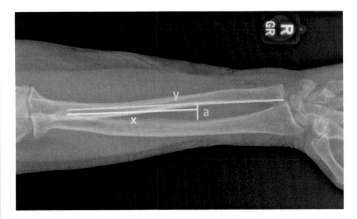

Fig. 1. Method used to determine the length and location of the maximal radial bow. The distance from the radial tubercle to the most ulnar part of the distal radius is represented as "y." Moreover, "a" represents the distance in mm from line "y" to the point of maximum radial bow. The location of the maximum radial bow is expressed as a percentage, calculated as (x/y) * 100.

progressive healing on radiographs within a 3-month period is a commonly used guideline.[7] Patients with a nonunion typically present with persistent pain at the fracture site and radiographs will show lack of bony consolidation over time. For ease of discussion, nonunions can be categorized into septic and aseptic nonunions. Aseptic nonunions can be further classified as atrophic, oligotrophic, or hypertrophic. An atrophic nonunion has minimal to no callus formation, leading to motion at the fracture site. Causes are typically due to the biological environment, although sometimes they may lack mechanical stability. Hypertrophic nonunions have abundant callus and fibrous tissue; however, this fails to mature and consolidate, usually due to high strain in the fracture environment.

Infected nonunions are suspected in cases where patients with risk factors such as immune compromise or a history of an open, contaminated fracture. A combination of serum white blood-cell count (WBC), erythrocyte sedimentation rate (ESR), and C-reactive protein (CRP) that exceed established limits can predict up to a 100% probability of infection, with ESR and CRP tests as the best predictors of infection.[8] Cultures are obtained at the time of surgery to confirm the diagnosis. These fractures require thorough debridement of the infected bone and tissue, including the removal of any existing hardware, as well as prolonged antibiotic treatment.

Malunions

Malunions are fractures that have healed but disrupt the radio–ulnar relationship. These may present as limitations in range of motion, or instability at the PRUJ or DRUJ. Angular deformities occur after residual angulation of the radius and/or ulna after healing. Axial rotational deformities affect the alignment of the PRUJ or DRUJ. A

thorough evaluation should be performed to determine the parameters that require correction and adequately plan corrective osteotomies. The goal of corrective surgery is to restore anatomic alignment and allow for early postoperative rehabilitation.

Heterotopic Ossification

Heterotopic ossification (HO) is characterized by the formation of skeletal bone in extraosseous sites with severe cases resulting in ankylosis.[9] Radioulnar synostosis is a specific instance of HO characterized by a bony bridge between the radius and the ulna. Risk factors include high-energy fractures, injury to the IOM, and patients with head injuries.[10] Prophylaxis in the form of either nonsteroidal anti-inflammatory drugs (NSAIDs) or low-dose radiation is also recommended in patients with earlier HO formation or high-risk factors.

Resection is indicated in cases where forearm motion is limited. There is currently no consensus on resection method and the use of interposition grafts.[11] **Fig. 2** shows commonly affected forearm regions and treatment recommendations.[9]

Refracture

Patients may seek hardwareremoval due to symptomatic hardware. Incidence of refracture after hardware removal of diaphyseal forearm fixation ranges from 1.0% to 22% and can occur either through a screw hole track or at the site of the original fracture.[12–15] It has been suggested that forearm plates should not be removed for at least 2 years following fixation.[16] In addition, it is advised against removing hardware when 4.5-mm plates are used given the incidence of refracture with this larger implant size when compared with the use of 3.5-mm plates.[2]

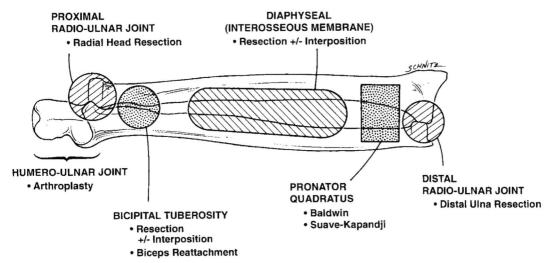

Fig. 2. Six regions of the forearm affected by HO along with suggested surgical treatments. (*From* Hastings H, Graham TJ. The classification and treatment of heterotopic ossification about the elbow and forearm. Hand Clin. 1994;10(3):417-437; with permission.)

EVALUATION
History and Physical Examination

A thorough but targeted history can identify relevant information about the original injury. Noting whether a fracture was open or resulted in segmental bone loss may help guide future treatment and workup. Functional status is important, as well as a timeline of pain and limitations. Earlier medical history should also be investigated to determine if there are factors that could limit healing; for example, a history of smoking, radiation to the area, or poor vascular status may require interdisciplinary teams to revise the nonunion.

Physical examination should focus on documenting baseline range of motion and comparing it to the contralateral side. Location of scars should also be evaluated, as well as factors concerning for infection such as a sinus tract or erythema.

Imaging

Plain radiographs allow for an overall assessment of forearm alignment, as well as evaluation of the fracture site. Standard views include posteroanterior (PA) and lateral views of the forearm in neutral rotation. A fracture is typically considered united when 3 out of 4 cortices on orthogonal imaging show healing.[17] Rotation can also be evaluated in plain radiographs. The radial styloid and the bicipital tuberosity should be approximately 180° from each other in a PA radiograph and the coronoid process and ulnar styloid should also be 180° from each other in a lateral view. Contralateral plain radiographs are useful in cases where

preoperative templating is required. Imaging of the elbow and wrist is obtained if there is concern for DRUJ or PRUJ malalignment. Computed tomography (CT) may be required to evaluate the nonunion site if radiographs are not sufficient, or to evaluate malrotation. To evaluate rotation, the CT images are typically obtained of the bilateral upper extremities in both pronation and supination. A CT angiogram may be useful to evaluate vascular status of the extremity, especially if vascularized bone grafts are planned. MRI with contrast can be helpful in the cases of infection to further delineate the extent of bony involvement and if any fluid collections are present.

Laboratory Studies

A complete blood count with differential and inflammatory markers should be obtained in patients presenting with nonunion to evaluate for infection. Thyroid and parathyroid hormone function should also be evaluated, as well as nutritional status through a comprehensive metabolic panel and vitamin D levels. The latter are especially important in cases of atrophic nonunion, where underlying causes must be corrected to allow for optimal healing.

TECHNIQUES
Autologous Bone Graft

Autologous bone graft has the advantage of histocompatibility and can include cancellous or cortical bone. Cancellous graft contains osteoconductive, osteoinductive, and osteogenic properties. Cortical grafts are mainly used in cases where structural support is needed. Major complications of autologous bone graft have been reported in up to 8.6% of patients and include infection, sensory nerve damage, and wound healing complications.[18]

Most commonly, cancellous autograft is obtained from the iliac crest, or from femur or tibia with the use of the reamer-irrigator-aspirator system (RIA, Synthes, Westchester PA).

Vascularized Bone Graft

Vascularized bone grafts can be used to reconstruct segmental defects in areas of scarred or infected tissue with poor vascular supply. Common donors for reconstruction in the forearm include free vascularized grafts harvested from the fibula or from the medial femoral condyle (MFC).

The free vascularized corticoperiosteal graft harvested from the MFC was originally described by Doi and Sakai to treat nonunions of the upper extremity.[19] It is associated with low donor site morbidity, has a reliable vascular supply from the medial genicular artery or descending genicular vessels, and provides a pliable construct ideal for nonunions of the forearm with small bony defects.

The free fibular autograft is a good option for larger bone defects (6 cm or more) that require stiffer constructs.[20] Chen and colleagues[21] described the use of an osteocutaneous fibular flap for reconstruction after traumatic loss of the radius with scar formation. These can provide diaphyseal bone segments up to 15 cm.[22] The peroneal artery is harvested with the required length of bone and anastomosed to the upper extremity vasculature, and a skin paddle may be obtained in cases where additional soft tissue coverage is needed.

Induced Membrane Technique

The induced membrane technique allows for bridging of larger bone defects and can be used in cases of infection. In the first stage, the bone and surrounding fibrous tissue are debrided. A cement spacer is inserted in the bony defect and temporary stabilization is applied. The second stage is usually performed 6 weeks after the initial stage. Previous incisions are opened, and the induced membrane is carefully incised to remove the cement spacer. Autograft is then inserted into the bony defect and can be either cancellous bone or cortical bone depending on the size needed. Final fixation is then performed. Forearm bone defects of up to 12 cm have been successfully treated with this technique.[23]

Corrective Osteotomies

Meticulous planning is necessary to successfully correct malalignment. The contralateral extremity should be evaluated with imaging to correctly restore ulnar variance and radial bow. Physiologic variations of up to 35° of torsion for the radius and 20° of torsion for the ulna have been described and should be considered when planning for corrective procedures.[24]

The ulna is typically approached through the subcutaneous approach and the radius is approached through the volar Henry approach. If both bones are malaligned, the ulna can be osteotomized first to reestablish forearm alignment. In cases where both bones require osteotomy before alignment of the ulna, it is recommended that the radius be corrected first; if this results in adequate passive motion, the ulna does not need to be corrected.[25]

Three-dimensional analysis is a useful tool in planning for corrective osteotomies. This can be combined with patient-specific instrumentation in order to obtain accuracy in angular correction.[26] CT scans of both extremities are used to obtain a template from the unaffected side and characterize the defects requiring correction in the operative extremity, and eventually postprocessed to produce 3D images.

CLINICAL OUTCOMES
Aseptic Nonunions

Several retrospective studies have evaluated revision of aseptic nonunions with positive results, both in terms of union rates and patient-reported functional outcomes.

Lapcin and colleagues treated aseptic forearm nonunions in 26 patients treated with iliac crest autograft and 3.5-mm locking compression plates (LCP), which resulted in union an average of 6 months after the procedure. Satisfactory or excellent results were obtained in 88% of patients.[27] A retrospective study performed by Regan and colleagues[28] in 23 patients with forearm fracture nonunions found that 91% healed after revision fixation was performed with a 3.5-mm LCP and either cancellous iliac crest bone graft or iliac crest aspirate. Similarly, Ring and colleagues[29] treated 35 forearm fracture nonunions with 3.5-mm LCPs and autogenous cancellous bone graft and achieved union 6 months after revision ORIF, with 66% of patients having satisfactory or excellent results. More recently, Kloen and colleagues[30] treated 51 forearm nonunions with open reduction and autograft in cases where it was deemed necessary, achieving a 100% union rate with

79% of patients having satisfactory or excellent results.

Allograft has also led to satisfactory results. Faldini and colleagues[31] compared 20 patients that underwent forearm nonunion repair with fibular cortical autograft with 14 patients that received homologous cortical bone allograft; all patients healed their nonunions and had satisfactory forearm function.

Septic Nonunions

Perna and colleagues[32] described a 2-stage treatment of infected nonunions in 18 patients, which resulted in healing an average of 5 months after the second-stage procedure, with 83% of patients having excellent or satisfactory functional results. The first stage included the removal of current hardware, debridement of the nonunion site, and application of an antibiotic-coated cement spacer in some cases. Cultures were obtained and external temporary fixation was performed. Targeted antibiotic therapy was completed, and patients underwent the second step of revision once infection was resolved. During the second stage, new plate osteosynthesis was performed along with homologous bone graft strut and intercalary allograft. Similarly, Prasarn and colleagues[33] reported resolution of all infections in a series of 15 patients who underwent serial debridements followed by definitive fixation within 14 days with tricortical iliac crest graft as needed and 6 weeks of intravenous antibiotic treatment.

Jupiter and colleagues reviewed 9 patients who had segmental defects of the radius, 4 of which had active infection. After debridement of the wound and antibiotic treatment, a vascularized osteoseptocutaneous fibular autograft was performed to address the bony defect. At an average follow-up of 24 months, all 4 of the cases with active infection showed union at the proximal and distal junctions of the bone-graft function.[34]

Management of Bone Defects

Walker and colleagues utilized the induced-membrane or Masquelet technique to reconstruct segmental defects in 9 patients with either acute or nonhealing forearm fractures. The first stage consisted of either internal or external spanning fixation and placement of a cement spacer placement for a median bony defect of 4.7 cm. At the second-stage procedure, the cement spacer was removed and replaced with bone graft obtained via RIA or iliac crest. All patients achieved union by final follow-up.[35]

Adani and colleagues[36] reported a 92% success rate with vascularized fibular grafts in patients with an average of 8.4 cm segmental bone defects following forearm trauma.

Corrective Osteotomies

Trousdale and colleagues[25] found that in a series of 27 patients who underwent corrective osteotomies, patients managed within 12 months after the initial injury gained an average of 79° of motion compared with 30° in those patients managed after 12 months. Complications included loss of motion due to HO formation, and instability of the DRUJ.

CLINICAL CASES
Case #1: Treatment of a Chronic Hypertrophic Ulnar Shaft Nonunion with Revision Open Reduction and Internal Fixation and Autograft

Case presentation

A 50-year-old male patient, employed as a construction worker, presented with a right ulna nonunion following a gunshot wound 15 years earlier treated with intramedullary fixation. They had recently noted increasing pain and motion at the fracture site (**Fig. 3**). Physical examination was notable for full elbow range of motion, supination to 50°, pronation to 40° and gross motion at the fracture site. The extremity was otherwise neurovascularly intact. The patient initially underwent removal of the ulna IM rod and operative cultures at the time were negative.

Six weeks after the removal of hardware, the patient underwent revision fixation. Autograft was obtained from the iliac crest and the ulna was approached through a longitudinal incision along the subcutaneous border. The nonunion was debrided of fibrous tissue to healthy bleeding bone and autograft was placed into the fracture site. A 3.5-mm compression plate was then contoured and applied in compression mode. Six cortices of fixation were obtained proximal and distal to the fracture, and the extremity was immobilized in a sugar tong splint. Four weeks postoperatively, the patient was transitioned to a removable splint and radiographs showed interval healing. Four months postoperatively, the patient was noted to have callus formation at the ulna; however, it was deemed slow to consolidate (**Fig. 4**). The patient was restricted to a 5-lbs weight-bearing limit and was prescribed a bone stimulator. Six months postoperatively, the patient had improvement in their elbow pain and had returned to work. Most recent imaging obtained 8 months postoperatively showed progressive consolidation with no loosening of the hardware (**Fig. 5**).

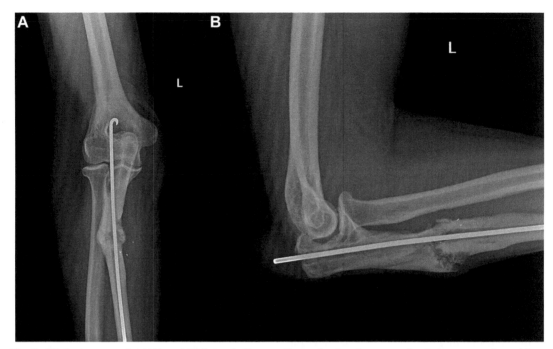

Fig. 3. (*A*) Anteroposterior (AP) and (*B*) lateral elbow radiographs showing a proximal ulnar nonunion with an intramedullary rod across the ulna.

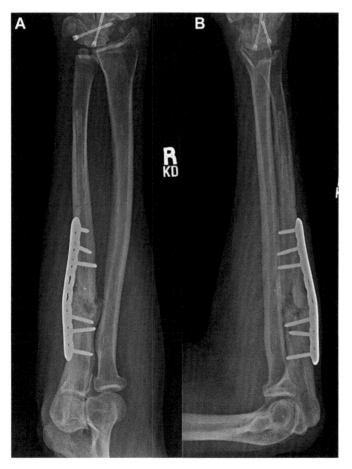

Fig. 4. (*A*) AP and (*B*) lateral radiographs of the right forearm obtained 4 months after revision ORIF of the proximal ulna, showing callus formation and limited consolidation. Patient had also undergone ipsilateral scaphoid excision and 4-corner fusion at the time of ulnar ORIF revision.

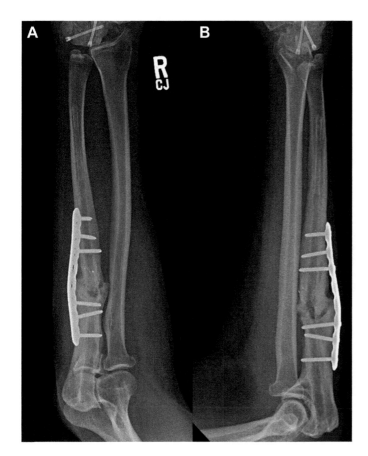

Fig. 5. (A) AP and (B) lateral radiographs of the right forearm obtained 8 months after revision fixation of the ulna. At the time, the patient had resolution of pain at the fracture site.

Discussion

The patient presented with a chronic hypertrophic nonunion after intramedullary fixation of a proximal ulnar shaft fracture 15 years prior. Given the acute worsening of pain and difficulty maintaining his job, the patient was indicated for hardware removal and revision fixation.

The patient's surgery was performed in stages, which allowed us to exclude infection as a cause for their nonunion. Once cultures from the first stage of surgery were negative, we proceeded with revision fixation. Given an appearance consistent with a hypertrophic nonunion, goals of fixation were to increase mechanical stability. After adequate debridement of the nonunion and ensuring adequate blood supply to the fracture ends by visualizing bleeding bone, a plate was placed in compression mode to obtain primary stability. In cases where additional stability is required but the soft tissue status limits the size of the incision, a second plate could be added to obtain 6 to 8 total cortices of fixation total. We also recommend provisionally fixing the plate spanning the fracture after a reduction is obtained and gently ranging the forearm to ensure there will be no mechanical blocks to motion.

The patient was diagnosed with delayed healing due to persistent pain at the fracture site and provided with a bone stimulator. Although studies have suggested a potential benefit from electromagnetic field stimulation in delayed union of long bone fractures, there is insufficient evidence to provide guidelines for current practices.[37] However, we think that is a reasonable additional conservative option before proceeding with further interventions. If an immobilization device is to be used on the extremity, it must permit direct contact to the skin at the time of stimulator use.

Case #2: Ulnar Shaft Fracture Fixation Complicated by Formation of Heterotopic Ossification

Case presentation

A 60-year-old female patient suffered a fall from standing height and presented with a distal third ulnar shaft fracture (**Fig. 6**). Past medical history was significant for rheumatoid arthritis, psoriasis, and previous wound dehiscence following earlier surgeries. The fracture was initially treated with cast immobilization but the patient ultimately

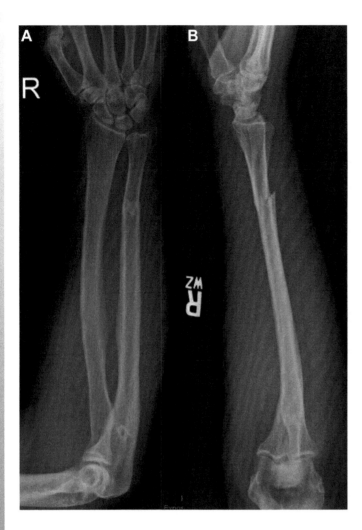

Fig. 6. (*A*) PA and (*B*) lateral radiographs of the right forearm showing a distal third ulnar shaft fracture.

pursued surgical management due to poor tolerance of the cast. The ulna was approached through its subcutaneous border and fixed with compression plating.

Six months after the initial surgery, the patient's forearm had 30° of supination and 50° of pronation, and she felt limited in performing activities of daily living. Imaging showed a healed fracture

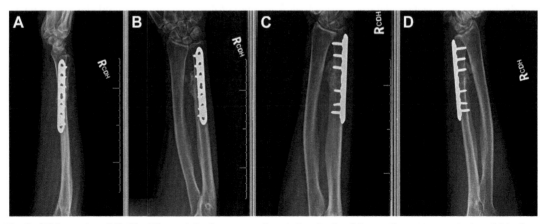

Fig. 7. (*A*) Lateral and (*B–D*) oblique right forearm radiographs obtained 6 months postoperatively, which show union at the fracture site and formation of HO around the fracture site.

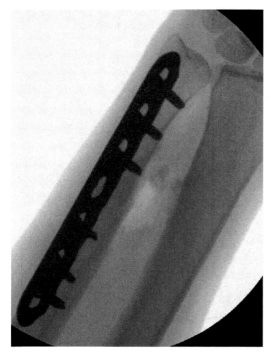

Fig. 8. Fluoroscopic image of the right forearm obtained immediately after HO excision.

and HO at the level of the fracture (**Fig. 7**). At that time, the patient underwent HO excision through a combined dorsal and volar approach centered over the IOM (**Fig. 8**). The patient was started on 25 mg of indomethacin 3 times per day for HO prophylaxis.

Two months after HO excision, imaging showed new heterotopic bone (**Fig. 9**). The patient continued occupational therapy while continuing indomethacin. She underwent repeat HO excision 6 months after the most recent surgery given discomfort and continued limitations in range of motion. The patient was started on celecoxib due to earlier poor tolerance of indomethacin and referred to a radiation oncologist for preoperative radiation. During the second HO excision, the approach was performed through a dorsal incision to minimize wound complications. Her postoperative course was complicated by drainage from the incision and delayed healing, which resolved with oral antibiotics and local wound care.

Three months after their second HO excision, the patient had 50° of pronation and supination, pain had resolved, and they were satisfied with the clinical outcome. Imaging showed no additional bony overgrowth (**Fig. 10**).

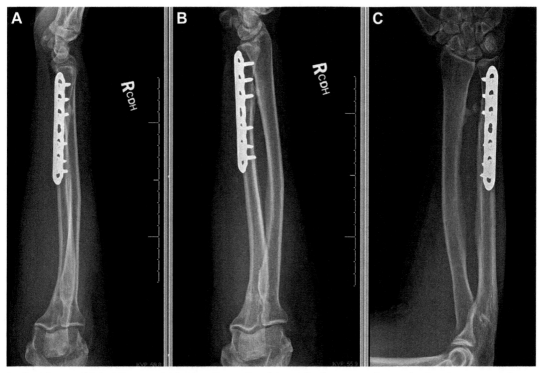

Fig. 9. (*A*) Lateral (*B*) oblique and (*C*) PA radiographs of the right forearm radiographs showing new HO formation 2 months after undergoing HO excision.

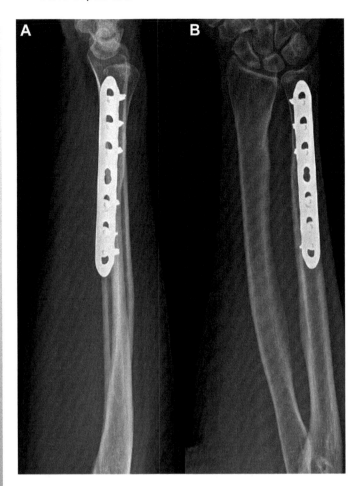

Fig. 10. (*A*) Lateral and (*B*) PA radiographs showing no recurrence of HO at most recent follow-up.

Discussion

Traditionally, ulnar shaft fractures with less than 50% displacement are considered to have stable surrounding soft tissue and amenable to closed treatment.[38] In this case, the patient was unable to tolerate cast immobilization and desired surgical management.

The decision to excise HO surgically must be balanced with the time it takes for the growth to be metabolically stable, which is typically 1 year, and the risk of progression and limited functionality for the patient.[9] Preoperative or postoperative low-dose radiotherapy targeted to the area of treatment can be considered in cases where patients have a known history of formation of ectopic bone.[9] In this case, the patient had a history of wound healing complications, and therefore did not undergo radiation until their second HO excision. In cases where radiotherapy is planned, we recommend counseling the patient regarding potential wound healing complications. Steps should be taken intraoperatively to minimize damage to the IOM, such as careful placement of retractors and the number and length of incisions should be minimized.

There is no consensus in the literature regarding the optimal NSAID to use as HO prophylaxis in forearm fractures, although the use of celecoxib and indomethacin has been described.[10] We recommend starting indomethacin 1 day before surgery and continuing therapy for 2 months postoperatively. In patients with high-risk factors or recurrent HO, we recommend preoperative referral to a radiation specialist for consideration of low-dose radiation.

SUMMARY

Forearm fractures can result in complications that range from refracture, nonunion, malunion, and infection. Despite the high union rates that have been seen since the introduction of 3.5-mm LCP for the fixation of operative fractures, complications can lead to pain and limited range of motion resulting in limitations in work and activities of daily living.

Each case requires a thorough investigation of the causes for failure to tailor treatment. Atrophic nonunions require improvement in bony biology, whereas hypertrophic nonunions require revision fixation with additional mechanical stability. Malunions that result in dysfunction require corrective osteotomies. Additional complications include soft tissue complications that result in a range of motion limitations such as HO or synostosis.

In addition to plain radiographs, we recommend obtaining serum WBC, ESR, and CRP in patients who present for nonunion; if there is concern for infection, removal of hardware, debridement, and treatment with targeted antibiotics should be completed before undergoing definitive fixation.

CLINICS CARE POINTS

- Obtain imaging of the forearm, as well as the wrist and elbow. A chronic Essex-Lopresti injury may limit motion requires a concurrent reconstructive procedure.
- Restoration of the radial bow is essential to restore forearm motion and function.
- Obtain intraoperative imaging of the DRUJ and examine its stability; DRUJ instability can also limit rotation and may require a separate reconstructive procedure.
- In the case of nonunion, evaluate inflammatory markers. Cases of infection require serial debridement and antibiotic treatments to cure the infection before revision fixation.
- If provisional stability is required in a contaminated wound, consider using a plate coated in antibiotic cement if an external fixator is not desirable.
- Iliac crest is considered the gold standard for autograft; however, RIA has recently gained popularity due to the higher volume of autograft that can be obtained and avoidance of cutaneous nerve disturbances that can be seen with iliac crest harvest.
- RIA can be especially useful in the second stage of a Masquelet reconstruction.
- Evaluate segmental bone loss after adequate debridement: for defects less than 2 cm, iliac crest bone autograft is an adequate option. Defects ranging from 2 to 5 cm are left to the discretion of the surgeon. Defects that are 5 cm or larger may require Masquelet or a free fibula transfer.
- Patients at high risk of HO formation should be placed on prophylactic therapy with a nonsteroidal anti-inflammatory agent and/or undergo radiotherapy to the area to be treated.

DISCLOSURES

D.J. Bozentka: Axogen principal investigator.

REFERENCES

1. Hadden WA, Reschauer R, Seggl W. Results of AO plate fixation of forearm shaft fractures in adults. Injury 1983;15(1):44–52.
2. Chapman MW, Gordon JE, Zissimos AG. Compression-plate fixation of acute fractures of the diaphyses of the radius and ulna. J Bone Jt Surg 1989;71-A(2):159–69.
3. Matejëiê A, Ivica M, Tomljenoviê M, et al. Forearm shaft fractures: results of ten-year follow-up. Acta Clin Croat 2000;39(3):147–53.
4. Schemitsch EH, Richards RR. The effect of malunion and functional outcome after plate fixation of fractures of both bones of the forearm in adults. J Bone Jt Surg 1992;74-A(7):1068–78.
5. Matthews LS, Kaufer H, Garver DF, et al. The effect on supination-pronation of angular malalignment of fractures of both bones of the forearm. J Bone Jt Surg 1982;64(1):14–7.
6. Goldfarb CA, Ricci WM, Tull F, et al. Functional outcome after fracture of both bones of the forearm. J Bone Jt Surg 2005;87-B(3):374–9.
7. Richard MJ, Ruch DS, Aldridge JM. Malunions and nonunions of the forearm. Hand Clin 2007;23(2):235–43.
8. Stucken C, Olszewski DC, Creevy WR, et al. Preoperative diagnosis of infection in patients with nonunions. J Bone Jt Surg 2013;95-A(15):1409–12.
9. Hastings H, Graham TJ. The classification and treatment of heterotopic ossification about the elbow and forearm. Hand Clin 1994;10(3):417–37.
10. Osterman AL, Arief MS. Optimal management of post-traumatic radioulnar synostosis. Orthop Res Rev 2017;9:101–6.
11. Dohn P, Khiami F, Rolland E, et al. Adult post-traumatic radioulnar synostosis. Orthop Traumatol Surg Res 2012;98(6):709–14.
12. Deluca PA, Lindsey RW, Ruwe PA. Refracture of bones of the forearm after the removal of compression Plates. J bone Jt Surg 1988;70(9):1372–6.
13. Labosky DA, Cermak MB, Waggy CA, et al. Forearm fracture plates: to remove or not to remove. J Hand Surgery, Am. 1990;15(2):294–301.
14. Hidaka S, Gustilo RB. Refracture of bones of the forearm after plate removal. J Bone Jt Surg 1984;66-A(8):1241–3.
15. Leung F, Chow S-P. A prospective, randomized trial comparing the limited contact dynamic compression plate with the point contact fixator for forearm fractures. J Bone Jt Surg 2003;85-A(12):2343–8.
16. Heim U. Forearm and hand/mini-implants. In: Muller M, Allgower M, Schneider R, et al, editors.

Manual of internal fixation: techniques recommended by the AO-ASIF group. 3rd edition. Berlin: pringer; 1991. p. 453–84.

17. Wildemann B, Ignatius A, Leung F, et al. Non-union bone fractures. Nat Rev Dis Prim 2021;7(1):1–21.

18. Younger E, Chapman M. Morbidity at bone graft donor sites. J Orthoapedic Trauma 1989;3(3):192–5.

19. Doi K, Sakai K. Vascularized periosteal bone graft from the supracondylar region of the femur. Microsurgery 1994;15(5):305–15.

20. Stevanovic M, Gutow AP, Sharpe F. The management of bone defects of the forearm after trauma. Hand Clin 1999;15(2):299–318.

21. Chen Z-W, Yan W. The study and clinical application of the osteocutaneous flap of fibula. Microsurgery 1983;4(1):11–6.

22. Dell P, Sheppard J. Vascularized bone grafts in the treatment of infected forearm nonunions. J Hand Surg Am 1984;9(5):653–8.

23. Lauthe O, Gaillard J, Cambon-Binder A, et al. Induced membrane technique applied to the forearm: Technical refinement, indications and results of 13 cases. Orthop Traumatol Surg Res 2021; 107(8):1–6.

24. Dumont CE, Nagy L, Ziegler D, et al. Fluoroscopic and magnetic resonance cross-sectional imaging assessments of radial and ulnar torsion profiles in volunteers. J Hand Surg Am 2007;32(4):501–9.

25. Trousdale RT, Linscheid RL. Operative treatment of malunited fractures of the forearm. J Bone Jt Surg 1995;77(6):894–902.

26. Singh S, Andronic O, Kaiser P, et al. Recent advances in the surgical treatment of malunions in hand and forearm using three-dimensional planning and patient-specific instruments. Hand Surg Rehabil 2020;39(5):352–62.

27. Lapcin O, Arikan Y, Yavuz U, et al. Evaluation of outcomes in aseptic non-unions of the forearm bones in adults treated with LCP and autograft. Ulus Travma ve Acil Cerrahi Derg 2016;22(3):283–9.

28. Regan DK, Crespo AM, Konda SR, et al. Functional outcomes of compression plating and bone grafting for operative treatment of nonunions about the forearm. J Hand Surg Am 2018;43(6):564.e1–9.

29. Ring D, Allende C, Jafarnia K, et al. Ununited diaphyseal forearm fractures with segmental defects: plate fixation and autogenous cancellous bone-grafting. J Bone Jt Surg 2004;86-A(11):2440–5.

30. Kloen P, Wiggers JK, Buijze GA. Treatment of diaphyseal non-unions of the ulna and radius. Arch Orthop Trauma Surg 2010;130(12):1439–45.

31. Faldini C, Traina F, Perna F, et al. Surgical treatment of aseptic forearm nonunion with plate and opposite bone graft strut. Autograft or allograft? Int Orthop 2015;39(7):1343–9.

32. Perna F, Pilla F, Nanni M, et al. Two-stage surgical treatment for septic non-union of the forearm. World J Orthop 2017;8(6):471–7.

33. Prasarn ML, Ouellette EA, Miller DR. Infected non-unions of diaphyseal fractures of the forearm. Arch Orthop Trauma Surg 2010;130(7):867–73.

34. Jupiter J, Gerhard H, Guerrero J, et al. Treatment of segmental defects of the radius with use of the vascularized osteoseptocutaneous fibular autogenous graft. J Bone Jt Surg Am 1997;79(4):542–50.

35. Walker M, Sharareh B, Mitchell SA. Masquelet reconstruction for posttraumatic segmental bone defects in the forearm. J Hand Surg Am 2019; 44(4):342.e1–8.

36. Adani R, Delcroix L, Innocenti M, et al. Reconstruction of large posttraumatic skeletal defects of the forearm by vascularized free fibular graft. Microsurgery 2004;24(6):423–9.

37. Griffin XL, Costa ML, Parsons N, et al. Electromagnetic field stimulation for treating delayed union or non-union of long bone fractures in adults. Cochrane Database Syst Rev 2011;13(4):CD008471.

38. Dymond J. The treatment of isolated fractures of the distal ulna. J Bone Jt Surg Br 1984;66-B(3):408–10.

Managing Difficult Problems in Small Joint Arthroplasty
Challenges, Complications, and Revisions

Steven L. Moran, MD*, Marco Rizzo, MD

KEYWORDS

- Arthroplasty • Proximal interphalangeal joint • Metacarpophalangeal joint • Carpometacarpal joint
- Silicone • Pyrocarbon • Complications

KEY POINTS

- Most finger joint arthroplasties in the United States are either constrained silicone implants or non-constrained pyrocarbon implants.
- The most common complications following silicone arthroplasty include implant fracture/failure, recurrent deformity, and instability. Revision arthroplasty can be managed with replacement of silicone implant, converting to a pyrocarbon arthroplasty, or converting to a fusion.
- The most common complications following pyrocarbon arthroplasty can include recurrent deformity, limitation of motion, squeaking, and pain. Revision arthroplasty can be managed with reconstruction of stabilizing soft tissue structures, replacement, and upsizing of pyrocarbon implant, converting to a silicone arthroplasty, or converting to a fusion.
- Although pain relief is expected with proximal interphalangeal (PIP) arthroplasty, improvement in motion is less predictable. In addition, reoperations to improve motion have been largely unsuccessful. Tempering patient expectations preoperatively will help minimize disappointment and need for reoperation if stiffness results.
- Thumb base arthroplasty is less frequent than metacarpophalangeal or PIP arthroplasty, but may be indicated for high demand and younger patients with sparing of the scapho-trapezial-trapeziod (STT) joint. Complications have included dislocation, pain, STT arthritis, and fracture. These complications can be managed with implant removal and converting to trapeziectomy, addressing STT arthritis, or implant revision.

 Video content accompanies this article at http://www.hand.theclinics.com.

INTRODUCTION

Small joint arthroplasty is a well-established procedure for the hand and wrist and has been shown to provide reliable pain relief with improvement in motion and hand function.[1–7] Silicone implants were designed in the 1960s and have remained the gold standard for metacarpophalangeal (MCP) and proximal interphalangeal (PIP) arthroplasty.

Despite its long history, hand and finger arthroplasty has not obtained the same success as hip or knee arthroplasty; outcome studies have identified problems with implant fracture and maintenance of finger function. Silicone implants were not designed as true joint replacement, but rather a spacer around which the finger may pivot. Capsule formation around the silicone creates stability, but implant fracture and functional

Department of Orthopedics, Mayo Clinic, 200 First Street SW, Rochester, MN 55905, USA
* Corresponding author. 12th Floor Mayo Building, 200 First Street SW, Rochester, MN 55905.
E-mail address: steven@mayo.edu

Hand Clin 39 (2023) 307–320
https://doi.org/10.1016/j.hcl.2023.02.006

hand.theclinics.com

deterioration are inevitable. Complications with silicone arthroplasty of the MCP and PIP inspired new arthroplasty designs consisting of non-constrained and semi-constrained implants made of different metals, plastics, and pyrocarbon.[3,8–12] Today, within the United States, silicone implants and pyrocarbon non-constrained arthroplasties are the predominant devices used for small joint arthroplasty. Each of these devices has their advantages and unique problems.

Despite the problems seen with specific implants, the management of arthroplasty complications can salvage joint function, reduce patients' pain, and improve patient satisfaction. Alternatives to arthroplasty include joint fusion; however, fusion is unappealing to many patients, particularly for the joints on the ulnar aspect of the hand, where absence of flexion limits grip strength and impairs hand mechanics. To preserve motion and prevent joint fusion, an understanding of the causes of arthroplasty failure and its correction is a valuable component of any hand surgeon's practice. In this article, the authors share their collective experience with the management of the complications associated with silicone and pyrocarbon arthroplasty for the hand and fingers.

METACARPOPHALANGEAL ARTHROPLASTY
Silicone

The long-term outcomes of silicone arthroplasty have been well-documented.[13–15] In 2003, Goldfarb and Stern published on 208 implants in 52 hands of patients with rheumatoid arthritis. Patients were followed for an average of 14 years postoperatively; 63% of implants were broken at the time of final follow-up and an addition 22% were deformed. Motion tended to revert toward preoperative values over time, with recurrence in ulnar drift and MCP extension deficits. Bone shortening and erosion was seen in most patients.[14] Trail and colleagues examined 1336 MCP joint silicone arthroplasties and found similar findings with a fracture rate of 66% at 17 years follow-up. The investigators found that previous thumb carpometacarpal (CMC) replacement and thumb metacarpalphalangeal (MP) joint fusion were associated with a significantly higher rate of revision. PIP joint replacement was associated with a higher chance of same finger MCP joint arthroplasty failure. Improvements in implant survival rates were seen with crossed intrinsic transfer, realignment of the wrist, and soft tissue balancing. Despite high rates of implant fracture, overall reported revision rate was 5.7%.[15] Recently, Notermans and colleagues found that those patients with better MCP motion tended to have higher rates of complications; one

would expect that greater motion correlates with higher repetitive stain to the implant and soft tissue constraints.[16]

Thus, when performing silicone arthroplasty, one must inform the patient of potential late problems; however, Burgess and colleagues have shown that MCP arthroplasty revision can provide high levels of patient satisfaction. In their evaluation of revision silicone arthroplasty in 18 patients with 62 implants, revision provided excellent pain relief, and most patients were pleased with their results. Objective results, however, showed little improvement in arc of motion and ulnar drift.[17]

Pyrocarbon MCP arthroplasties were designed as an alternative to metal and silicone small joint arthroplasty. Pyrocarbon has an elastic modulus equivalent to cortical bone; this has allowed the implant to be used as a hemiarthroplasty. In addition, it is biologically inert—minimizing the risk of wear and potential risk of particulate-related inflammation or osteolysis. Finally, its articular surface has exceptional resistance to wear. The implants for MCP replacement are designed as non-constrained anatomic implants; thus, they require precise placement with preservation of the native collateral ligaments for stability. These soft tissue requirements are usually deficient in patients suffering from inflammatory arthroplasty and may not be intact in those suffering from post-traumatic or osteoarthritis. So, patient selection is the first critical step to avoid postoperative complications.

Most large survival studies with the use of pyrocarbon implants for inflammatory and degenerative arthritis have shown excellent pain relief and preservation of joint function.[18,19] Long-term predictors of complications include smoking status, age at time of implantation, and profession. Thus, the placement of an implant in younger active patients may necessitate revision. The most common complications include subsidence and instability.

Cook and colleagues reported a 70% 16-year of implant survival for the early PyroCarbon implant design. The patients in that study, the majority of whom had rheumatoid artritis (RA), had good outcomes.[18] A study by Parker and colleagues reported decrease pain, a decrease in extension, lag and improved grip and pinch strength. Patients with inflammatory arthritis had a greater incidence of joint subluxation and dislocation.[19] Cummings and colleagues found that rates of implant survivorship at 5 and 10 years to be 90% and 81%, respectively; however, 15% of arthroplasties underwent revision at a mean 5 years postoperatively. Rates of implant survival following reoperation were 85%, 84%, 76%, and 68%, at 1, 2 5, and 10 years respectively.

Pain improved, arc of motion improved, appositional and oppositional strength all improved after surgery.[20] Finally, Wagner and colleagues reviewed 128 revision arthroplasties in 64 patients. Fifty of these revisions were for non-constrained implants and 78 were for silicone implants. The 5- and 10-year survival rates following revision were 81% and 79%. Preserved motion and pain relieve were seen in the majority of silicone and pyrocarbon revision patients. These articles suggest that attempts to revise MCP joint arthroplasty, while complicated, have an excellent chance of providing the patient with long-term preservation of function and pain relief.[21]

Finally, postoperative radiographic changes do not always correlate with functional problems or pain. Subluxation, if asymptomatic can be observed. Fractured implants may remain for years without becoming symptomatic. Although an honest discussion needs to occur with the patient regarding the status of their implants, we let pain and loss of function guide therapy in these cases.

Pearls for Success

There are many things which can be done preoperatively to improve the long-term survival of MCP implants. For RA patients, careful patient selection is a key; patients with active disease or poor soft tissues may be better suited for a fusion or a constrained silicone implant. In addition, stabilization of the wrist to correct radial deviation of the carpus can limit the tendency for recurrent ulnar drift within the fingers. For wrist stabilization, we prefer tendon transfers or partial fusions. We are quick to use cross-intrinsic transfers to help provide ligamentotaxis to stabilize poor soft tissues.[15,22,23] For the index finger, where the standard cross-intrinsic transfer cannot be used, the EIP may be used to stabilize the index finger by locating it to the radial side of the proximal phalanx or by attaching it to the insertion of the first dorsal interosseus muscle.

The most frequent acute complication following MCP pyrocarbon arthroplasty is that of joint dislocation or subluxation.[21] This complication is often the result of incompetent or injured collateral ligaments. Late instability may develop from implant subsidence in cases of osteoporosis or in cases of ongoing soft tissue deterioration as in RA. Early dislocation may be resolved by upsizing the implant and revising the soft tissues (Fig. 1). Such cases of late subsidence can be minimized

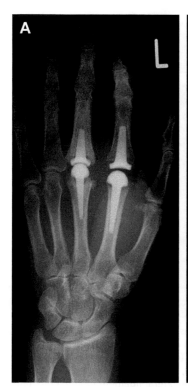
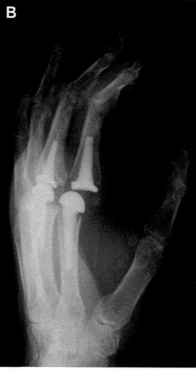
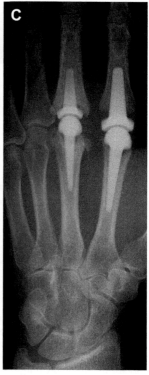

Fig. 1. (*A*, *B*) AP and oblique radiographs of a case of early postoperative subluxation of an MCP pyrocarbon implant due to the partial resection of collateral ligament origin at the level of the metacarpal neck. In this case, stability was restored by upsizing both the distal and proximal components in conjunction with soft tissue reconstruction. (*C*) Two-year postoperative AP radiograph showing joint stability.

by properly sizing implants at initial operation and the liberal use of impaction bone grafting into the metacarpal. PyroCarbon MCP component sizing is usually limited by the size of the proximal phalangeal component. In addition, proximal and distal components cannot be mismatched in size as it may produce edge wear to the implant. Thus, there will be times when the metacarpal component may be undersized for the metacarpal shaft. In such cases, impaction grafting may allow for a tighter press fit and mitigate against future subsidence. If instability persists, or a larger implant is not possible, then attempts should be made to reconstruct the collateral ligaments. The authors have found that the use of a horizontal mattress stich with a 2 to 0 or 0 braided suture placed before the final implant is placed can

provide excellent support for early motion (Videos 1 and 2). In recurrent cases or those cases where there are poor soft tissues, the use of a suture tape through bone tunnels can be used to resolve instability (**Fig. 2**); however, conversion to a constrained silicone design offers the best chance for postoperative stability.

In Wanderman and colleagues' study of over 800 MCP arthroplasties (which included silicone, pyrocarbon, and surface replacement), acute dislocation requiring intervention was seen in 4% of cases. Almost 80% of revision cases were due to soft tissue deficiency; however, soft tissue stabilization procedures alone had only a 28% success rate in achieving a stable MCP joint, whereas revision arthroplasty had a 71% success rate. Subgroup analysis showed an 86% success

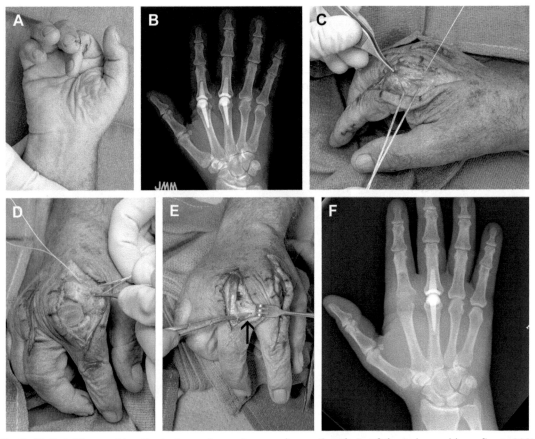

Fig. 2. (*A–F*) A 65-year old patient who underwent pyrocarbon arthroplasty of the index and long finger MCP joints for OA. (*A*) Patient presented with severe radial instability of index and clinical instability of long finger. AP radiograph (*B*) shows the rotation of proximal phalanx of index finger. (*C–E*) At the time of surgery, the index finger radial collateral ligament origin and insertion were compromised, necessitating a change to a silicone implant for the index finger. Suture tape was used to reconstruct radial collateral ligament of the index finger. (*E*) The long finger was revised and stabilized with collateral ligament stitch and cross-intrinsic transfer from the index ulnar lateral band. (*E*) Arrow points to the portion of the ulnar lateral band being transferred to proximal phalanx of long finger to complete the cross-intrinsic transfer. (*F*) AP radiographs at 12 months following surgery showing stable result.

rate for silicone revisions and a 43% success rate with non-constrained revisions. The 5-year survival for silicone revision was 80% and only 36% for non-constrained implants.[24]

Joint overstuffing, while less frequent, can result in limited extension and tendency toward flexion deformity or volar subluxation. To avoid oversizing the arthroplasty, the surgeon should check range of motion at the time of initial joint placement; in an appropriately tensioned joint, the MCP joint should allow for 15° to 20° of hyperextension. If this is not possible it is likely the joint is too tight. In these cases, additional bone may need to be resected or the implants can be downsized (**Fig. 3**).

Fracture at the time of implantation or revision implantation can also occur in cases of osteoporotic bone. In such cases, it is safe to proceed with implantation as the stem often extends beyond the fracture line. In more significant cases, a suture or small gauge wire can be used as a cerclage to reestablish cortical stability to allow

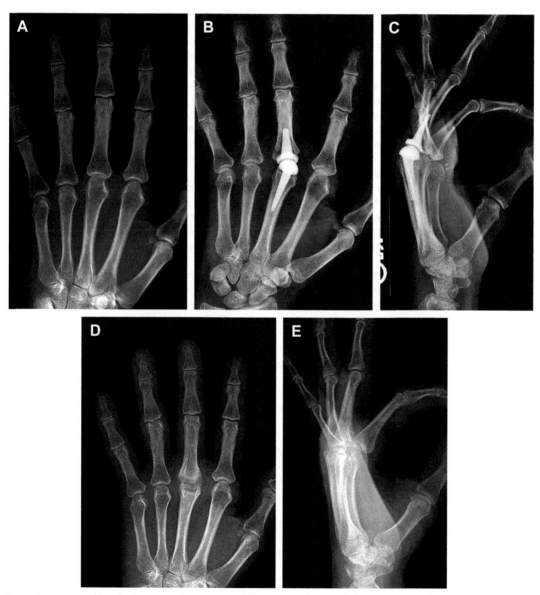

Fig. 3. (*A–E*) A 63-year-old woman who was treated for MCP arthritis of her middle finger of the left hand. (*A*) She underwent pyrocarbon MCP arthroplasty and at 6 months (*B, C*) demonstrated ulnar deviation and limited extension secondary (at least in part) to overstuffing the joint. This was remedied with a revision to silicone and radial collateral plication, extensor centralization with intrinsic release. (*D, E*) Her radiographs at 16 months post-revision.

for implant placement. Patients with intraoperative fractures are delayed in motion protocols by 2 to 4 weeks depending on the postoperative imaging. In Wagner and colleagues' article examining over 800 MCP arthroplasties, fracture occurred in 3% of primary and secondary arthroplasties. No case was aborted, and all fractures healed during follow-up. The 2- and 5-year survival rates were 96% and 80%, a rate which did not differ from patients who did not experience fracture. Fracture was associated with an increased risk of postoperative instability, so augmentation of the collaterals at the time of closure should be considered.[25]

PROXIMAL INTERPHALANGEAL ARTHROPLASTY

The PIP joint is historically more susceptible to instability and deformity following arthroplasty than the MCP joint. The PIP has fewer tendinous and muscular constrains, and arthritis can often create coronal plane deformities which can be difficult to correct with arthroplasty. Currently, there are two popular implants in the United States are silicone and pyrocarbon. Surface replacement (SR)-PIP (Small Bone Innovations, Morrisville, PA) implants are no longer available in most centers, and their management will not be covered in this article. Silicone interposition implants consist of one-piece flexible, stemmed, hinged elastomer spacers that can be used in all digits after resection arthroplasty of the PIP joint. As in the MCP joint, the implant does not function as a true joint but rather a spacer that is stabilized by a fibrous capsule, which develops around the implant. The success of PIP implant arthroplasty largely depends on the condition of the surrounding soft tissues including the collateral ligaments, tendons, and volar plate. When these structures are preserved, implant arthroplasty has a higher success rate; when they are not, patients should be counseled on the benefits of fusion over attempts at arthroplasty.

The major complications from PIP arthroplasty continue to be implant failure, instability, and loss of motion.[26] The reported incidence of implant fracture with silicone arthroplasty is variable, ranging from 5% to 44%, and rotational malalignment and lateral deviation may occur with longer follow-up.[27,28] Takigawa and colleagues reviewed 70 implants with an average follow-up of 6.5 years and reported pain relief in 70%, improvement in extension, but no change in total active motion of the PIP joint. Complications included fractures in 15% of the implants, and nine joints required revision.[28]

Lin and colleges reviewed their experience of 69 PIP silicone arthroplasties done through a volar approach. There was an improvement in the extension deficit from 17° to 8° but no improvement in overall arc of motion. A complete resolution of preoperative pain was noted in 67 of 69 joints, and complications were observed in 12 joints, including five implant fractures and three cases of implant malrotation.[29] Pettersson and colleagues compared newer silicone implants with a traditional silicone implant design and found better patient satisfaction but otherwise similar results.[30] Despite the complications, silicone remains the benchmark for newer surface replacement implants such as pyrocarbon.[31]

The results of pyrolytic carbon arthroplasty for PIP joint replacement have been the subject of several recent studies. Wagner and colleagues published the largest and most comprehensive study to date. A total of 170 consecutive PIP Pyro-Carbon joint replacements were performed in 90 patients. Fifty-four percent of patients in this study suffered from osteoarthritis (OA). The minimum follow-up was 2 years and the mean follow-up was 5.2 years. The joint range of motion remained unchanged at 41°; mean grip strength also remained unchanged following surgery. Pain was significantly improved in 87% of patients. Despite the improvement in pain relief and maintenance of motion, implant removal was required in 21% of implants, and 33% required some form of revisional surgery. Subsidence was seen in over 50% of implants with 36% of implants displaying signs of progressive instability at final follow-up. Young age has been found to correlate with higher complication rates.[27]

Watts and colleagues reviewed the outcomes of 97 PIP arthroplasty with a minimum 2-year follow-up. Thirteen percent of digits required a revision at an average of 15 months postoperative. There were no significant differences in the preoperative and postoperative range of motion. Overall joint survivorship was 85% during the 2 year follow-up.[32] In a follow-up to this study, Dickson and colleagues looked at 51 implants, all in cases of noninflammatory arthritis. The average follow-up was 103 months, and all arthroplasties were performed in the index or long finger PIP joint. At final follow-up, the mean arc of motion was 54° and there was no difference in grip strength between the operative and nonoperative side. The mean DASH score was 29, but patients displayed excellent pain relief and satisfaction with the procedure. The average survival of the implant remained consistent with Watt's original study and was 88% over a 10-year period.[33]

More recently, Vitale and colleagues compared the outcomes between index finger fusion and pyrocarbon arthroplasty of the PIP joint. They evaluated 79 patients in total, with the arthroplasty group being followed for 6 years. Arthroplasty patients maintained preoperative motion and had improvement in oppositional pinch strength. There were no differences in pain relief, satisfaction, or Michigan Hand Questionnaire scores between treatment groups; however, the arthroplasty group had a higher risk of complications.[34]

Branam and colleagues have published a study comparing the outcomes of pyrolytic carbon implants with silicone implants for PIP arthroplasty. This retrospective study compared the outcomes of 19 PyroCarbon implants with 23 silicone implants. Although differences in final motion arc and pain relief were statistically insignificant, coronal plane deformity was more prevalent and more pronounced in patients who had silicone arthroplasty.[35] More recently, Förster and colleagues published a large meta-analysis of 1868 PIP arthroplasties, which included pyrocarbon, silicone, and metal-polyethylene implants. The study found complication rates to be similar between implant types at 10% to 14%. Silicone implants tended to display greater finger deviations (3%)

and instability (2%) compared other types of implants; however, reoperation is less frequent with silicone arthroplasty.[36] It seems that each implant has its own advantages and disadvantages, and the superiority of one implant over another has yet to be determined.

More recently, the idea of hemiarthroplasty for management of PIP joint arthritis has become a due to the favorable alternative to total joint replacement, due to the wear characteristics of pyrocarbon on cartilage and bone. Pettersson and colleagues reviewed 42 fingers in 38 patients undergoing PIP joint hemiarthroplasty. Although there was a significant improvement in DASH and visual analog pain scales, there was no significant change in grip, pinch, or range of motion. Over the 4.6-year follow-up, only four joints required revision for failure.[37]

Our present indications for PIP arthroplasty are primarily limited to oligoarticular RA patients with good disease control or those with OA or post-traumatic arthritis. Hemiarthroplasty is used if reasonable joint congruity can be created on the middle phalanx. Hemiarthroplasty, in our

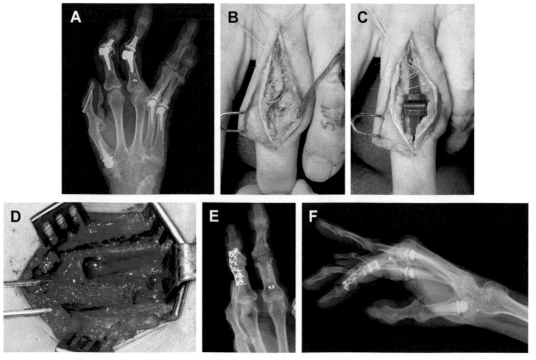

Fig. 4. (A–F) A 58-year-old patient with previously placed SR-Avanta implants for RA with the development of severe hyperextension deformity of index and long finger PIP. (A) AP radiograph of hand. The removal of implants resulted in a fracture of long finger proximal phalanx (B) in addition to substantial bone loss at index. Long finger was converted to silicone with aid of cerclage suture in the proximal phalanx (C). Index finger was fused with aid of iliac crest strut (D) placed into medullary canal of proximal and middle phalanx and then plated (E). (D) Bone strut in forceps overlying iliac crest donor site. (E, F) AP and lateral radiographs of 6 months after surgery with stable finger function.

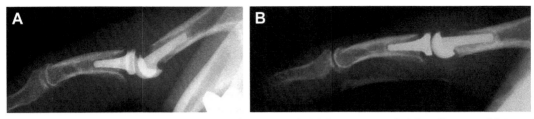

Fig. 5. (*A, B*) PIP hyperextension may occasionally be managed with long-term oval eight splint wear. (*A*) Lateral radiograph of hyperextension deformity which was corrected using an oval eight splint being worn full time for 6 months. (*B*) Lateral radiograph (without splint) at 1 year from beginning treatment. Note that change in stem position of proximal phalanx over time.

experience, has fewer long-term complications than total PIP arthroplasty. Total pyrocarbon arthroplasty is reserved for younger or more active patients with stable soft tissues.[38] A revision of the pyrocarbon can be attempted once, but after this, the authors have found that moving to silicone can provide motion with fewer complications.[26] In cases of excessive bone loss, multiple revisions or infection the authors move to PIP fusion. When converting an arthroplasty to fusion, the authors have found that iliac crest bicortical graft can be fashioned as an intramedullary strut to span the

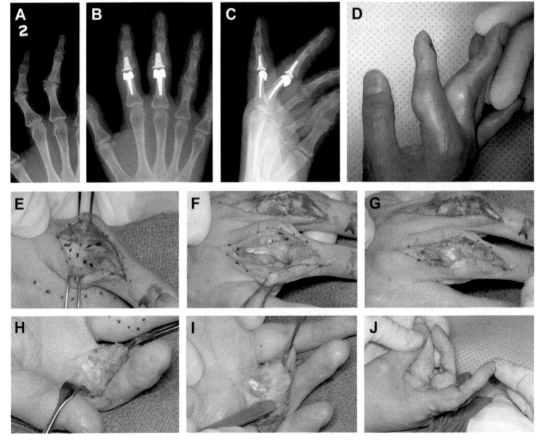

Fig. 6. A 55-year-old woman with PIP arthritis of the index and middle fingers who was treated initially with silicone PIP arthroplasty (*A*). She went on to have instability and implant fracture and was revised to metal-plastic SRA implants (*B, C*). She went through rehabilitation but failed to gain motion and ended up with fixed swan neck deformities (*D*). Through a combined V-Y lengthening of the extensor (*E–G*) and superficialis hemitenodesis (*H, I*), the swan neck deformity is corrected allowing maintenance of the implant and more functional position of the fingers (*J*).

arthroplasty site and allow for stable fixation with plates, pins, or screws (**Fig. 4**).

Common postoperative complications can include joint hyperextension (**Fig. 5**). Hyperextension, if untreated, will usually result in implant failure and joint squeaking. Squeaking has been shown to result from increasing load across the pyrocarbon surface.[39] The temporary resolution of squeaking is possible with saline or hyaluronic acid injections around the implant, but permanent resolution usually requires addressing the joint hyperextension. Hyperextension can be managed nonoperatively with the use of oval eight splints and PIP flexion splints with the goal of creating a limited flexion contracture. If this is unsuccessful, joint revision is usually required. The use of a hemi-superficialis tenodesis can prevent swan necking; however, we have not found tenodesis procedures effective and prefer to convert patients to silicone implants.

Flexion contracture, if significant, can be debilitating for the patient. In these cases, attempts at tenolysis can be attempted. Reoperation to improve motion has a guarded prognosis. Thus, in many cases, conversion to silicone or fusion may be necessary to prevent recurrent contracture (**Fig. 6**). Thankfully, in many of these cases, the joint is pain free, so patients may choose to live with their limited motion rather than undergo fusion.

Intraoperative fractures can also occur, particularly when removing older surface replacement implants which are osseointegrated. Wagner and colleagues evaluated 382 consecutive PIP arthroplasties. Intraoperative fracture was found to occur in 5% of arthroplasties. Risks for fracture were RA and lower body mass index (BMI). The average follow-up was 5.2 years with implant survival rate without surgery following intraoperative fracture being 76% and 64% at 2 and 5 years, respectively. There was no difference in survival rates to those who did not suffer and intraoperative fracture.[40] As in cases of metacarpal fractures, suture cerclage can be used to salvage the bone and allow arthroplasty to proceed (see **Fig. 4**).

In Wagner and colleagues' study of 75 consecutive PIP revisions, two-thirds or these patients had a history of prior PIP trauma (**Fig. 7**). Revision cases had a 5-year survival rate of 70%. Although complication rates were high, pain relief was

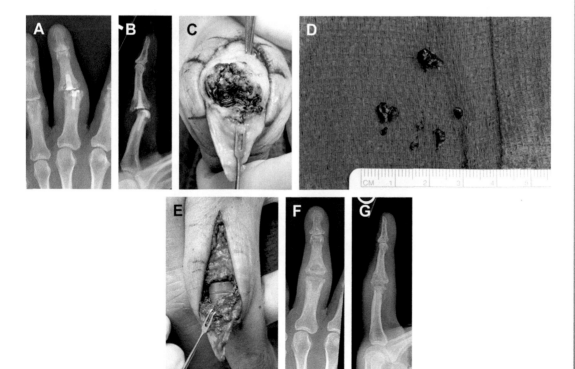

Fig. 7. A 44-year-old patient who underwent pyrocarbon PIP arthroplasty for post-traumatic arthritis of long finger. He reportedly did well and then developed progressive limitation of motion and deviation of the digit. (*A, B*) At the time of presentation, patient demonstrated implant fracture on AP and lateral radiographs. Intraoperatively, a significant amount of graphite-stained tissue was appreciable (*C, D*). He was revised to a silicone implant (*E*). At 6 months post-revision his radiographs (*F, G*) demonstrated stable implant and alignment with a 50° arc of PIP motion. In addition, his PIP hyperextension was corrected.

excellent. Instability was associated with worse long-term outcomes following revision. Pyrocarbon implants were found to have higher complication rates than silicone.[26]

Several investigators have tried to evaluate the benefits of the volar or dorsal approach in decreasing complications associated with PIP arthroplasty.[29,41] Herren and Simmen report that the volar approach was associated with fewer complications, although there was not a significant difference.[42] Their findings suggest that the volar approach may be beneficial if collateral ligament integrity is critical, as in cases of pyrocarbon arthroplasty. In Yamamoto's systematic review of 40 papers, they found that silicone implants placed through a volar approach showed the best arc of motion, with less extension lag and fewer complications after surgery among all the

implant designs and surgical approaches.[43] More recent reports have failed to show any differences between complications or outcomes using a dorsal or volar approach.[44] The authors would agree that the volar approach may reduce extensor lag by preserving the central slip attachment, but dorsal osteophytes may be hard to visualize, and bone cuts can be technically difficult. For OA, the authors prefer the dorsal approach with reattachment of the central slip and revision arthroplasty; the authors prefer to use the same incisions used for the primary surgery if possible.

CARPOMETACARPAL ARTHROPLASTY

Trapezium prosthetic arthroplasty has been used to treat basal joint arthritis of the thumb for decades. Implant arthroplasty seeks to preserve joint

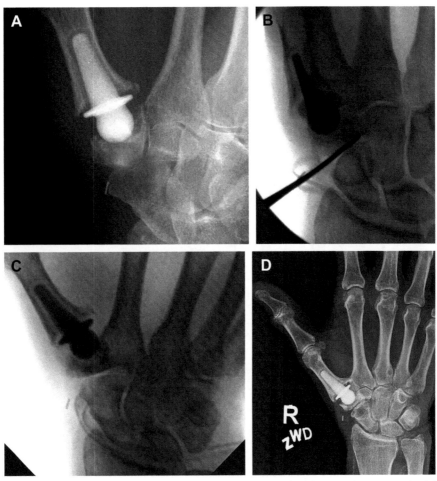

Fig. 8. A 63-year old patient who underwent pyrocarbon CMC hemiarthroplasty. Eighteen months following implantation the patient complained of pain over the palmar STT region. Radiographs revealed STT arthritis (A). Interpositional arthroplasty was performed at STT joint with resection of arthritis surface and placement of interpositional dermal allograft. (B, C) Intraoperative radiographic images of dermal allograft placement. (D) Thumb and wrist 8 years following procedure with a stable CMC and asymptomatic STT joint.

biomechanics, prevent metacarpal subsidence, and improve thumb stability. Unfortunately, prosthetic CMC arthroplasty has had a problematic history. Early metal implant designs, used primarily in Europe, had a high incidence of aseptic cup loosening, metallosis, and dislocation.[45,46] Newer designs, which have avoided metal on metal articulations, have shown more promise with failure rates running between 4% and 11%.[46–49] If these newer arthroplasties fail, they can be converted to a trapeziectomy with or without suspension-plasty by separating the trapezial base from metacarpal stem. The trapezial component is then removed with the trapezium.[50]

Within the United States, the use of hemiarthroplasty with metal or pyrocarbon has gained popularity. These implants still have complication rates which are higher than primary trapeziectomy.[51] Subluxation is the most common complication that may be encountered after hemiarthroplasty and is the primary cause of implant failure. In series of 54 thumb CMC joints undergoing pyrocarbon hemiarthroplasty, De Aragon reported that 10 of the 15 early failures were due to metacarpal

subluxation or dislocation; the investigators attributed this to the creation of a shallow trapezial cup.[52]

Symptomatic subluxation rates have decreased with the use of a second-generation pyrocarbon implants. In a series of 47 patients who underwent CMC pyrocarbon hemiarthroplasty, only 3.5% needed revision for instability. In this series, the most common reason for revision or implant removal was the development of scaphoid-trapezium-trapezoid (STT) arthritis.[51] Other rare complications have included infection, aseptic loosening, and trapezial fracture; these complications may warrant implant removal and conversion to complete trapeziectomy.[52]

The potential complication of subluxation or dislocation is best mitigated in the operating room during the initial procedure. The trapezial cup should be roughly one-third of the depth of the trapezium. In addition, once the implant has been seated into the central socket in the trapezium the implant should remain reduced as the thumb is taken through a full range of motion, before capsular closure. If dislocation occurs,

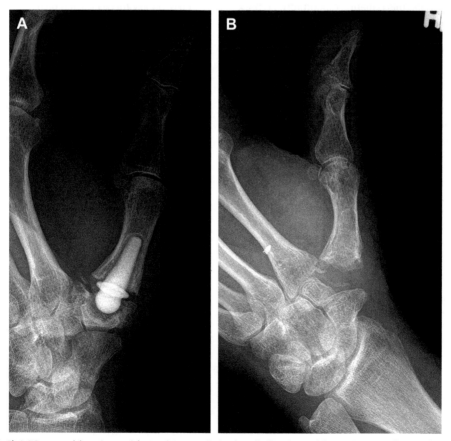

Fig. 9. (*A, B*) A 58-year-old patient with persistent pain in thumb despite stable CMC pyrocarbon arthroplasty and no evidence of STT arthritis. (*A*) Patient was converted to a trapeziectomy with Thompson suspension-plasty 18 months following index procedure. (*B*) A stable thumb at 2 years and patient is now symptomatic.

verify that there has been adequate metacarpal base resection, attempt to use a larger implant, and verify that the cup has been placed central within the trapezium. A strong capsuloligamentous reconstruction will then prevent postoperative instability and dorsal subluxation.

Postsurgical acute or subacute dislocation is managed most effectively by returning to the OR and deepening the cup within the trapezium and then using a braided 2 to 0 suture in a figure of eight fashion through drill holes in the trapezium and metacarpal base. This creates a dorsal brace against any further dorsal dislocation. Maintaining the implant's position during the early capsular healing phase can be facilitated with the use of a Kirschner wire if necessary.

The late development of STT arthritis has been noted to occur in 5% of patients over a follow-up period of 16 years. The development may represent unrecognized preexisting arthritis, ongoing pantrapezial instability, or potential "overstuffing" the joint, which may exacerbate degenerative changes at the scaphotrapezial joint. Regardless of etiology, the authors have found two reliable ways to manage this patient's discomfort: (1) proximal trapezial resection with interpositional arthroplasty or (2) trapeziectomy and some form of metacarpal suspension (**Fig. 8**).

In a study of 176 implants, Zelenski found that the most common reason for implant removal was due to the development of STT arthritis or unresolved pain. The removal of a pyrocarbon CMC implant and subsequent trapeziectomy successfully relieved pain in patients in whom pyrocarbon arthroplasty had failed (**Fig. 9**). After revision, patients lost some abduction motion but had similar strength compared with those who underwent primary trapeziectomy.[53] Similar findings were reported by Kaszap, showing that thumb function following the removal of CMC arthroplasty is equivalent to those patients undergoing primary trapeziectomy.[50]

SUMMARY

Implant arthroplasty of the MCP, PIP, and CMC joints remains a means of preserving motion and function for patients with inflammatory and osteoarthritis, but complications will be inevitable. The best way of minimizing complications in small joint arthroplasty is choose the right patients and adhere to meticulous surgical technique. Pyrocarbon has become the major alternative to silicone and offers the potential for long-term implant survival; however, these implants require intact soft tissue constraints. Postoperative instability and dislocation can be managing with revisional surgery that focuses on the stabilization of the soft tissues or conversion to silicone implants before considering joint fusion. The ultimate solution to problems associated with small joint arthroplasty will come with advancements in implant design, until then surgeons should familiarize themselves with salvage techniques.

SUPPLEMENTARY DATA

Supplementary data related to this article can be found online at https://doi.org/10.1016/j.hcl.2023.02.006.

REFERENCES

1. Swanson AB. Flexible implant resection arthroplasty. Hand 1972;4:119–34.
2. Swanson AB. Flexible implant arthroplasty for arthritic finger joints: rationale, technique, and results of treatment. J Bone Joint Surg 1972;54A:435–55.
3. Blair WF, Shurr DG, Buckwalter JA. Metacarpophalangeal joint arthroplasty with a metallic hinged prosthesis. Clin Orthop 1984;184:156–63.
4. Wilson YG, Sykes PJ, Niranjan NS. Long-term follow-up of Swanson's Silastic arthroplasty of the metacarpophalangeal joints in rheumatoid arthritis. J Hand Surg 1993;18B:81–91.
5. Chung KC, Kostis SV, Kim HM. A prospective outcomes study of Swanson metacarpophalangeal joint arthroplasty for the rheumatoid hand. J Hand Surg 2004;29A:646–53.
6. Beckenbaugh RD, Dobyns JH, Linscheid RL, et al. Review and analysis of silicone-rubber metacarpophalangeal implants. J Bone Joint Surg Am 1976; 58:483–5.
7. Bravo CJ, Rizzo M, Hormel KB, et al. Pyrolytic carbon proximal interphalangeal joint arthroplasty: results with minimum two-year follow-up evaluation. J Hand Surg 2007;32:1–11.
8. Walker PS, Erkman MJ. Laboratory evaluation of a metal-plastic type of metacarpophalangeal joint prosthesis. Clin Orthop 1975;112:340–56.
9. Beckenbaugh RD. The development of an implant for the metacarpophalangeal joint of the fingers. Acta Orthop Scand 1999;70:107–8.
10. Beckenbaugh RD. Pyrolytic carbon implants. In: Simmen BR, Allieu Y, Lluch A, et al, editors. Hand arthroplasties. London: Martin Dunitz; 2000. p. 323–7.
11. Doi K, Kuwata N, Kawai S. Alumina ceramic finger implants: a preliminary biomaterial and clinical evaluation. J Hand Surg 1984;9:740–9.
12. Linscheid RL, Murray PM, Vidal MA, et al. Development of a surface replacement arthroplasty for proximal interphalangeal joints. J Hand Surg [Am] 1997; 22:286–98.
13. Boe C, Wagner E, Rizzo M. Long-term outcomes of silicone metacarpophalangeal arthroplasty: a

longitudinal analysis of 325 cases. J Hand Surg Eur 2018;43:1076–82.

14. Goldfarb CA, Stern PJ. Metacarpophalangeal joint arthroplasty in rheumatoid arthritis. J Bone Joint Surg 2003;85:1869–78.

15. Trail IA, Martin JA, Nuttall D, et al. Seventeen-year survivorship analysis of silastic metacarpophalangeal joint replacement. J Bone Joint Surg Br 2004; 86:1002–6.

16. Notermans BJW, Lans J, Arnold D, et al. Factors Associated With Reoperation After Silicone Metacarpophalangeal Joint Arthroplasty in Patients With Inflammatory Arthritis. Hand (NY) 2020;15:805–11.

17. Burgess SD, Kono M, Stern PJ. Results of revision metacarpophalangeal joint surgery in rheumatoid patients following previous silicone arthroplasty. J Hand Surg Am 2007;32:1506–12.

18. Cook SD, Beckenbaugh RD, Redondo J, et al. Long-term follow-up of pyrolytic carbon metacarpophalangeal implants. J Bone Joint Surg Am 1999;81:635–48.

19. Parker W, Moran SL, Hormel KB, et al. Nonrheumatoid metacarpophalangeal joint arthritis. Unconstrained pyrolytic carbon implants: Indications, techniques and outcomes. Hand Clin 2006;22: 183–93.

20. Cummings PE, Claxton MR, Wagner ER, et al. Outcomes of Pyrocarbon Arthroplasty in Metacarpophalangeal Joints Affected by Rheumatoid Arthritis. Hand 2022. online ahead of print.

21. Wagner ER, Houdek MT, Packard B, et al. Revision Metacarpophalangeal Arthroplasty: A Longitudinal Study of 128 Cases. J Am Acad Orthop Surg 2019;27:211–8.

22. Clark DI, Delaney R, Stilwell JH, et al. The value of crossed intrinsic transfer after metacarpophalangeal silastic arthroplasty: a comparative study. J Hand Surg Br 2001;26:565–7.

23. Dell PC, Renfree KJ, Below Dell R. Surgical correction of extensor tendon subluxation and ulnar drift in the rheumatoid hand: long-term results. J Hand Surg Br 2001;26:560–4.

24. Wanderman N, Wagner E, Moran S, et al. Outcomes Following Acute Metacarpophalangeal Joint Arthroplasty Dislocation: An Analysis of 37 Cases. J Hand Surg Am 2018;43:289. e1-.e6.

25. Wagner ER, RVr Demark, Wilson GA, et al. Intraoperative periprosthetic fractures associated with metacarpophalangeal joint arthroplasty. J Hand Surg Am 2015;40:945–50.

26. Wagner ER, Luo TD, Houdek MT, et al. Revision Proximal Interphalangeal Arthroplasty: An Outcome Analysis of 75 Consecutive Cases. J Hand Surg Am 2015;40:1949–19455.e1.

27. Wagner ER, Weston JT, Houdek MT, et al. Medium-Term Outcomes With Pyrocarbon Proximal Interphalangeal Arthroplasty: A Study of 170 Consecutive Arthroplasties. J Hand Surg Am 2018;43:797–805.

28. Takigawa S, Meletiou S, Sauerbier M, et al. Long-term assessment of Swanson implant arthroplasty in the proximal interphalangeal joint of the hand. J Hand Surg [Am] 2004;29:785–95.

29. Lin HH, Wyrick JD, Stern PJ. Proximal interphalangeal joint silicone replacement arthroplasty: clinical results using an anterior approach. J Hand Surg [Am] 1995;20:123–32.

30. Pettersson K, Wagnsjö P, Hulin E. NeuFlex compared with Sutter prostheses: a blind, prospective, randomised comparison of Silastic metacarpophalangeal joint prostheses. Scand J Plast ReConstr Surg Hand Surg 2006;40:284–90.

31. Bales JG, Wall LB, Stern PJ. Long-term results of Swanson silicone arthroplasty for proximal interphalangeal joint osteoarthritis. J Hand Surg Am 2014;39: 455–61.

32. Watts AC, Hearnden AJ, Trail IA, et al. Pyrocarbon proximal interphalangeal joint arthroplasty: minimum two-year follow-up. J Hand Surg Am 2012;37:882–8.

33. Dickson DR, Nuttall D, Watts AC, et al. Pyrocarbon Proximal Interphalangeal Joint Arthroplasty: Minimum Five-Year Follow-Up. J Hand Surg Am 2015; 40:2142–8.e4.

34. Vitale MA, Fruth KM, Rizzo M, et al. Prosthetic Arthroplasty Versus Arthrodesis for Osteoarthritis and Posttraumatic Arthritis of the Index Finger Proximal Interphalangeal Joint. J Hand Surg Am 2015;40: 1937–48.

35. Branam BR, Tuttle HG, Stern PJ, et al. Resurfacing arthroplasty versus silicone arthroplasty for proximal interphalangeal joint osteoarthritis. J Hand Surg Am 2007;32:775–88.

36. Forster N, Schindele S, Audigé L, et al. Complications, reoperations and revisions after proximal interphalangeal joint arthroplasty: a systematic review and meta-analysis. J Hand Surg Eur 2018;43:1066–75.

37. Pettersson K, Amilon A, Rizzo M. Pyrolytic carbon hemiarthroplasty in the management of proximal interphalangeal joint arthritis. J Hand Surg Am 2015;40:462–8.

38. Wagner ER, Robinson WA, Houdek MT, et al. Proximal Interphalangeal Joint Arthroplasty in Young Patients. J Am Acad Orthop Surg 2019;27:444–50.

39. Davis C, Thoreson AR, Berglund L, et al. Investigation of squeaking in pyrolytic carbon proximal interphalangeal joint implants. J Med Dev Trans ASME 2014;8. UNSP 014508.

40. Wagner ER, Van Demark R, Kor DJ, et al. Intraoperative Periprosthetic Fractures in Proximal Interphalangeal Joint Arthroplasty. J Hand Surg Am 2015; 40:2149–54.

41. Drake ML, Segalman KA. Complications of small joint arthroplasty. Hand Clin 2010;26:205–12.

42. Herren DB, Simmen BR. Palmar approach in flexible implant arthroplasty of the proximal interphalangeal joint. Clin Orthop Relat Res 2000;371:131–5.

43. Yamamoto M, Malay S, Fujihara Y, et al. A Systematic Review of Different Implants and Approaches for Proximal Interphalangeal Joint Arthroplasty. Plast Reconstr Surg 2017;139:1139e–51e.

44. Tranchida GV, Allen ST, Moen SM, et al. Comparison of Volar and Dorsal Approach for PIP Arthroplasty. Hand (N Y) 2021;16:348–53.

45. Søndergaard L, Konradsen L, Rechnagel K. Long-term follow-up of the cemented Caffinière prosthesis for trapezio-metacarpal arthroplasty. J Hand Surg Br 1991;16:428–30.

46. Vitale MA, Taylor F, Ross M, et al. Trapezium prosthetic arthroplasty (silicone, Artelon, metal, and pyrocarbon). Hand Clin 2013;29:37–55.

47. Bellemère P, Lussiez B. Thumb Carpometacarpal Implant Arthroplasty. Hand Clin 2022;38:217–30.

48. Logan J, Peters SE, Strauss R, et al. Pyrocarban Trapeziometacarpal Joint Arthroplasty-Medium-Term Outcomes. J Wrist Surg 2020;9:509–17.

49. Smeraglia F, Barrera-Ochoa S, Mendez-Sanchez G, et al. Partial trapeziectomy and pyrocarbon interpositional arthroplasty for trapeziometacarpal osteoarthritis: minimum 8-year follow-up. J Hand Surg Eur 2020;45:472–6.

50. Kaszap B, Daecke W, Jung M. Outcome comparison of primary trapeziectomy versus secondary trapeziectomy following failed total trapeziometacarpal joint replacement. J Hand Surg Am 2013;38(5): 863–71.e3.

51. Vitale MA, Hsu CC, Rizzo M, et al. Pyrolytic Carbon Arthroplasty versus Suspensionplasty for Trapezial-Metacarpal Arthritis. J Wrist Surg 2017; 6:134–43.

52. Martinez de Aragon JS, Moran SL, Rizzo M, et al. Early outcomes of pyrolytic carbon hemiarthroplasty for the treatment of trapezial-metacarpal arthritis. J Hand Surg Am 2009;34:205–12.

53. Zelenski NA, Rizzo M, Moran SL. Outcomes of Secondary Trapeziectomy Following Carpometacarpal Pyrocarbon Prosthetic Arthroplasty. J Hand Surg Am 2022;47:429–36.

Carpometacarpal Joint Pathology in the Thumb and Hand
Evaluation and Management of Difficult Conditions

Bilal Mahmood, MD[a], Warren C. Hammert, MD[b],*

KEYWORDS

- Carpometacarpal arthritis • Arthroplasty • Revision • Trapezium • Subsidence • Impingement
- Instability • Trapezoid

KEY POINTS

- Thumb carpometacarpal (CMC) arthroplasty, consisting of trapeziectomy with or without suspensionplasty, ligament reconstruction, and/or tendon interposition is well proven with largely good outcomes and high patient satisfaction.
- For persistent symptoms following thumb CMC arthroplasty, one must first identify the cause of continued pain and dysfunction and come up with a revision surgery to address these problems.
- Data on revision surgeries are sparse and often combine a heterogeneous group of surgical techniques. Improvement is common following revision surgery, but typically results are not as good as primary surgery.

INTRODUCTION

Thumb carpometacarpal (CMC) arthritis is widely prevalent, with about 40% of women 80 years of age or older with radiographic evidence.[1] The prevalence increases to over 90% in both women and men in their 90s.[2] It is one of the joints most commonly affected by osteoarthritis, only second to the distal interphalangeal joints in the upper extremity.[3] The goal of treating thumb CMC arthritis is to provide pain relief, while maximizing stability, mobility, and strength. Various treatment options have included metacarpal osteotomy, arthrodesis, implant arthroplasty, and trapezium excision (with or without ligament reconstruction [LR] and/or tendon interposition [TI] or with suspensionplasty).

ANATOMY AND PATHOPHYSIOLOGY

The thumb CMC joint is a saddle shaped joint, inherently unstable, which allows for circumduction and opposition. The metacarpal articular surface is 34% smaller in diameter than the articulating surface of the trapezium.[4] Owing to the inherent instability from bony geometry, the soft tissues are critically important. There are 16 ligaments that help stabilize the joint, with the anterior oblique (palmar "beak"), dorsoradial, and dorsal intermetacarpal ligaments discussed most often.[3] All play an important role, however, as does the dynamic stabilization provided by the surrounding muscles and tendons (Abductor Pollicis Longus [APL], Extensor Pollicis Longus [EPL], Extensor Pollicis Brevis [EPB], Flexor Pollicis

The authors have nothing to disclose.
[a] Department of Orthopaedic Surgery, University of Rochester, 601 Elmwood Avenue, Box 665, Rochester, NY 14642, USA; [b] Department of Orthopaedic Surgery, Duke University Medical Center, 5601 Arringdon Park Drive, Suite 300, Morrisville, NC 27560, USA
* Corresponding author.
E-mail address: warren.hammert@duke.edu

Hand Clin 39 (2023) 321–329
https://doi.org/10.1016/j.hcl.2023.02.007
0749-0712/23/© 2023 Elsevier Inc. All rights reserved.

Longus [FPL], Flexor Pollicis Brevis [FPB], Abductor Pollicis Brevis [APB], adductor pollicis, and opponens pollicis). From pinch to maximum grasp, the thumb CMC joints force is 12 to 20 times the applied load, with the volar half of the articular surface seeing the highest forces. Patients involved in manual labor or with repetitive thumb use have a 12-fold increased risk of thumb CMC arthritis.[5] Post-traumatic arthritis following articular fractures may also contribute and patients with ligamentous laxity and a higher Beighton score also have a higher incidence of thumb CMC arthritis and radiographic changes.[3]

PHYSICAL EXAMINATION

Patients with thumb CMC arthritis often describe throbbing or aching pain at the base of the thumb, particularly within the thenar eminence. They commonly gesture with their contralateral hand, grasping the symptomatic thumb and thenar muscles, almost as if stabilizing or immobilizing their symptomatic joint. Advanced thumb CMC arthritis may present with an adduction contracture at the CMC joint and compensatory thumb Metacarpophalangeal joint (MCP) hyperextension. On examination, tenderness and crepitus may be palpated at the thumb CMC joint. The grind test involves placing an axial load to the thumb CMC joint through the thumb metacarpal. This will elicit pain and often crepitus. Pinch strength testing may also be helpful and serve as a baseline during treatment. It is important to recognize the association of carpal tunnel syndrome occurring in 30% of patients with thumb CMC arthritis.[4]

IMAGING

Plain radiographs are the mainstay for diagnosing thumb CMC arthritis on imaging. These may be posterior Anterior (PA), lateral, and oblique views of the thumb or hand. A true PA, or Robert view, is obtained with the shoulder flexed and in internal rotation with the wrist hyperpronated. Some patients may find this position difficult to obtain. In addition, a 30° stress view of the thumbs can allow visualization of all the trapezial articulations (trapezial first metacarpal, scaphotrapezial, trapezial-trapezoid, and trapezial-second metacarpal). The most widely used staging system on radiographs was described by Eaton (**Table 1**).

TREATMENT

Treatment is largely based on the extent of symptoms the patient presents with as many can be managed nonoperatively. Immobilization, which may be hand or forearm-based orthosis, is often

Table 1 Eaton classification	
Eaton Classification	**Radiographic Findings of Thumb CMC**
Stage 1	Normal or slight widening
Stage 2	Mild joint narrowing with osteophytes formation of <2 mm
Stage 3	Marked joint narrowing with osteophyte formation of 2 mm or more
Stage4	Stage 3 plus STT arthritis

one of the first treatment options. Patients may try using topical or oral nonsteroidal antiinflammatory drug (NSAIDs). Outpatient hand therapy and home exercises focusing on thenar and first dorsal interosseous strengthening helps with stabilization of the thumb CMC joint. Corticosteroid injections are widely used as well, with 89% of hand surgeons using these as part of nonoperative management.[6]

When nonoperative management fails to provide an adequate amount of relief, a multitude of surgical options are available. For Eaton stage I disease, with largely normal radiographic findings, possible procedures include CMC arthroscopy, metacarpal extension osteotomy, or volar LR.

More commonly, patients with persistent symptoms after nonoperative management also have Eaton stage II–IV disease. The radiographic appearance is not directly correlated to symptoms, with some patient having advanced radiographic changes and no symptoms and others having minimal radiographic changes and substantial symptoms. Over the course of the last few decades, the surgical gold standard for Eaton stage II–IV disease has included trapeziectomy with or without LR, TI, both (LRTI), or suture suspensionplasty. Evidence does not support one technique over the other in comparing these, although the LRTI is often viewed as having potential long-term benefits.[7,8] CMC arthrodesis is an option often reserved for younger patients as it is associated with greater pinch strength and has reported satisfaction rates between 60% and 100%.[9,10] Rates of nonunion range from 8% to 21%. Data on arthroplasty with silicone implants note high complication rates, and data on newer implants and total joint prostheses remain sparse.

COMPLICATIONS AND REVISIONS

Our focus for the remainder of this review will be on the evaluation and management of failed thumb

CMC arthroplasty, defined as persistent symptoms following surgery. Primary thumb CMC arthroplasty is considered highly successful with mostly good and excellent outcomes noted in the literature.[7,11,12] Revision rates are noted to be less than 3%, although there remains a deficiency in literature on failures and revision procedures.[13,14] Failure of thumb CMC arthroplasty may be due to a variety of reasons. It is helpful to divide these into neurogenic and non-neurogenic causes (**Box 1**). Non-neurogenic causes of failure include thumb metacarpal and scaphoid impingement due to subsidence, thumb metacarpal-trapezoid impingement, TI graft extrusion, incomplete trapeziectomy, untreated/unrecognized STT arthritis or MCP instability, FCR tendinopathy, and infection.[14,15] Other causes that are also non-neurogenic, but may be related to untreated diagnoses included carpal tunnel syndrome, trigger thumb, and de Quervain's tenosynovitis. Neurogenic causes of failure include injury to the superficial radial sensory or lateral antebrachial cutaneous nerve branches, which could lead to chronic regional pain syndrome (CRPS).

Nonoperative measures are a viable option in treating complications of thumb CMC arthroplasty. In the cases of untreated diagnoses such as carpal tunnel syndrome, trigger thumb, or de Quervain's tenosynovitis, splinting or injections may help symptoms resolve. FCR tendinopathy developing after CMC arthroplasty can be treated conservatively with immobilization and corticosteroid injections. When nonoperative management fails or is not a viable option and revision surgery is chosen, both the cause of failures along with the primary procedure performed are vital to understand before a revision procedure.[13]

EVALUATION

A thorough evaluation of patient complaints and symptoms is vital in treating persistent symptoms after thumb CMC arthroplasty. Short of a major complication in the early postoperative period, such as infection or tendon extrusion, waiting to see what symptoms persist after 6 months of recovery is appropriate. Pain within this time frame is often temporary, and radiographs may exaggerate the amount of subsidence and impingement.[14] Substantial pain lasting beyond 6 months generally requires further work up and intervention.

Mechanical or non-neurogenic causes of pain are often described as a continued deep ache, grinding, or feelings of instability. Work up includes obtaining radiographs, which may show subsidence leading to metacarpal impingement on the scaphoid or trapezoid. Subsidence is often asymptomatic and not an indication for revision, thus radiographs findings need to be correlated with the physical examination.[4] Radiographs may also demonstrate unaddressed STT arthritis or incomplete trapezium resection. Residual pinch or grasp weakness may be due to unaddressed MCP instability with continued MCP hyperextension resulting in pain and weakness (**Fig. 1**). This can occur with a failure to address or correct hyperextension of greater than 10° at the MCP

Box 1
Causes of thumb carpometacarpal arthroplasty failure

Neurogenic

- Superficial sensory radial neuritis/neuroma
- Lateral antebrachial cutaneous nerve neuritis
- Chronic regional pain syndrome

Non-neurogenic

- Thumb metacarpal-scaphoid impingement from subsidence
- Thumb metacarpal-trapezoid impingement
- Untreated/unrecognized STT arthritis
- Incomplete trapeziectomy
- Tendon interposition graft extrusion
- Failed implant (synovitis, loosening, implant extrusion)
- MCP instability/arthritis
- FCR tendinopathy
- Infection

Miscellaneous/Associated Diagnoses

- Carpal tunnel syndrome
- De Quervain's tenosynovitis
- Trigger thumb

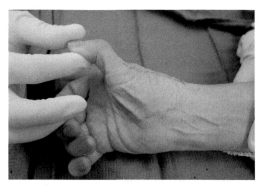

Fig. 1. Clinical photograph showing an adduction contracture and MCP joint instability/hyperextension.

joint.[16] FCR tendinopathy can be diagnosed on examination, with tenderness palpated along its course and brought up by pain on resisted flexion of the FCR on examination. This has been reported in up to 25% of patients following APL suspensionplasty and often occurs 2 to 10 months follow surgery.[17]

Neurogenic pain is challenging to treat. It is often diffuse and poorly defined by the patient. They may describe burning, hypersensitivity, and swelling. Cases of a specific injury to the superficial sensory radial nerve may result in sensory deficit, and a positive Tinel sign may indicate a developing neuroma.

SURGICAL REVISIONS

If nonoperative options have not adequately relieved symptoms following thumb CMC arthroplasty, one can consider revision surgery. As mentioned, both the cause of symptoms and the initial surgical technique are important in determining the options available for revision surgery.

Metacarpal Subsidence with Metacarpal-Scaphoid Impingement

Although rare, symptoms from metacarpal subsidence and metacarpal-scaphoid impingement can occur following trapeziectomy with or without LR, TI, or both (LRTI). Specific revision options depend on the initial procedure. In cases where the FCR is still available, a traditional LRTI with FCR autograft is a primary option. Care must be taken in revision surgery when approaching through the prior incision to carefully dissect nerve branches that may be encased in scar. Residual interposition debris needs to be excised with the aid of fluoroscopy, and the first metacarpal stability is tested. One goal of the revision procedure is to stabilize and align the base of the first metacarpal with the base of the second metacarpal.

If the FCR is not available, the APL and ECRL are reliable options. The APL can be used with a distally based slip, passed through the radial/volar thumb metacarpal base, exiting dorsal/ulnar and suture back to itself. The ECRL can be used as a distally based slip and can be passed dorsal to volar through the second metacarpal base, exiting in a region very close to the FCR insertion (**Fig. 2**). The ECRL slip may be passed around the APL insertion and back onto itself or passed through the thumb metacarpal base in a similar manner to an LRTI (**Fig. 3**). Determining what tendon to use as part of a revision surgery comes down to availability and prior surgery.

An adjunct to a revision as described above is using a suture button suspensionplasty of the first

metacarpal to the second metacarpal. For this, the first and second metacarpal bases are brought into appropriate alignment and pinned based on the suture button (Mini TightRope: Arthrex, Naples, FL) guide. Fluoroscopy is used to confirm appropriate alignment before suture and button placement. With use of the tightrope, care must be taken to check passive motion, pistoning, and any proximal impingement before tying the knots. A similar adjunct to a tightrope is the use of percutaneous K-wire (0.054 or 0.062) fixation of the thumb metacarpal to the index metacarpal for 4 weeks along with immobilization.[18] This tends to keep the metacarpal suspended, but it may flex and additional methods to keep the metacarpal extended may be helpful as extending the metacarpal will decrease the MCP hyperextension.

Thumb Metacarpal-Trapezoid Impingement

Impingement of the thumb metacarpal base and trapezoid is a rare diagnosis, but has been shown in certain cases using advanced imaging. Technetium-99m methylene diphosphonate bone scintigraphy (^{99m}Tc MDP), single-photon emission computed tomography (CT), and standard CT scans have been used to demonstrate this impingement.[15] For most, a CT scan can be used to confirm diagnosis and may show abutment and erosion at the point of contact (see **Fig. 3**). This has been described in prior revision arthroplasties where Burton noted resecting the lateral aspect of the trapezoid at the time of revision arthroplasty due to intraoperative findings of impingement.[19] When tenderness is localized to the base of the thumb and index finger metacarpals, one should have a high degree of suspicious for metacarpal-trapezoid impingement, particularly when standard imaging does not identify a reason for continued pain or dysfunction. This can however occur concurrently with subsidence as well.

As with the case for metacarpal-scaphoid impingement, revision surgery depends on the initial surgery. If metacarpal-trapezoid impingement is in part due to subsidence, then the same revision options as described above remain. In addition, resection of the lateral aspect of the trapezoid at the time of revision arthroplasty can resolve symptoms.

In case where further attempts at a soft tissue reconstruction are not possible, excision of the trapezoid with fusion of the index and middle finger metacarpal bases to the capitate is an option in the case of thumb metacarpal-trapezoid impingement. The technique is described by Renfree and Roarke, with an initial dorsal incision

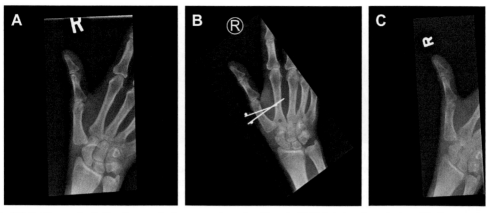

Fig. 2. (A) Radiographs following an index procedure for thumb CMC joint arthroplasty with ligament reconstruction using APL showing subsidence which was symptomatic. (B) Revision ligament reconstruction using ECRL with temporary pinning. (C) Radiographs 3 months after surgery.

made from the radial styloid to the base of the index metacarpal.[15] The trapezoid is excised piecemeal through this incision, and the articulating facets of the index finger metacarpal base and capitate are decorticated and fused using a 3.4 mm headless screw. The interspace between the index and middle finger metacarpals is also decorticated as is the middle finger CMC joint and fixed with staples (**Fig. 4**).[15]

Scaphotrapezial Trapezoidal Arthritis (STT) Arthritis

Untreated or unrecognized STT arthritis results in continued scaphoid-trapezoid (ST) arthritis following a basal joint arthroplasty. The diagnosis may be evident on radiographs showing ST

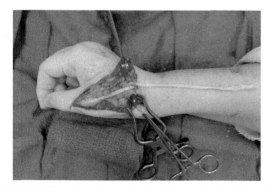

Fig. 3. Clinical photograph showing a distally based split ECRL to be used for reconstruction with a 26-gauge wire through the trapezial space and through the base of the index metacarpal prior to passing the split ECRL dorsal to volar through the index metacarpal base. The EPL tendon is the other tendon visualized as this case involved the use of a previous incision and exposure extended for an MCP joint arthrodesis.

arthritis and can be correlated with tenderness on examination. Revision for untreated ST arthritis involves resection of either the distal scaphoid or proximal trapezoid, with advocates for both procedures. An osteotome or sagittal saw can be used to remove the bone, and an interpositional graft is placed. This can be tendon, dermis, or allograft and secured using a suture anchor in the trapezoid to prevent extrusion.[14] Again, the revision surgery depends on the initial surgery. If a portion of the FCR is available, this may be used for the interpositional graft. Residual osteophytes particularly at the base of the thumb metacarpal should be resected as these can cause pain with grip.

Instability of the Thumb Metacarpal

A recurring theme in revision surgery is to suspend and stabilize the thumb metacarpal, and the possibility of no available soft tissue options is an uncommon but possible scenario. Patients in this category may also have a failed implant or suture button fixation. In these challenging cases a fusion of the first metacarpal base to the second metacarpal base can provide stability. Surgery involves exposing the bases of the first and second metacarpals and elevating a portion of the ECRL. A bur and rongeurs are used to expose cancellous bone and a 2.0-mm T-plate is used to compress across the fusion site (**Fig. 5**). Our preference is to perform the arthrodesis between thumb and index metacarpal for stability when soft tissues are not likely to be effective. We avoid attempts to fuse the metacarpal to the scaphoid as this further shortens the thumb and if successful would cause the thumb to move with the scaphoid throughout wrist movement.

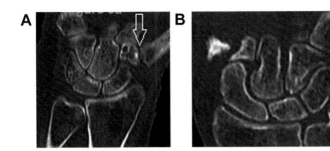
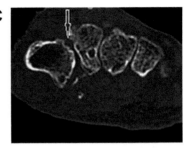

Fig. 4. CT scan showing thumb metacarpal-trapezoid impingement (*A*), erosion (*B*), and an axial view demonstrating abutment (*C*). Arrows indicates area of impingement between thumb metacarpal and trapezoid. (*From* Renfree KJ, Roarke MC. Thumb Metacarpal-Trapezoid Impingement as an Etiology of Pain After Trapeziectomy and Basal Joint Soft Tissue Arthroplasty: A Case Series. J Hand Surg Am. 2021L46(1):931.e1-e6; with permission.)

Incomplete Excision of the Trapezium

Building on the above challenges, when planning on revision surgery for an incomplete trapezium resection, a plan for addressing subsidence, impingement, and instability must also be considered. The principles described above will determine options for revision LR, possible percutaneous pinning or suture button fixation, or osseous procedures. Careful consideration of all potential causes of pain on preoperative evaluation can guide one, but intraoperative evaluation may also show additional pathology that needs to be addressed.

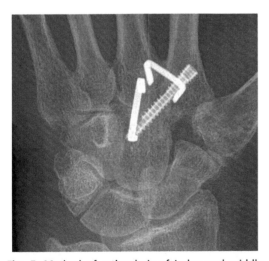

Fig. 5. Method of arthrodesis of index and middle finger CMC joints after excision of trapezoid. (*From* Renfree KJ, Roarke MC. Thumb Metacarpal-Trapezoid Impingement as an Etiology of Pain After Trapeziectomy and Basal Joint Soft Tissue Arthroplasty: A Case Series. J Hand Surg Am. 2021L46(1):931.e1-e6; with permission.)

Herniated Tendon Interposition Graft

Similar to above, revision surgery for excision of a herniated TI graft requires an intraoperative evaluation and the possible revision LR or adjunct procedures. Once again, the specifics of the initial surgery determine the available options as described above. A slip of the FCR can be used if available, or the APL or ECRL may be used for LR. Adjuncts including pinning or suture button fixation may also be used.

Thumb Metacarpal phalangeal joint (MCP) Pathology

Unaddressed/unrecognized thumb MCP instability or arthritis can be symptomatic in isolation or in combination with failure at the base of the metacarpal. In cases of missed MCP arthritis, the standard of care is to address this during revision surgery with an MCP arthrodesis. Multiple options exist for this, including tension band wiring, intramedullary devices, plate fixation, headless compression screws, and so forth. Care is taken to perform the arthrodesis in approximately 20° to 25° of flexion for optimal functional grasp and power grip. This is the same treatment for MCP joint hyperextension greater than 30° (**Figs. 6** and **7**). In case of thumb MCP hyperextension less than 30° that remains symptomatic and require revision surgery, a soft tissue procedure such as a volar capsulodesis is performed.

Failed Implant Arthroplasty

Implant arthroplasty for thumb CMC arthritis has failed to gain traction due to complications of loosening, synovitis, implant subsidence, and dislocations. Implant arthroplasty has failure rates an order of magnitude greater (1.7–4.5 per 100 procedure-years) than those of non-implant arthroplasty failure rates (0.23–0.52 per 100

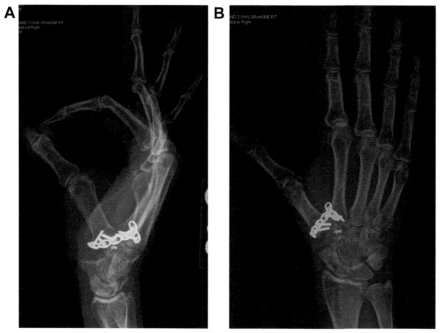

Fig. 6. PA (*A*) and Lateral (*B*) radiographs of a first to second metacarpal arthrodesis procedure using a 2.0-mm locking T-plate in compression mode. (*From* Hess DE, Drace P, Franco MJ, Chhabra AB. Failed Thumb Carpometacarpal Arthroplasty: Common Etiologies and Surgical Options for Revision. J Hand Surg Am. 2018;43(9):844-52; with permission.)

procedure-years), as noted by Ganhewa and colleagues[20] Revision surgery for a failed implant arthroplasty involves removing the implant and performing a debridement and synovectomy as necessary. A complete trapeziectomy is performed and an appropriate suspensionplasty or LR option can be used. Kaszap and colleagues reported outcomes of secondary trapeziectomy following a failed implant arthroplasty to have similar outcomes to a primary trapeziectomy.[21]

Neuroma

The superficial sensory branch of radial nerve (SSRN) and its branches may be injured during thumb CMC surgery. The initial management for nerve-related pain is with hand therapy and pain management. The treating hand therapist will use desensitization techniques, and neuromodulating medications such as gabapentin may be helpful. If symptoms continue for greater than 6 months or there is evidence of a non-progressing Tinel

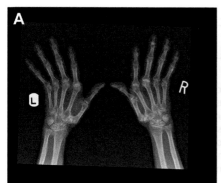
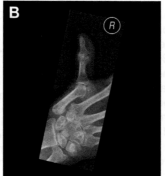
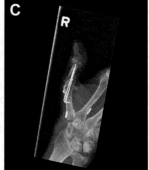

Fig. 7. (*A*) Radiographs before index surgery for right thumb CMC arthroplasty with tendon interposition. (*B*). Postoperative subsidence with metacarpal-scaphoid impingement and MCP joint instability with hyperextension greater than 30°. (*C*) Postoperative radiographs following revision surgery with an MCP arthrodesis and revision CMC arthroplasty with suture button.

sign, surgical exploration is considered. Careful dissection is performed to free up the SSRN from any scar. If a neuroma is identified, it can be resected and the nerve reconstructed with conduit or allograft. The treating surgeon may also consider target muscle reinnervation or regenerative peripheral nerve interface following resection of the neuroma if a distal nerve for reconstruction is not identified.

Chronic Regional Pain Syndrome

CRPS presents with pain, swelling, erythema, decreased range of motion, and stiffness. In acute cases, there may be hyperhidrosis, and in subacute cases of symptoms greater than 3 months, one may notice skin dryness, atrophy, and cyanosis.[14] Radiographs will show disuse osteopenia. In chronic cases, joint contractures can develop. Surgery should be avoided in patients with active CRPS, unless an underlying nerve compression, such as carpal tunnel syndrome is identified. Hand therapy should be initiated early, and judicious use of oral steroids may be considered. A referral to pain management is recommended.

OUTCOMES

Appropriate management of revision surgery for thumb CMC arthritis involves a careful evaluation of the cause of failure combined with the specifics of the index surgery and then the treating surgeon can determined the options for the revision surgery. Resection arthroplasty with or without LR, TI, or both has been considered a successful and reliable procedure. Thus, data on outcomes of revisions in challenging situations are limited.

The few studies evaluating outcomes have done so by combining a variety of index surgeries with a variety of revision surgeries. The Conolly and Rath evaluation system has been used to address functional outcomes.[22] For this score, pain relief, motion, and strength were used to categorize results as good, fair, or poor. Conolly and Rath reviewed 17 patients with failed CMC arthroplasty and noted good results in 53%, fair results in 18% and poor results in 29%. Of note, 12 out of 17 patients had undergone an implant arthroplasty as an index procedure. In 2006, Cooney and colleagues reviewed 17 revisions performed for mechanical pain from 1988 to 2000 and noted good results in 76%, fair results in 12%, and poor results in 12%.[13] Papatheodorou and colleagues reviewed 32 patients with revision primarily due to subsidence and noted good results in 84% and fair results in 16%.[23]

Sadhu and colleagues compared revision thumb CMC arthroplasty to primary cases and noted general worse patient-reported outcomes, pain scores, as well as high rates of depression, even with similar pinch strength, grip strength, and motion.[24] Although revision surgery can improve symptoms, a successful initial surgery has outcomes that revision procedures are unlikely to match. Thus, patient expectations should be managed appropriately. It is important to once again note of the variety of index and revision procedures performed in these studies, and thus, specific comparisons of techniques cannot be made.

SUMMARY

The core principles of thumb CMC arthroplasty complications and revisions are to (1) identify the specific cause of failure and source of symptoms, (2) review what was performed in the initial surgery and identify options for revision surgery, (3) proceed with revision surgery with an appropriate plan and backup plan to correct problem while creating a stable base for the thumb. Several surgical options exist, and there is no one approach that is used in all scenarios. If the index surgery was performed elsewhere, obtaining the operative report is important to determine the initial technique for suspensionplasty or LR. If no soft tissue reconstruction options remain, suture button suspension/fixation, distraction arthroplasty without a soft tissue reconstruction, or arthrodesis to the index metacarpal base can be all considered. The specific surgery performed is also based on patient factors, functional levels, and goals. The literature is sparse on outcomes of specific revision surgeries, but as a whole, good to fair results are achieved for a majority of patients undergoing revision thumb CMC arthroplasty. However, these results are worse than those of a successful primary surgery.

CLINICS CARE POINTS

- In considering failure of thumb CMC arthroplasty, we recommend proceeding with caution during the first 6 months. Pain during this time may be temporary, and subsidence and impingement based early radiographs can be over diagnosed and are rarely symptomatic.
- Distinct untreated diagnoses, such as carpal tunnel syndrome, trigger thumb, and de Quervain's tenosynovitis, can treated independently beginning with standard nonoperative treatment.

- If considering thumb metacarpal-trapezoid impingement, a CT scan can show abutment and erosion not evident on plain radiographs.

- Distally based slips of the FCR, APL, and ECRL are considered the main soft tissue reconstruction options available.

- Using adjunct fixation, such as temporary thumb to index metacarpal K-wire pinning or suture button stabilization, are additional non-arthrodesis techniques to consider.

- Good outcomes can be achieved for a majority of patients undergoing revision thumb CMC arthroplasty.

- Managing patient expectations is an important component of revision thumb CMC arthroplasty.

REFERENCES

1. Wilder FV, Barrett JP, Farina EJ. Joint-specific prevalence of osteoarthritis of the hand. Osteoarthr Cartil 2006;14(9):953–7.

2. Becker SJE, Briet JP, Hageman Michiel GJ S, et al. Death, taxes, and trapeziometacarpal arthrosis. Clin Orthop Relat Res 2013;471(12):3738–44.

3. Weiss AC, Goodman AD. Thumb basal joint arthritis. J Am Acad Orthop Surg 2018;26(16):562–71.

4. Murray P. Treatment of the osteoarthritis hand and Thumb. In: Wolfe S, Pederson W, Kozin S, et al, editors. Green's operative hand surgery. Vol 1. 8th ed; 2022. p. 409–37.

5. Fontana L, Neel S, Claise J, et al. Osteoarthritis of the thumb carpometacarpal joint in women and occupational risk factors: A Case–Control study. J Hand Surg Am 2007;32(4):459–65.

6. Wolf JM, Delaronde S. Current trends in nonoperative and operative treatment of trapeziometacarpal osteoarthritis: A survey of US hand surgeons. J Hand Surg Am 2012;37(1):77–82.

7. Vermeulen GM, Slijper H, Feitz R, et al. Surgical management of primary thumb carpometacarpal osteoarthritis: A systematic review. J Hand Surg Am 2011;36(1):157–69.

8. Wajon A, Vinycomb T, Carr E, et al. Surgery for thumb (trapeziometacarpal joint) osteoarthritis. Cochrane Database Sys Rev 2017;2017(4).

9. Piacenza A, Vittonetto D, Rossello MI, et al. Arthrodesis versus arthroplasty in thumb carpometacarpal osteoarthritis: Impact on maximal voluntary force, endurance, and accuracy of pinch. J Hand Surg Am 2022;47(1):90.e1–7.

10. Lansinger YC, Lehman TP. Nonunion following trapeziometacarpal arthrodesis with plate and screw fixation. J Hand Surg Am 2015;40(11):2310–4.

11. Elfar JC, Burton RI. Ligament reconstruction and tendon interposition for thumb basal arthritis. Hand Clin 2013;29(1):15–25.

12. Huang K, Hollevoet N, Giddins G. Thumb carpometacarpal joint total arthroplasty: A systematic review. J Hand Surg Eur 2015;40(4):338–50.

13. Cooney WP, Leddy TP, Larson DR. Revision of thumb trapeziometacarpal arthroplasty. J Hand Surg Am 2006;31(2):219.e1–9.

14. Hess DE, Drace P, Franco MJ, et al. Failed thumb carpometacarpal arthroplasty: Common etiologies and surgical options for revision. J Hand Surg Am 2018;43(9):844–52.

15. Renfree KJ, Roarke MC. Thumb metacarpal-trapezoid impingement as an etiology of pain after trapeziectomy and basal joint soft tissue arthroplasty: A case series. J Hand Surg Am 2021; 46(10):931.e1–6.

16. Armbruster EJ, Tan V. Carpometacarpal joint disease: Addressing the metacarpophalangeal joint deformity. Hand Clin 2008;24(3):295–9.

17. Low TH, Hales PF. High incidence and treatment of flexor carpi radialis tendinitis after trapeziectomy and abductor pollicis longus suspensionplasty for basal joint arthritis. J Hand Surg Eur 2014;39(8): 838–44.

18. Munns JJ, Matthias RC, Zarezadeh A, et al. Outcomes of revisions for failed trapeziometacarpal joint arthritis surgery. J Hand Surg Am 2019;44(9): 798.e1–9.

19. Burton R. Complications following surgery of the basal joint of the thumb. Hand Clin 1986;2(2):265–9.

20. Ganhewa AD, Wu R, Chae MP, et al. Failure rates of base of thumb arthritis surgery: A systematic review. J Hand Surg Am 2019;44(9):728–41.e10.

21. Kaszap B, Daecke W, Jung M. Outcome comparison of primary trapeziectomy versus secondary trapeziectomy following failed total trapeziometacarpal joint replacement. J Hand Surg Am 2013;38(5): 863–71.e3.

22. Conolly WB, Rath S. Revision procedures for complications of surgery for osteoarthritis of the carpometacarpal joint of the thumb. J Hand Surg Eur 1993; 18(4):533–9.

23. Papatheodorou LK, Winston JD, Bielicka DL, et al. Revision of the failed thumb carpometacarpal arthroplasty. J Hand Surg Am 2017;42(12):1032.e1–7.

24. Sadhu A, Calfee RP, Guthrie A, et al. Revision ligament reconstruction tendon interposition for trapeziometacarpal arthritis: A case-control investigation. J Hand Surg Am 2016;41(12):1114–21.

Wrist and Distal Radioulnar Joint Arthroplasty
Maximizing Results in Difficult Conditions

Amit Gupta, MD, FRCS[a,b,]*, Luis Scheker, MD[c]

KEYWORDS

• Wrist arthritis • Total wrist arthroplasty • DRUJ • Distal radioulnar joint arthroplasty

KEY POINTS

- Satisfactory results can be attained with total wrist arthroplasty (TWA), in patients with rheumatoid arthritis or osteoarthritis. Improvements in newer generation of implants have allowed for this.
- Patients have been noted to have improvement in function, pain, grip strength, and satisfaction with TWA.
- Distal radioulnar joint (DRUJ) arthroplasty is an option that should be considered in patients with DRUJ instability or arthritis, along with other reconstructive options.

TOTAL WRIST ARTHROPLASTY

Traditional management of wrist arthritis consists of proximal row carpectomy, partial carpal fusions, or, in the event of pancarpal arthritis, total wrist fusion. Although proximal row carpectomy and partial wrist fusions preserve some motion at the wrist while relieving pain symptoms, the quality of results obtained from these procedures is not predictable or optimal in many instances. Total wrist fusions are credited with universal pain relief at the expense of wrist motion. However, critical analysis of the results of total wrist arthrodesis shows that the results are not always consistent with what has been claimed and that pain relief is unpredictable at best. In a study, 14 of 22 patients who had undergone wrist arthrodesis had residual pain, and 4 of these patients had severe pain 6 years later.[1] In another study, only 6 of 36 patients remained pain-free 4 years after wrist arthrodesis.[2]

Moreover, many patients do not like loss of motion in their wrists. In a study of wrist arthrodesis, only 40% of patients were satisfied at 1 year.[3] In another study, 100% of patients who had wrist arthrodesis indicated that they would have a procedure performed so they could move their wrists again.[1]

Management of hip, knee, ankle, and shoulder joints has evolved from arthrodesis to arthroplasty. The wrist joint is following the same pattern of evolution with the advent of reliable designs.

Indications

The major indication of TWA is rheumatoid arthritis (RA).[4] Traditionally, wrist arthroplasty is recommended for rheumatoid wrists when wrist damage is extensive and there is severe bone loss and gross soft-tissue imbalances (**Fig. 1**). These situations set up the arthroplasty for failure. For a successful arthroplasty, good bone stock and soft-tissue balance are essential.

Osteoarthritis (primary) is a good indication for wrist replacement[4] because there is good bone mass for insertion of the implant and good soft

[a] Department of Orthopedic Surgery, University of Louisville, Louisville, KY, USA; [b] Louisille Arm & Hand, Louisville, KY, USA; [c] Plastic and Reconstructive Surgery, University of Louisville School of Medicine, Glenview, KY, USA
* Corresponding author.
E-mail address: handoc@bellsouth.net

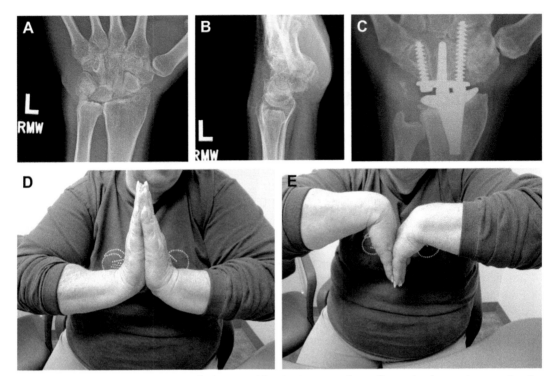

Fig. 1. (*A–E*). A 65-year-old patient with rheumatoid wrist. Preoperative radiographs show osteoporosis, ulnar translocation of carpus and midcarpal arthritis with VISI deformity of the left wrist. (*A* and *B*). Postoperative radiograph shows placement of ReMotion TWA (*C*). Clinical photograph shows excellent range of motion at 1 year postoperative. The left wrist is the operated site (*D* and *E*).

tissues for balance and function. Indications will increase in number when TWA results become predictable.

Posttraumatic arthritis is a controversial indication for wrist arthroplasty because there are more "conservative" options such as limited wrist fusions. However, the quality of results of wrist arthroplasty surpasses that of scaphoid excision and 4-corner fusion.

More controversial indications are failed proximal row carpectomies (**Fig. 2**) and failed 4-corner fusions.

Surgical Technique

The implant insertion is done with a dorsal longitudinal approach[4]. Two retinacular flaps are elevated, one based radially and the other ulnarly. A distally based dorsal capsular flap is elevated. Now precision-guided technology instruments are used to accurately insert the implant, particularly to precisely center the capitate/third metacarpal axis to the central longitudinal axis of the radius. The lunate spacer is inserted into the lunate fossa and is used to assemble and position the radial block over the Lister tubercle. The radial block is fixed to the radius with 2 thick Kirschner

wires (K-wires) that are bent out of the way. The radiolucent marker is fixed to the radial block, and the wrist is imaged in 2 planes to confirm that the marker is aligned to the long axis of the radius in both planes. Now the carpal cutting guide is assembled into the radius block, and the distal "tang" is positioned over the third metacarpal. The carpus is resected along the guide, taking care not to damage the palmar capsule. The cutting guide and the resected carpals (part of the scaphoid, lunate, and triquetrum) and the tips of the capitate and hamate are removed, and the burr guide is inserted into the radial block. Next, the articular surface of the radius is contour burred after hyperflexing the wrist. The burring removes the articular cartilage and exposes the subchondral bone. The burr guide is now removed, and the radial drill guide is inserted into the radius block. The radial drill guide is appropriately positioned, and a reduction is performed. If the joint seems too loose, a plus-size polyethylene ellipse is selected. The definitive radial component is impacted in, with some impact grafting if necessary. The carpal component is inserted into the capitate, and the screw drill guides are used to aim the drill for the second metacarpal on the radial side and the fourth metacarpal on the ulnar side.

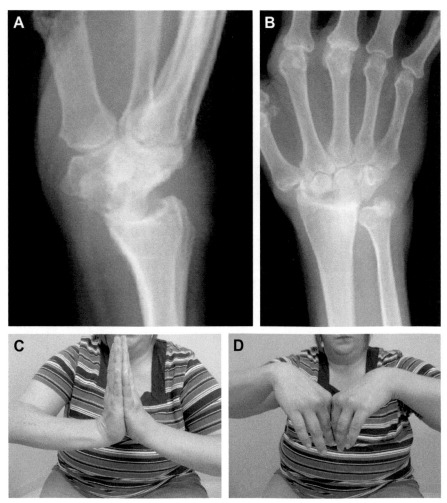

Fig. 2. (*A–D*). A 45-year-old patient who had a failed proximal row carpectomy with severe radio capitate arthritis and volar translocation of carpus (*A* and *B*). Clinical photograph shows excellent range of motion at 2 years postoperative (*C* and *D*).

After the screw lengths are measured, screws are inserted. The ulnar screw should not cross the carpometacarpal (CMC) joint and should remain in the hamate. The radial screw crosses the second CMC joint, and the tip is positioned ideally in the base of the second metacarpal. Although the screws are being tightened sequentially, care is taken to avoid rotating the carpal plate. Now an appropriate polyethylene insert is snap-fitted onto the carpal component, and the joint is reduced. The wrist is imaged in 2 planes to confirm proper insertion of the components. At this point, a small osteotome is used to remove some of the cartilage between the capitate and the hamate and other carpal bones, and these spaces are packed with cancellous graft harvested from the excised carpus. The dorsal capsule is repaired with nonabsorbable sutures. The radially based retinacular flap is positioned over the capsule to prevent any portion of the metal radial rim from abrading the extensor tendons. The ulnar-based retinacular flap is closed over all the extensor tendons except the extensor pollicis longus, which is left in an extraretinacular position. Now the tourniquet is released, hemostasis obtained, and skin closure performed in routine fashion. The wrist is put in a well-padded plaster splint and kept well elevated during the postoperative period.

In certain situations, modifications are needed. For rheumatoid wrists with bone loss, it may be necessary to cross the CMC joints with the central carpal peg and the 2 carpal screws. For bone deficiency, additional bone grafting may be necessary. For poor bone quality, I recommend using a small amount of cement with the radial and carpal components. For soft-tissue imbalance, tendon

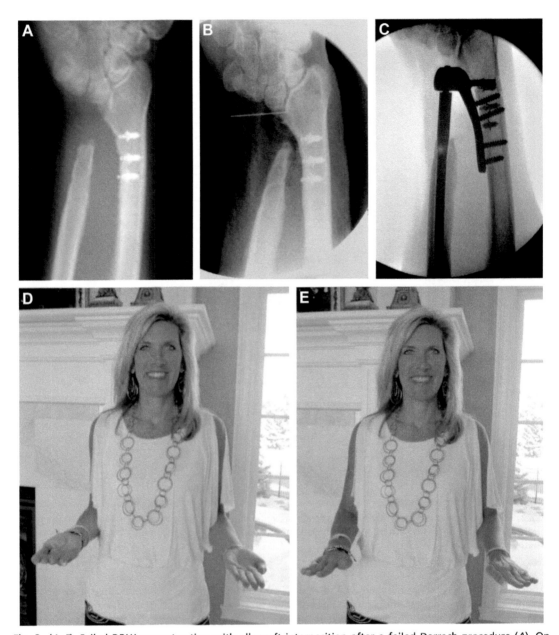

Fig. 3. (A–E). Failed DRUJ reconstruction with allograft interposition after a failed Darrach procedure (A). On load bearing, there is radioulnar impingement (B). Successful Scheker total DRUJ replacement arthroplasty (C). Clinical photograph shows excellent range of motion postoperatively (D and E).

transfers may be necessary at time of arthroplasty. For capsular deficiency, the palmar capsule may be reinforced with cadaveric fascia lata. The dorsal capsule can be reconstructed with a retinacular flap.

In revising a failed proximal row carpectomy to wrist arthroplasty, it is first necessary to obtain sufficient "space" for the implant. After the joint is exposed, 2 laminar spreaders are used to distract the carpus from the radius. This maneuver may

also be necessary in conversion of a wrist arthrodesis to arthroplasty. In failed proximal row carpectomy and failed scapholunate advanced collapse revisions, the missing scaphoid can be replaced by harvesting the pisiform through a separate palmar incision. With the pisiform held in the space normally occupied by the scaphoid, the radial carpal screw is inserted. In all these situations, the dorsal capsule should be reconstructed with a retinacular flap.[3]

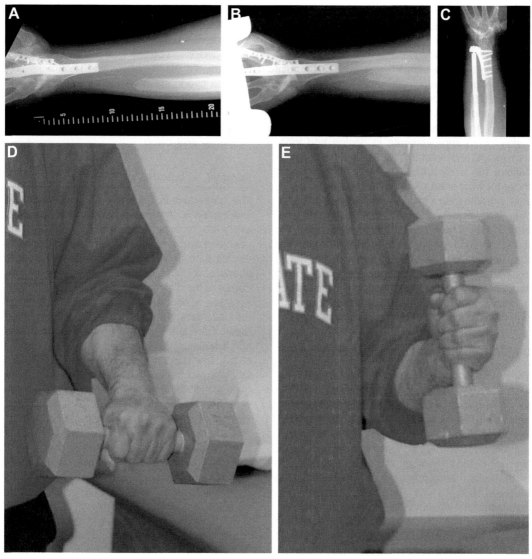

Fig. 4. (*A–E*). Failed ultrashort Darrach procedure (*A*). On load bearing, there is radioulnar impingement (*B*). Successful Scheker total DRUJ replacement arthroplasty (*C*). Clinical photograph shows excellent range of motion postoperatively (*D* and *E*).

Postoperative Care

The patient comes to the office 5 to 7 days after surgery. If the swelling is manageable, an orthoplast splint is fashioned for the wrist and finger motion, and gentle active wrist motions are encouraged. Formal physical and occupational therapy with digital motion, wrist motion, and edema-reducing protocols is started 10 days to 2 weeks after surgery. It typically takes 4 to 6 months to gain optimal range of motion (ROM) and strength.

Outcomes

Cooney and colleagues[5] studying ReMotion (Stryker, Kalamzoo, MI) total wrist implants reported a 97% survival at 6 years. Herzberg and colleagues[6] in 2012 reported on ReMotion Total Wrist implants in 129 RA and in 86 non-RA patients. The survival rate of the implant for patients with RA was 96% and 92% for non-RA patients. There were improvements in visual analog scale, Quick DASH, and grip strength in both groups.

Similar results were also reported by other authors with ReMotion total wrist implant in 65 wrists with follow-up of 5 to 9 years.[7]

SUMMARY

Bunnell wrote, "A painless stable wrist is the key to hand function." Up until now, to make the wrist stable, we have had to make it stiff too. However, this does not have to be the case. The bar for functional motion at the wrist is very low. As estimated by Palmer and colleagues,[8] a functional wrist requires only 30° extension, 5° wrist flexion, 10° radial deviation, and 15° ulnar deviation. The question in the year 2023 is: can we consistently and safely provide such ROM to our patients' wrists without resorting to a destructive procedure like wrist fusion? With improvements in design and long-term results showing that these designs work, indications for wrist arthrodesis will decrease and those for wrist arthroplasty will increase.

In a article critically analyzing wrist arthroplasties, Berber and colleagues[9] concluded that wrist arthroplasty had evolved considerably from the first-generation implants to current prostheses that appear to have better survival and lower complication profiles. Patients are experiencing improvement in physical function, satisfaction, pain control, and grip strength. Furthermore, wrist arthroplasty is maintaining range of motion.

DISTAL RADIOULNAR JOINT ARTHROPLASTY

The functional importance of the distal radioulnar joint (DRUJ) has been ignored and misunderstood for a long time, resulting in the distal ulna being amputated, fused, and modified such that its function disappeared, leaving the patient with considerable disability. Historically, it was Claude Bernard in 1851[10] who published on the resection of the ulnar head, followed by others including Moore in 1880.[11] Thirty years later, Darrach[12] proposed that the resection be made subperiosteal. The failures of the available techniques led Kapandji whose chief was Sauvé to perform a fusion of the distal ulnar radio joint with resection of a segment proximal to the head of the of the ulna and create a pseudarthrosis at that point to maintain pronation and supination.[13] However, the problem of instability of the end of the ulna persisted although at a more proximal level. In the 80s and the 90s, interest in distal ulnar radio joint increased, with studies that have allowed us to better understand kinematics, biomechanics, and anatomy.[14–21] These studies resulted in a better understanding and a reasoned therapeutic approach to the clinical problems that affect the DRUJ.

Pathologic conditions that affect DRUJ include arthritic problems of inflammatory, degenerative, and traumatic origin, genetic conditions such as Madelung deformity, Ehlers-Danlos syndrome, and sports conditions such as epiphyseal arrest of the distal radius found in the gymnast. The innumerable techniques[22–30] that attempt to solve the problems of the DRUJ available in the literature is an indicator of the lack of a definitive solution to this problem that not only cause pain and functional disability but can also significantly depress the patient's quality of life and health-like social function (work, sports activities, relationship with friends and family), physical function, vitality, and even mental functional state. The patient is unable to return to work further affecting the patient's economic well-being.

Surgical Technique

The procedure is generally accomplished under axillary block. An iodine plastic wrap is used to avoid contact between the implant (the stem specially) and the skin. A tourniquet is applied for visualization. A 10-cm longitudinal incision in the shape of a hockey stick is made along the ulnar border of the distal forearm, in the interval between the fifth and sixth dorsal compartments, 8 cm over the distal forearm and 2 cm oblique from ulnar to radial. Care is taken to avoid damage to the sensory branch of the ulnar nerve. The skin and subcutaneous flap are elevated from the forearm fascia up to the radial wrist extensors. A rectangular ulnar-based fascia/retinacular flap is created with enough width to cover the head of the implant; it includes the most proximal 3 mm of the extensor retinaculum. This flap will be used later to create a buffering barrier between the prosthesis and the extensor carpi ulnaris (ECU). The dissection is continued between the extensor digiti quinti minimi and the ECU until the ulna is encountered, and the extensor digiti quinti minimi is elevated from the ulna and the interosseous membrane for at least 8 cm. The sensory branch of the posterior interosseous nerve is divided to avoid avulsion of the nerve from the thumb extensors when placing an elevator between the extensor mass and the radius. The ECU tendon sheath is opened completely up to its insertion at the base of the fifth metacarpal. This avoids pressure of the tendon against the distal end of the implant. The remaining head of the ulna, if present, is then excised at a level just proximal to the cartilage or where the DRUJ would have been. At this stage, the radial attachment of the triangular fibrocartilage, if found intact, is left undisturbed. If left in situ, this structure can provide a barrier between the prosthesis and the carpal bones. The ulnar shaft is then retracted volarly, thus ensuring access to the radius. The interosseous membrane is elevated from the radius along the distal 8 cm of the interosseous crest. The radial trial plate is then placed over the interosseous crest of the radius, and its volar border is aligned with the volar surface of the radius. Care is taken to ensure that at least 3 mm of the sigmoid notch lies distal to the end of the plate. Depending on the anatomy encountered, the distal radius may require contouring. Often the volar lip of the sigmoid notch has to be removed with a saw blade or a medium-size burr ball to create a flat surface to ensure proper seating of the radial plate. After the position of the trial plate has been deemed appropriate—meaning parallel to the volar shaft of the radius and at least 3 mm proximal to the end of the radius—a 1.4-mm (0.054-in.) K-wire is inserted in 1 of the holes at the distal end of the trial as well as the most proximal hole. An image intensifier is used to check the position of the trial, both in anteroposterior and lateral positions. If no adjustment is needed, a 2.5-mm drill bit is used with the provided guide to drill the screw hole at the oval opening, the proper screw length is gauged, the hole is tapped, and the appropriate length 3.5-mm screw is placed. The image intensifier is used again to confirm plate positioning and proper screw length. With confirmation of the length of the screw and good plate contact with the bone, the distal K-wire is removed, and the hole for the radial peg is drilled with appropriate drill bit. When the surgeon is satisfied, the trial component is removed and replaced with the prosthesis radial component. If necessary, a soft mallet is used to achieve good contact between the radial plate and the ulnar border of the radius. After the last screw is placed in position, a final check of the radial plate to confirm screw length and position is performed with the image intensifier. Attention is now turned to the ulna. With the forearm fully pronated, a measuring device with an appropriate color ball (blue for a large implant and black for a small implant and screwed until the ball and the metal lip of the measuring device are in good contact) fitting into the hemisocket of the radial component is seated, and the ulna is juxtaposed against its shaft. This enables the surgeon to assess the exact amount of ulna to be resected. After final resection of the distal ulna, a 2.3-mm (0.090-in) guide wire is inserted into the ulnar medullary canal to act as a centralizer for a cannulated drill bit of the predetermined size. It is important that the guide wire surpass the length of the drill bit to avoid penetrating the ulnar cortex. The cannulated drill bit is introduced for a length of 11 cm. Next, a medullary broach of appropriate size is inserted into the canal to bevel the distal ulna and plane its distal end. The medullary canal is now thoroughly irrigated, and the stem of the ulnar component is introduced. The ultra high molecular weight (UHMW) polyethylene ball is placed over the distal peg or pivot, and the ulnar

component is positioned within the hemisocket of the radial component. Finally, the other half of the radial socket or cover is positioned and secured with a transverse screw. The image intensifier is once again used to confirm adequacy of the overall position. Full range of motion is confirmed. The fascia/retinacular flap is placed between the prosthesis and the ECU tendon and sutured to the radius. This prevents tenosynovitis of the ECU and provides a cushion over the implant, especially for a patient with little subcutaneous adipose tissue. The tourniquet is released, and complete hemostasis is secured. The skin is then closed with interrupted sutures and a bulky soft dressing is applied.

Postoperative Protocol

The wound is kept dry and clean in a bulky soft dressing for 2 weeks, at which time the skin sutures are removed. Immediate full range of motion is encouraged. Lifting is allowed as soon as the patient has recovered from the anesthetic and after full recovery is limited to 20 lbs (9 kg). In vitro testing showed that ultimate load to failure was between 67 to 84 kgs at an average of 169 lbs (76 kg), at which point the highly polished peg and the end of the ulna stem bent. By limiting lifting to 20 lbs (9 kg) we have a margin of safety of 7 times.

Results

Our combined cases surpass 400 patients; of those, 263 have more than 5 years follow-up, and 128 had more than 2 procedures before the total DRUJ was implanted. The average preoperative grip strength measured with a dynamometer (Jamar II, Jamar Dynamometer, Boling Brook, IL) was 38.3 lbs (17.4 kg) on the affected side and 70 lbs (32 kg) on the opposite side. The postoperative grip strength increased to a mean of 44.5 lbs (20.2 kg) on the operated side. Mean postoperative grip strength, evaluated with a dynamometer (Jamar II, Jamar Dynamometer), was 63.4% of the contralateral unaffected side. Before surgery, patients could lift an average of 2.6 lbs (1.2 kg) with the affected side, limited by pain; after surgery, they were able to lift an average of 11.6 lbs (5.3 kg). Patients subjectively scored preoperative pain on a scale from 0 to 5 at an average of 3.8, and postoperative pain at a mean of 1.3. Mean pronation was 79° (range 15°–90°) and mean supination was 72° (range 30°–90°) at final follow-up. Seventy percent of our patients have had at least 1 previous procedure; some had failed "ulna stabilization" with tendon sling procedures, allograft tendon interposition (**Fig. 3**), Ultra short Darrach procedure

(**Fig. 4**) and failed ulnar head replacement. Of this group of patients, 1 had 14 previous procedures. Most of these patients have been incapacitated for a prolonged period because of pain. This has led to a lack of use, causing muscle atrophy in both the arm and the forearm. For this reason, these previously operated patients were often weaker than those who received the device as their first procedure or those on whom the replacement was performed shortly after the failed previous procedure. Rampazzo and colleagues[31] noticed while evaluating those patients with implants aged younger than 40 years that when the implant was performed primarily, the results were much better in regards of postoperative pain, strength, and speed of recovery, Postoperative complications were seen in 26 cases. Two patients had low-degree soft tissue infection that resolved with antibiotic treatment. Both patients had multiple previous operations. Two patients had ECU tenosynovitis due to the implant being too large. We now have a smaller implant for those cases. This was successfully treated by creating a fascial flap that was interposed between the implant and the ECU tendon. A fascial flap is now performed routinely at the initial implantation surgery. Eight patients had ectopic bone formation around the distal ulna and were treated successfully with surgical excision. This ectopic calcification was caused by the bone marrow scaping around the original stem that had no extended collar. Now the stem has a 1-cm extended collar, where the ulnar canal is sealed and no other cases of ectopic bone have been seen. Of the patients with ectopic bone formation, 6 patients had ECU tendinitis that settled after excision of the ectopic bone. One patient, on 1-year follow-up x-rays, was noticed to have some ulna resorption in the distal segment of the ulna where she had an ulna shortening 6 months before the replacement arthroplasty. At present, the ulna stem remains well secured and she is symptom free.

At the time of this writing, longest follow-up with the Aptis DRUJ prosthesis is 15 years. No prosthesis had to be removed because of excessive wear, loosening, or material failure. There have been 4 implants removed because of unknown preoperative allergies, 3 to nickel and 1 to cobalt chrome, and an additional 3 due to late infections. Those with allergies had replacement implants made of titanium. Those with infections were treated by removing the implants, extensive curettage and bone substitute with antibiotic inserted in the defects, replacing the implants 3 to 6 months later. Galvis and colleagues[32] reported excellent recovery in cases of RA with ruptured tendons. The Aptis DRUJ prosthesis is an alternative to the other salvage procedures that allows full range of motions as well as the ability to grip and lift weights encountered in daily living.

CLINICS CARE POINTS

- New generation total Wrist Arthroplasty provides a promising new method to preserve wrist range of motion.
- Distal Radioulnar joint replacements are helpful in challenging patients with destroyed distal radioulnar joints.

REFERENCES

1. Adey L, Ring D, Jupiter JB. Health status after total wrist arthrodesis for post traumatic arthritis. J Hand Surg Am 2005;30(5):932–6.
2. De Smet L, Truyen J. Arthrodesis of the wrist for osteoarthritis: outcome with a minimum follow-up of 4 years. J Hand Surg Br 2003;28(6):575–7.
3. Rauhaniemi J, Tiusanen H, Sipola E. Total wrist fusion: a study of 115 patients. J Hand Surg Br 2005;30(2):217–9.
4. Gupta A. Total wrist arthroplasty. Am J Orthop 2008;37(8 Suppll):12–6.
5. Cooney W, Manuel J, Froelich J, et al. Total wrist replacement: a retrospective comparative study. J Wrist Surg 2012;01(02):165–72.
6. Herzberg G, Boeckstyns M, Sorensen A, et al. "Remotion" total wrist arthroplasty: preliminary results of a prospective international multicenter study of 215 cases. J Wrist Surg 2012;1(1):17–22.
7. Boeckstyns MEH, Herzberg G, Merser S. Favorable results after total wrist arthroplasty: 65 wrists in 60 patients followed for 5–9 years. Acta Orthop 2013;84(4):415–9.
8. Palmer AK, Werner FW, Murphy D, et al. Functional wrist motion: a biome- chanical study. J Hand Surg Am 1985;10(1):39–46.
9. Berber O, Garagnani L, Gidwani S. Systemic review of total wrist arthroplasty and arthrodesis in wrist arthritis. J Wrist Surg 2018;17(7):424–40.
10. Bernard CH, Huette CH. In: Buren WHV, Isaacs CE, editors. Illustrated manual of operated surgery and surgical anatomy. New York: HBailliere; 1857.
11. Moore EM. Three cases illustrating luxation of the ulna in connection with Colles' fracture. Med Record 1880;17:305.
12. Darrach W. Forward dislocation at the inferior radioulnar joint with fractures of the lower third of radius. Ann Surg 1912;56:801.
13. Sauvé L, Kapandji M. Nouvelle technique de traitement chirurgical des luxations récidivantes isolées

de l'extrémité inférieure du cubitus. J Chir 1936;7: 589.

14. Palmer AK, Werner FW. The triangular fibrocartilage complex of the wrist- anatomy and function. J Hand Surg 1981;6A:153–72.

15. Palmer AK, Werner FW. Biomechanics of the distal radioulnar joint. Clin Orthop 1984;187:26–35.

16. Thiru RG, Ferlic DC, Clayton ML, et al. Arterial anatomy of the triangular fibrocartilage of the wrist and its surgical significance. J Hand Surg 1986;11(2):258–63.

17. Mikic ZD. Detailed anatomy of the articular disc of the distal radioulnar joint. Clin Orthop 1989;245: 123–32.

18. Chidgey LK. Histologic Anatomy of the Triangular Fibrocartilage. Hand Clinic 1991;7:249–62.

19. Acosta R, Hnat B, Scheker LR. Distal radio-ulnar ligament motion during supination and pronation. J Hand Surg 1993;18B:502–5.

20. Hagert CG. The distal radioulnar joint in relation to the whole forearm. Clin Orthop 1992;275:56–64.

21. Linscheid RL. Biomechanics of the distal radioulnar joint. Clin Orthop 1992;275.

22. Kessler I, Hecht O. Present application of the Darrach procedure. Clin Orthop 1970;72:254–60.

23. Tsai TM, Stillwell JH. Repair of chronic subluxation of the distal radioulnar joint (ulnar dorsal) using flexor carpi ulnaris tendon. J Hand Surg 1984;9B:289–94.

24. Bowers WH. Distal radio-ulnar joint arthroplasty: the hemi-resection interposition. J Hand Surg 1985;10A: 169–72.

25. Watson HF, Ryu J, Burgess RC. Matched distal ulnar resection. J Hand Surg 1986;11A:812–7.

26. Breen TF, Jupiter JB. Extensor carpi ulnaris and flexor carpi ulnaris tenodesis of the unstable distal ulna. J Hand Surg 1989;14A:612–7.

27. Leslie BM, Carlson G, Ruby LK. Results of ECU tenodesis in rheumatoid wrist undergoing a distal ulnar resection. J Hand Surg 1990;15A:547–51.

28. Sanders RA, Frederick HA, Hontas R. The Sauvé-Kapandji procedure: a salvage operation for the distal radio-ulnar joint. J Hand Surg 1991;19A: 1125–9.

29. Tsai TM, Shimizu H, Adkins P. a modified extensor carpi ulnaris tenodesis with Darrach procedure. J Hand Surg 1993;18A:697–702.

30. Scheker LR, Severo A. Ulnar shortening for the treatment of early Post-traumatic osteoarthritis at the distal Radioulnar joint. J Hand Surg 2001;26B(1): 41–4.

31. Rampazzo A, Gharb BB, Brock G, et al. Functional outcomes of the aptis-scheker distal radioulnar joint replacement in patients under 40 years old. J Hand Surg Am 2015;40(7):1397–403.

32. Galvis EJ, Pessa J, Scheker LR. Total joint arthroplasty of the distal radioulnar joint for rheumatoid arthritis. J Hand Surg Am 2014;39(9):1699–704.

Revision Arthroplasty in the Challenging Elbow

Ryan C. Xiao, MD[a], Zina Model, MD[b], Jaehon M. Kim, MD[a], Neal C. Chen, MD[c],*

KEYWORDS

• Elbow arthroplasty • Revision • Fracture • Infection • Periprosthetic • Loosening

KEY POINTS

• Primary total elbow arthroplasty has a lower survivorship than total hip and total knee arthroplasty.
• The most common indications for revision total elbow arthroplasty are loosening, infection, and periprosthetic fracture.
• Challenges of revision total elbow arthroplasty include the management of soft tissue, preservation of bone stock, and management of concurrent infection or fracture.

INTRODUCTION

The number of total elbow arthroplasties (TEA) performed has been growing, most commonly in the setting of inflammatory arthritis but also with increasing use for distal humerus fractures and posttraumatic arthropathy.[1] National database registries from Scandivania, the United Kingdom, Australia, and New Zealand have witnessed a similar rising trend in the incidence of revision TEA, paralleling the increase in primary TEA.[1]

Compared with total knee and hip arthroplasties, TEA demonstrates a high rate of complications and less predictable survivorship.[2–5] Where primary hip and knee arthroplasties can expect upwards of 95% survivorship at 10 years, the Norwegian national database demonstrated a survivorship of 81% in primary TEA.[2] Though TEA implant designs and surgical techniques have improved since its inception, the complication rate ranges from 11% to 38%.[3] A recent systematic review examining modern semiconstrained implants found a complication rate of 60.7%, skewed in part due to the increased prevalence of trauma as the indication for primary TEA.[6] Similarly in long-term follow-up, Peretta el al found an

overall 41% rate of revision following primary TEA, with a 57% rate of revision for TEA performed for trauma compared to 27% for TEA performed for inflammatory arthritis.[7]

Modern TEA implants most commonly require revision secondary to implant loosening, infection, and periprosthetic fracture.[3,6] Revision TEA presents its own unique challenges, notably consideration of soft tissue handling in the multiply-operated elbow, triceps management, preservation of bone stock, and management of concurrent infection or fracture. Identifying the central problem helps guide treatment and likely improves outcomes. In this review, we will discuss preoperative evaluation of the failed elbow arthroplasty, surgical approaches, techniques for revision, outcomes, and complications following revision total elbow arthroplasty.

PREOPERATIVE EVALUATION (WHAT IS THE PROBLEM?)
Aseptic Loosening

Aseptic loosening is the most common indication for revision total elbow arthroplasty. A systematic review examining 2,939 TEA demonstrated a

The authors, their immediate families, and any research foundations with which they are affiliated have not received any financial payments or other benefits from any commercial entity related to the subject of this article.

[a] Department of Orthopaedic Surgery, Mount Sinai Hospital, 425 West 59th Street, New York, NY 10019, USA; [b] Department of Orthopaedic Surgery, Massachusetts General Hospital, 55 Fruit Street, Boston, MA 02114, USA; [c] Hand Fellowship Program, Department of Orthopaedic Surgery, Massachusetts General Hospital, Hand and Arm Center, 55 Fruit Street, Boston, MA 02114, USA
* Corresponding author.
E-mail address: NCHEN1@PARTNERS.ORG

Hand Clin 39 (2023) 341–351
https://doi.org/10.1016/j.hcl.2023.03.001
0749-0712/23/© 2023 Elsevier Inc. All rights reserved.

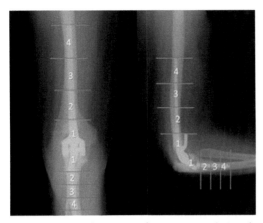

Fig. 1. Radiographic zones for TEA osteolysis. The radiographic zone 1 starts with the periarticular portion of the implant and then moves outwards as zones 2 through 4 divide the remaining implant stem into thirds. (*From* Lee H, Vaichinger AM, O'Driscoll SW. Component fracture after total elbow arthroplasty. J Shoulder Elbow Surg. 2019;28(8):1449-1456; with permission.)

13.7% incidence of loosening over a 16 year period in linked TEA designs and a 10.1% incidence of loosening in unlinked designs.[8] It is theorized that the generation of polyethylene and metallic particulate debris in the TEA incites a biologic reaction leading to histiocyte and giant cell-mediated osteolysis.[9] However, that concept is debated, as some authors feel that third body wear is the primary mode of failure. Morrey suggests that fracture may lead to third body wear and that some designs with precoating are susceptible to aseptic loosening.[10]

The Mayo classification describes radiographic loosening based on the comparison of immediate and successive postoperative radiographs, assessing the width of a radiolucent line at the bone-cement interface and degree of involvement around the bone-cement interface.[11] Ranging from types I to V, type I loosening includes the presence of lucency less than one mm in width and involving less than half of the total bone cement interface while type V involves radiolucency greater than 2 mm in width and encompassing the entirety of the bone-cement interface with gross tilt or subsidence of the implant.[11] The location of osteolysis in TEA creates 4 zones for the humeral component and 4 for the ulnar component, based on both anteroposterior and lateral radiographic views (**Fig. 1**).

More recently, Gandhi and colleagues[12] proposed a radiographic methodology to determine implant loosening, indicated by the presence of at least one of the 4 following criteria: progression of radiolucent widening, disruption of the cement mantle, migration of the implant components, and bead shedding. The aforementioned criteria demonstrated excellent reproducibility with the substantial interobserver agreement. All implants with 2 or more radiographic criteria of loosening and 93% of implants that met one of the criteria were found to be loose intraoperatively.

A preoperative bone scan is another tool to inform decision-making and can be helpful in determining if a prosthesis is loose. However, a bone scan is not diagnostic and should be interpreted with caution, as demonstrated by a 37% correlation between positive bone scan findings and intraoperative loosening.[13]

Infection

The incidence of infection following TEA ranges from 1.9% to 9%.[14,15] A recent systematic review noted 3.4% of TEAs complicated by deep infection.[3]

In the absence of obvious clinical symptoms, low-grade infection can be difficult to distinguish from aseptic loosening. More systemic signs of infection may be absent.[16] However, given the dearth of significant soft tissue coverage overlying the elbow implant, new onset or persistent elbow swelling, pain, loss of motion, wound drainage, and/or erythema should raise concern for an infectious etiology. Though the data remain limited, factors including diabetes,[17] obesity,[18] active tobacco use,[19] hypothyroidism,[19] and history of prior elbow operation[16] all may increase the risk of infection following TEA and may warrant increased scrutiny.

When imaging the potentially infected TEA, serial radiographs with the demonstration of progressive loosening, endosteal scalloping, and/or implant migration can suggest the presence of infection.[14,16] Use of further imaging with MRI or CT has limited clinical utility.

While elevated ESR and CRP can suggest infection, these values are frequently within normal limits and demonstrate inconsistent correlation with an infected TEA prosthesis.[14,15] Appropriate diagnostic threshold values for inflammatory markers have not been validated in the setting of periprosthetic elbow infection, and the concurrent presence of inflammatory arthritis can obscure the interpretation of elevated ESR and CRP values.[16,20]

If a high clinical suspicion for periprosthetic infection remains, the clinician should proceed to the aspiration of the elbow prosthesis. Achermann and colleagues[21] refer to the guidelines for periprosthetic knee infection and suggest the use of greater than 1700 leukocytes and 65% polymor-phonuclear cells as a threshold for making the diagnosis of periprosthetic elbow infection. Aspiration of the TEA yields variable culture sensitivities, ranging from 22% to 83%.[14,21] With sensitivities over 60% and specificities over 95% in the total shoulder literature, synovial alpha-defensin seems to provide promising clinical utility.[22,23] Synovial leukocyte esterase, IL-1beta IL-6, IL-8, and IL-10 all demonstrate better predictive value than convential ESR and CRP values but, as with synovial alpha defensin, the data lacks validation in the setting of total elbow arthroplasty.[23,24]

Despite the low negative predictive value of aspiration and the inconsistent ability to obtain a positive culture, isolation of an organism can confirm the diagnosis and guide antibiotic selection. The confirmation of suspected infection should be obtained by intraoperative cultures and pathology. Staphylococcus aureus remains the most common organism identified in the infected TEA, followed by staphylococcus epidermidis.[16,20] Less common organisms include C. Acnes, Corynebacterium, Enterobacter, and Streptococcus agalactiae.[16,20,21]

Periprosthetic Fractures

Periprosthetic fracture occurs in 3% of TEAs and can occur from direct trauma, cantilever bending of the components, stress fracture secondary to osteolysis or stress shielding, and poor patient compliance with activity restrictions.[3] Fractures occur most commonly around the humeral condyles of the TEA, followed by the proximal ulna.[25]

In the evaluation of periprosthetic elbow fractures, the Mayo classification emphasizes the consideration of 3 main factors: fracture location, implant stability, and quality of the remaining bone stock.[25] O'Driscoll and Morrey describe fractures as occurring in regions A through C; region A involving a periarticular fracture around the condyles or olecranon, region B a fracture of the shaft at the level of the implant stem, and region C a fracture in the diaphysis past the tip of the stem. Type B fractures are further subclassified as types 1 through 3; type 1 involves a well-fixed implant with good bone stock, type 2 involves an unstable implant with good remaining osseous support, and type 3 involves an unstable implant with significant osteolysis.[25]

When a patient has an ipsilateral shoulder and elbow arthroplasty, the bone between the implants is particularly vulnerable to fracture.[26,27] Multiple case reports describe a humeral fracture between an elbow and shoulder arthroplasty.[27–30]

PREOPERATIVE EVALUATION (COMPONENT PROBLEMS)
Soft Tissue Evaluation

Given the thin subcutaneous tissue overlying the elbow, management of soft tissue coverage in the revision setting can be challenging. Existing scars need to be evaluated carefully. It is helpful to know the age of the existing scars if possible. Narrow bridges between scars are vulnerable to skin necrosis. In general, the ratio of the width to the length of a skin bridge should be less than 1:4.

When preserved, the triceps muscle can provide supplemental coverage around the implant and may help mitigate the risk of infection.[31] In addition to providing an additional layer of coverage to the implant, the triceps plays an integral role in the function and outcome following TEA revision. However, a recent systematic review examining 4,825 TEAs noted a 3.5% incidence of triceps insufficiency in primary TEAs and a 22% incidence following revision TEA.[32] As gravity-assisted elbow extension can mask a dysfunctional elbow extensor mechanism, preoperative triceps insufficiency should be noted and addressed at the time of revision arthroplasty.[33]

Ulnar Neuropathy

In the preoperative evaluation, it is critical to assess both the function and location of the ulnar nerve. Prior operative reports should be obtained to determine the type of implant and the location of the ulnar nerve. Even if not transposed, distortion of normal elbow anatomy can make it difficult to identify the ulnar nerve in the setting of a revision TEA procedure. Though direct injury or laceration to the ulnar nerve is unusual, indirect trauma can occur and ulnar neuropathy arises in 2.9% of cases.[3] Most ulnar nerve palsies involve a sensory component and remain self-limited. In a retrospective review examining 1607 TEAs performed at a single institution, Rispoli and colleagues[34] noted a 0.5% incidence of ulnar neuropathy necessitating surgical neurolysis following TEA.

If a patient has clinical signs of ulnar neuropathy preoperatively, it is helpful to quantify the degree of neuropathy using electromyographic/nerve conduction velocity (EMG/NCV) studies. If EMG/NCV studies are equivocal, neuromuscular ultrasound may be beneficial.

When approaching the ulnar nerve, it is often helpful to identify the nerve in native tissue either proximal or distal to the prior surgical area. A nerve stimulator may also be helpful if scar is dense as it can be difficult to identify the nerve in the mulitply operated wound.

Implants

Early hinged TEA implant designs suffered from over-constraint. Without permissive laxity at the ulnohumeral joint, the rigid hinged articulation led to increased stresses at the bone-implant interface, resulting in early loosening and subsequent failure. Conversely, unconstrained unhinged designs placed an over-reliance on soft tissue constraints and suffered from instability and dislocation.[35] These implant designs have shown a historically higher incidence of complications, up to 62.9% and with rates of loosening from 33% to 70%.[36–38] As such, most surgeons utilize a semi-constrained implant with some degree of coronal plane laxity to balance the competing risks of instability and loosening. An anterior humeral flange attempts to reduce torsional forces at the implant and counteract posteriorly-directed stresses.

A linked semiconstrained implant features a central locking pin through an ulnohumeral hinge with +3.5 to −3.5 degrees of varus-valgus laxity in an effort to reproduce native elbow kinematics. Loosening and excessive bushing wear represent the most common modes of failure.[39,40] Bushing wear in the semiconstrained TEA designs can present as pain, squeaking, crepitus, or increased varus-valgus laxity at the elbow.[40] On stress radiographic views, a varus-valgus arc between 7 and 10 degrees indicates partial bushing wear and an arc greater than 10 degrees indicates complete wear.[40]

In response to the bushing wear, a newer TEA featuring a spherical articulation was designed to minimize complications from stresses at the ulnohumeral hinge and facilitate ease of bearing exchange.[41] While the Norwegian registry demonstrated promising 5-year survival rates with the spherical bearing TEA,[2] more recent literature shows a 76.8% survivorship at 10 years and relatively high rate of infection at 7.5%.[42] Biomechanical modeling suggests diminished stresses on the polyethylene bearing, but further studies are warranted to assess for meaningful clinical differences.[43]

In revision cases of early loosening and eccentric polyethylene wear, some surgeons advocate for the consideration of polyethylene exchange alone, though technique varies per implant design.

Bone Stock

Periprosthetic fracture, loosening, osteoporosis, infection, and stress shielding can all compromise bony integrity. Humeral bone stock can be classified as grades I through IV.[44] Grade I describes surface wear of the distal humerus with intact subchondral architecture. Grade II denotes loss of the trochlea but the preservation of the medial and lateral epicondyles. Grade III indicates the absence of either medial or lateral epicondyle. Grade IV describes bone loss of the distal humerus at or proximal to the olecranon fossa.[44] Evaluation of ulnar osseous integrity focuses on the proximal ulna and olecranon, loss of which can compromise the support of the ulnar stem and also correlates with triceps insufficiency.[45]

SURGICAL APPROACH

Though many approaches have been described for use in the TEA, the most commonly utilized include the triceps-sparing,[31,46] triceps-reflecting,[47,48] and triceps-splitting approaches.[49] For primary TEA, triceps-sparing approaches have gained favor as they mitigate the risks of triceps insufficiency.[46]

Triceps-Sparing

The triceps-sparing approach to the TEA retains the integrity of the triceps insertion and extensor mechanism of the elbow. Visualization and subsequent instrumentation can be a challenge, especially in revision TEA or contracted tissue. The approach starts with a posterior incision over the elbow down to the triceps fascia. Full-thickness medial and lateral flaps are developed and the ulnar nerve is identified and protected. From there, the elbow can be approached from both medial and lateral sides[31] or from a medial-only approach.[46]

Triceps-Reflecting

The triceps-reflecting approach detaches a portion of the triceps insertion from the olecranon. Starting with a posterior incision over the elbow, the ulnohumeral joint is approached from the medial side. After the protection of the ulnar nerve and elevation of the medial triceps along the medial intermuscular septum, the triceps is retracted laterally to allow the release of the triceps insertion from the olecranon. The remaining extensor mechanism is reflected laterally and the tip of the olecranon can be resected to visualize the trochlea. Release of the MCL allows access to the distal humerus for instrumentation.[47] Alternatively, a wafer of olecranon can be taken during the release of the triceps insertion, potentially facilitating bone-to-bone healing.[48]

Trans-Triceps (or Triceps-Splitting)

A posterior elbow incision is made with a midline split through the triceps. Visualization requires the release of the medial and lateral aspects of the triceps tendon from the underlying olecranon.

Dissection continues distally and involves subperiosteal elevation both medially and laterally of the proximal ulnar crest. MCL and LCL are released as needed.[49]

As an alternative, if the olecranon and triceps enthesis are in good condition, a proximally-based V-shaped cut can be made in the triceps. The V-shape provides more surface area than a transverse cut, maximizing contact for suture fixation and potential healing.

Management of Triceps Tendon Defects

Integrity of the olecranon process and quality of the triceps tendon determines the ability to successfully repair or reconstruct the extensor mechanism.[50] With an intact olecranon process and triceps tendon, tendon repair through olecranon bone tunnels has been described with good overall success.[50,51]

If the tendon quality is poor, a rotational anconeus muscle flap or achilles tendon allograft can be used for triceps tendon reconstruction.[50] Resorption of the olecranon process necessitates some form of bone grafting. A calcaneal bone graft with attached achilles tendon allograft has been used to reconstruct both triceps tendon and olecranon process.[50] Though used infrequently, these techniques can be useful in the right clinical situation.

Coverage Options

Tissue contracture, intra-operative swelling, and implant prominence can all impede the ability to achieve a primary tension-free closure and may necessitate the use of soft tissue flaps.[52]

For small defects at the tip of the elbow, the anconeus is described as an option; however, its blood supply can be injured during the initial exposure of the distal humerus, and its short pedicle limits its ability to provide anterior or medial elbow coverage.[53] In general, the flexor carpi ulnaris (FCU) flap can successfully cover most small defects as the ulnar artery has a number of perforators that supply the FCU.[53]

Larger soft tissue defects may require coverage with a pedicle latissimus dorsi flap or free flaps.[54] With its long pedicle and wide muscle base, the latissimus flap can provide coverage up to 150 cm². However, distal tip necrosis of the latissimus flap presents a known complication that occurs in 17% to 57% of cases.[54]

SPECIAL TECHNIQUES
Cement Removal

Goals of cemented component extraction include the preservation of existing bone stock and avoidance of stress risers. The techniques utilized for implant removal involve a combination of burrs, osteotomes, drills, an ultrasonic osteotome system, and an osteotomy with windows to access different segments of the bone-cement interface. Cortical perforation with extraction can cause cement extravasation during cementing of the final implant.

The first technique involves a combination of burrs, osteotomes, and drills to extract the implant. After exposing the bone-cement interface, a high-speed diamond-tipped burr can be used to disrupt the proximal bone-implant interface. Then thin, flexible osteotomes can be used to break up the interface distally. The use of a 2.0mm drill parallel to the implant or the use of a curette can assist in removing distal cement.

In cases of challenging implant removal, osteotomies, and cortical windows can be utilized to access the implant at different levels (**Fig. 2**). One approach involves using a sagittal saw to create a longitudinal split in the bone and disrupt the bone-cement interface along the entire length of the prosthesis. An extraction device can be attached and a reverse impactor used to free the implant from cement. Alternatively, if minimal cement resides at the tip of the stem, a window can be made proximal to the humeral stem. From this window, an impactor can be applied to the tip of the stem and impacted to break apart the proximal interface. If possible, it is helpful to keep the corners rounded to avoid a stress riser. Similarly, a window distal to the ulnar stem can be used to access the distal interface. If these windows are utilized, a new prosthesis needs to bypass this window by 2 cortical widths and caution should be taken to avoid cement extrusion.

Finally, a wider rectangular window can also be made. It is important to plan how to close a cortical window before its creation. Before creating a window, we place multiple 18 gauge wires deep to the periosteum around the humerus or ulna. After the window has been created and implant extracted, the window can be closed, allograft struts placed, and the 18 gauge wires tightened before cementation and final implant placement.

Though originally designed for revision hip and knee arthroplasty, ultrasonic devices can also be employed in revision total elbow arthroplasty for selective cement removal. However, the temperature increase in ultrasonic melting and removal of cement can cause thermal injury to adjacent nerves, and therefore it is recommended to identify and protect the radial and ulnar nerves while using the device in the humeral and ulnar canals respectively.[55] Fluoroscopic guidance is a

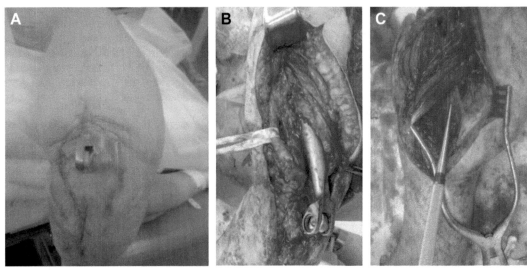

Fig. 2. Clinical photo before revision (*A*) and intra-operative photos demonstrating exposure and removal of implant (*B*) and use of a cortical window for cement and component extraction (*C*).

valuable aid to prevent the breach of the thinned humeral or ulnar cortices.

SPECIFIC SCENARIOS
Periprosthetic Infection and Aseptic Loosening

Treatment of periprosthetic complications total elbow arthroplasties includes single and two-stage revision, component retention, and resection arthroplasty. *S epidermidis* has been shown to cause the most virulent periprosthetic infection that fails single and two-stage revision, and may be an indication for resection arthroplasty.[20] Eyre-Brook and colleagues[56] demonstrated that single-stage revision can be successful in cases of presumed aseptic loosening based on clinical assessment, normal inflammatory markers, and negative aspiration even despite positive intraoperative cultures.

Single-stage revision is employed for aseptic revision, though there is some evidence of the efficacy of single-stage revision for septic loosening, with a success rate reported from 60 to 80% in small series.[14,20,57] Single-stage exchange involves removal of the implant, cement, and any infected or nonviable tissue, including synovial membrane and sinus tracts. Bone canals should be copiously irrigated. Canal preparation can be checked with fluoroscopy to limit the risk of cortical breach. If there is osteolysis at the tip of the stem or a cortical breach, the next length stem available should be used with antibiotic cement fixation. Careful wound closure to

minimize dead space and the use of minimal suture material can help with postoperative healing.

For 2-stage revision, the first stage involves the removal of prosthesis and nonviable tissue and the insertion of antibiotic spacer. There are numerous options for spacers, including a cement ball spacer, an antibiotic cement-coated bent Steinman pin, Ilizarov rod coated in antibiotic cement, and prosthesis of antibiotic-loaded acrylic cement (PROSTALAC).[58,59]

The author's preferred technique is a round antibiotic cement ball spacer placed in the void between the humerus and ulna. Cue ball arthroplasty is a described method of antibiotic spacer that allows for some functional motion of the elbow joint without a metal implant that risks biofilm formation. The technique involves one or multiple balls of antibiotic-impregnated cement implanted in the elbow to help maintain soft tissue tension and allow pain-free elbow range of motion (**Fig. 3**).[60] Care should be taken to avoid oversizing the ball. Postoperatively, patients are continued on appropriate antibiotics and monitored with serologic markers until the normalization of lab values, usually for at least 6 weeks. In the second stage surgery, infection control is confirmed with intraoperative frozen tissue samples before reimplantation ($\geq$ 5 neutrophils per high-powered field is a contraindication to reimplantation).[61] Again, stems need to be long enough to bypass cortical windows and areas of osteolysis.

Washout with component retention and polyethylene exchange is less commonly utilized for the management of periprosthetic infection. Streubel and colleagues reported on 23 patients and

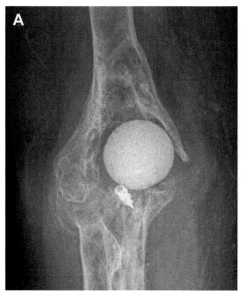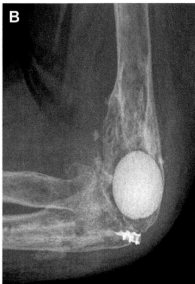

Fig. 3. AP (*A*) and lateral (*B*) postoperative radiographs demonstrating revision of TEA to cue ball arthroplasty.

Yamaguchi and colleagues described 14 patients with periprosthetic infection with well-fixed implants that were managed with multiple irrigation and debridement surgeries.[20,62] Streubel's series had a 4% failure rate[62] and Yamaguchi's series had a 50% failure rate.[20]

Periprosthetic Fracture

Analogous to the Vancouver classification for periprosthetic femur fractures, the Mayo Classification for periprosthetic elbow fractures[25] describes fractures based on location relative to the stem, implant stability, and quality of remaining bone stock (**Fig. 4**).

Type I fractures can usually be managed with plate fixation. Fractures of the distal humerus condyles in the setting of a linked prosthesis can be managed nonoperatively, while those in an unlinked prosthesis may require revision to a linked prosthesis. Olecranon fractures can be managed with plate fixation or tension band wiring.

Type II fractures of the humeral and ulnar stems with well-fixed stems can be stabilized with cerclage wires with or without cortical strut grafts as adjuncts. Allograft struts should extend proximally beyond the stem for the humerus and distal to the stem for the ulna. Fractures at the level of the stem with loose implants but good bone stock can be revised to a long stem implant bypassing the fracture by at least 2 cortical diameters and augmented with cortical strut grafts with cerclage wires.[44,63]

Type III fractures proximal to the humeral stem can be managed nonoperatively with Sarmiento

bracing in some cases, but closed treatment may go on to nonunion. Proximal fractures with well-fixed implants can be treated with compression plating with cerclage wiring through the plate and unicortical locking screws.[64]

Revision Arthroplasty with Bone Loss

In the setting of revision arthroplasty for both aseptic loosening with extensive osteolysis and periprosthetic fracture with poor bone stock, bone loss creates a challenge for reconstruction. Shortening the humerus by 2 to 3 centimeters is an option during revision; however, significant shortening can distort muscle and ligament tension, thereby impairing postoperative function.

Cortical strut allograft and cancellous autograft can fill smaller bone defects. Structural allograft-prosthetic composites are an option for large bone defects. In these revision settings, care must be taken to avoid lengthening or shortening the construct to balance soft tissue tension; preoperative radiographs of the entire upper extremity and of the contralateral extremity (if normal) can help with planning the length of the graft. Intraoperatively, trial placement of the prosthesis and allograft before cementing can help assess appropriate soft tissue tension.[65] Cementation can be performed as a single-stage or via two-stage technique, for which the implant is first cemented to the allograft and subsequently cemented into the host. Two-stage cementation is usually preferred as it is easier to control implantation and graft length can be modified before cementing into host bone.

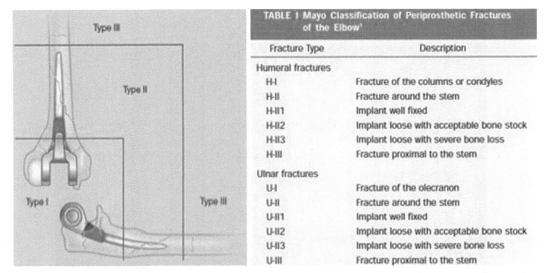

TABLE I Mayo Classification of Periprosthetic Fractures of the Elbow¹	
Fracture Type	Description
Humeral fractures	
H-I	Fracture of the columns or condyles
H-II	Fracture around the stem
H-II1	Implant well fixed
H-II2	Implant loose with acceptable bone stock
H-II3	Implant loose with severe bone loss
H-III	Fracture proximal to the stem
Ulnar fractures	
U-I	Fracture of the olecranon
U-II	Fracture around the stem
U-II1	Implant well fixed
U-II2	Implant loose with acceptable bone stock
U-II3	Implant loose with severe bone loss
U-III	Fracture proximal to the stem

Fig. 4. Mayo classification of periprosthetic elbow fractures. (*From* Aronowitz, Sanchez-Soto J. Elbow arthroplasty. In: Revell PA, ed Joint replacement technology. 2nd edn. Elsevier. 2014; 602-27; with permission.)

Plate fixation can augment allograft-host bone stability.

Impaction grafting has been shown to be a relatively reliable method for revision with bone loss.[66–68] For this technique, careful shaft preparation with implant and cement removal and debridement of metallosis and fibrinous tissue is performed, noting any cortical perforation or false tracks. Guidewires are then passed into the medullary canal, which is then widened with a cannulated flexible reamer. A cement restrictor is then placed down the canal followed by a trial stem as a spacer. The spacer should be slightly larger than the planned final implant. Allograft is then packed tightly around the spacer and impacted by removing and replacing the spacer multiple times to achieve stability of the packed bone. Then cement—either low viscosity cement or injecting when the cement is less viscous—is injected into the canal followed by final implants. The bone graft demonstrates varying ranges of incorporation at a follow-up; Rhee and colleagues[68] found radiographic evidence of resorption without clinical loosening in all of their cases, while Loebenberg had a 16% postoperative loosening rate requiring revision.[67]

Lastly, the ulnar component can be implanted into the radius as a salvage option for massive, unreconstructable ulnar bone defects. Although this construct does not allow for pronosupination, a review of 5 cases demonstrated that patients achieved stable elbows without distal component loosening.[69] This may be a better salvage option than either arthrodesis (which has high reoperation rates and low rates of union) or resection arthroplasty (which can result in instability).

OUTCOMES AND COMPLICATIONS

As the number of TEAs performed increases with broadened indications in a younger and more active patient population, the need for revision surgery also grows. The survival and complication rates following primary TEA are not as favorable as those for other joint arthroplasties, with a reported complication rate ranging from 20 to 40%.[3,7] Survival of TEA is longer in patients who receive a TEA for inflammatory arthritis than those for trauma indications such as unreconstructable elbow fractures and posttraumatic arthritis.[7,70] The most common indications for revision are aseptic loosening, infection, and periprosthetic fracture.[71]

Despite advances in implant technology and diagnostic tools, revision surgery continues to have a high complication rate. A systematic review of revision TEA literature found a 44% complication rate resulting in a 21.8% reoperation rate. However this also showed that outcomes data demonstrate significantly improved pain scores, patient-reported outcomes measures, and range of motion parameters compared to preoperatively.[71]

CLINICS CARE POINTS

- Rates of failure are highly variable across the literature for TEA.
- Ulnar neuropathy is a common accompanying condition that should be evaluated with the painful TEA.

- Take caution with thermal cement removal. The radial nerve is intimate with the humerus and is at risk of thermal injury.
- Revision surgery requires attention to the possibility of infection and attention to how much bone stock has been lost5. Resection arthroplasty is an option for cases of severe, irreconstructable bone loss.

FUNDING

Grants- This work was supported in part by the Jesse B. Jupiter, MD Fund/ Hanjorg Wyss Medical Foundation.

DISCLAIMERS

None.

GRANTS SUPPORTING THIS WORK

None.

REFERENCES

1. Macken AA, Prkic A, Kodde IF, et al. Global trends in indications for total elbow arthroplasty: a systematic review of national registries. EFORT Open Rev 2020; 5(4):215–20.
2. Krukhaug Y, Hallan G, Dybvik E, et al. A survivorship study of 838 total elbow replacements: a report from the Norwegian Arthroplasty Register 1994-2016. J Shoulder Elbow Surg 2018;27(2):260–9.
3. Welsink CL, Lambers KTA, van Deurzen DFP, et al. Total elbow arthroplasty: a systematic review. JBJS Rev 2017;5(7):e4.
4. Jauregui JJ, Banerjee S, Cherian JJ, et al. Early outcomes of titanium-based highly-porous acetabular components in revision total hip arthroplasty. J Arthroplasty 2015;30(7):1187–90.
5. Chaudhry H, MacDonald SJ, Howard JL, et al. Clinical outcomes and midterm survivorship of an uncemented primary total hip arthroplasty system. J Arthroplasty 2020;35(6):1662–6.
6. Parker P, Furness ND, Evans JP, et al. A systematic review of the complications of contemporary total elbow arthroplasty. Shoulder Elbow 2021;13(5): 544–51.
7. Perretta D, van Leeuwen WF, Dyer G, et al. Risk factors for reoperation after total elbow arthroplasty. J Shoulder Elbow Surg 2017;26(5):824–9.
8. Voloshin I, Schippert DW, Kakar S, et al. Complications of total elbow replacement: a systematic review. J Shoulder Elbow Surg 2011;20(1):158–68.
9. Goldberg SH, Urban RM, Jacobs JJ, et al. Modes of wear after semiconstrained total elbow arthroplasty. J Bone Joint Surg Am 2008;90(3):609–19.
10. Morrey BF. Modes of wear after semiconstrained total elbow arthroplasty. J Bone Joint Surg Am 2009; 91(2):487–8 [author reply: 488-9].
11. Ramsey ML, Adams RA, Morrey BF. Instability of the elbow treated with semiconstrained total elbow arthroplasty. J Bone Joint Surg Am 1999;81(1):38–47.
12. Gandhi MJ, Eyre-Brook AI, Gopinath P, et al. Reliability analysis of radiologic and intraoperative loosening in total elbow arthroplasty. J Shoulder Elbow Surg 2021;30(10):2401–5.
13. Holst DC, Angerame MR, Dennis DA, et al. What is the value of component loosening assessment of a preoperatively obtained bone scan prior to revision total knee arthroplasty? J Arthroplasty 2019;34(7S): S256–61.
14. Gille J, Ince A, González O, et al. Single-stage revision of peri-prosthetic infection following total elbow replacement. J Bone Joint Surg Br 2006;88(10): 1341–6.
15. Morrey BF, Bryan RS. Infection after total elbow arthroplasty. J Bone Joint Surg Am 1983;65(3):330–8.
16. Wolfe SW, Figgie MP, Inglis AE, et al. Management of infection about total elbow prostheses. J Bone Joint Surg Am 1990;72(2):198–212.
17. Pope D, Scaife SL, Tzeng TH, et al. Impact of diabetes on early postoperative outcomes after total elbow arthroplasty. J Shoulder Elbow Surg 2015; 24:348–52.
18. Griffin JW, Werner BC, Gwathmey FW, et al. Obesity is associated with increased postoperative complications after total elbow arthroplasty. J Shoulder Elbow Surg 2015;24:1594–601.
19. Somerson JS, Boylan MR, Hug KT, et al. Risk factors associated with periprosthetic joint infection after total elbow arthroplasty. Shoulder Elbow 2019;11(2): 116–20.
20. Yamaguchi K, Adams RA, Morrey BF. Infection after total elbow arthroplasty. J Bone Joint Surg Am 1998; 80(4):481–91.
21. Achermann Y, Vogt M, Spormann C, et al. Characteristics and outcome of 27 elbow periprosthetic joint infections: results from a 14-year cohort study of 358 elbow prostheses. Clin Microbiol Infect 2011; 17(3):432–8.
22. Unter Ecker N, Koniker A, Gehrke T, et al. What Is the Diagnostic Accuracy of Alpha-Defensin and Leukocyte Esterase Test in Periprosthetic Shoulder Infection? Clin Orthop Relat Res 2019;477(7): 1712–8.
23. Frangiamore SJ, Saleh A, Grosso MJ, et al. α-Defensin as a predictor of periprosthetic shoulder infection. J Shoulder Elbow Surg 2015;24(7):1021–7.
24. Frangiamore SJ, Saleh A, Grosso MJ, et al. Neer Award 2015: Analysis of cytokine profiles in the diagnosis of periprosthetic joint infections of the shoulder. J Shoulder Elbow Surg 2017;26(2): 186–96.

25. O'Driscoll SW, Morrey BF. Periprosthetic fractures about the elbow. Orthop Clin North Am 1999;30(2): 319–25.

26. Day JS, Lau E, Ong KL, et al. Prevalence and projections of total shoulder and elbow arthroplasty in the United States to 2015. J Shoulder Elbow Surg 2010;19(8):1115–20.

27. Inglis AE, Inglis AE Jr. Ipsilateral total shoulder arthroplasty and total elbow replacement arthroplasty: a caveat. J Arthroplasty 2000;15(1):123–5.

28. Mavrogenis AF, Angelini A, Guerra E, et al. Humeral fracture between a total elbow and total shoulder arthroplasty. Orthopedics 2011;34(4).

29. Carroll EA, Lorich DG, Helfet DL. Surgical management of a periprosthetic fracture between a total elbow and total shoulder prostheses: a case report. J Shoulder Elbow Surg 2009;18(3):e9–12.

30. Gill DR, Cofield RH, Morrey BF. Ipsilateral total shoulder and elbow arthroplasties in patients who have rheumatoid arthritis. J Bone Joint Surg Am 1999; 81:1128–37.

31. Pierce TD, Herndon JH. The triceps preserving approach to total elbow arthroplasty. Clin Orthop Relat Res 1998;354:144–52.

32. Meijering D, Welsink CL, Boerboom AL, et al. Triceps insufficiency after total elbow arthroplasty: a systematic review. JBJS Rev 2021;9(7).

33. Dachs RP, Fleming MA, Chivers DA, et al. Total elbow arthroplasty: outcomes after triceps-detaching and triceps-sparing approaches. J Shoulder Elbow Surg 2015;24(3):339–47.

34. Rispoli DM, Athwal GS, Morrey BF. Neurolysis of the ulnar nerve for neuropathy following total elbow replacement. J Bone Joint Surg Br 2008;90(10): 1348–51.

35. Kaufmann RA, D'Auria JL, Schneppendahl J. Total elbow arthroplasty: elbow biomechanics and failure. J Hand Surg Am 2019;44(8):687–92.

36. Park SE, Kim JY, Cho SW, et al. Complications and revision rate compared by type of total elbow arthroplasty. J Shoulder Elbow Surg 2013;22(8): 1121–7.

37. Dee R. Total replacement arthroplasty of the elbow for rheumatoid arthritis. J Bone Joint Surg Br 1972; 54:88–95.

38. Kudo H, Iwano K. Total elbow arthroplasty with a non-constrained surface replacement prosthesis in patients who have rheumatoid arthritis: A long-term follow-up study. J Bone Joint Surg Am 1990;72: 355–62.

39. Aldridge JM 3rd, Lightdale NR, Mallon WJ, et al. Total elbow arthroplasty with the Coonrad/Coonrad-Morrey prosthesis. A 10- to 31-year survival analysis. J Bone Joint Surg Br 2006;88(4):509–14.

40. Wright TW, Hastings H. Total elbow arthroplasty failure due to overuse, C-ring failure, and/or bushing wear. J Shoulder Elbow Surg 2005;14(1):65–72.

41. Hastings H 2nd, Lee DH, Pietrzak WS. A prospective multicenter clinical study of the Discovery elbow. J Shoulder Elbow Surg 2014;23(5):e95–107.

42. Borton ZM, Prasad G, Konstantopoulos G, et al. Mid- to long-term survivorship of the cemented, semiconstrained Discovery total elbow arthroplasty. J Shoulder Elbow Surg 2021;30(7):1662–9.

43. King EA, Favre P, Eldemerdash A, et al. Physiological loading of the coonrad/morrey, nexel, and discovery elbow systems: evaluation by finite element analysis. J Hand Surg Am 2019;44(1):61.e1–9.

44. Sanchez-Sotelo J, O'Driscoll S, Morrey BF. Periprosthetic humeral fractures after total elbow arthroplasty: treatment with implant revision and strut allograft augmentation. J Bone Joint Surg Am 2002;84(9):1642–50.

45. Burnier M, Nguyen NTV, Morrey ME, et al. Revision elbow arthroplasty using a proximal ulnar allograft with allograft triceps for combined ulnar bone loss and triceps insufficiency. J Bone Joint Surg Am 2020;102(22):2001–7.

46. Prokopis PM, Weiland AJ. The triceps-preserving approach for semiconstrained total elbow arthroplasty. J Shoulder Elbow Surg 2008;17(3):454–8.

47. Bryan RS, Morrey BF. Extensive posterior exposure of the elbow. A triceps-sparing approach. Clin Orthop Relat Res 1982;166:188–92.

48. Wolfe SW, Ranawat CS. The osteo-anconeus flap. An approach for total elbow arthroplasty. J Bone Joint Surg Am 1990;72(5):684–8.

49. Campbell WC. Incision for exposure of the elbow joint. Am J Surg 1932;15:65.

50. Celli A, Arash A, Adams RA, et al. Triceps insufficiency following total elbow arthroplasty. J Bone Joint Surg Am 2005;87(9):1957–64.

51. Sanchez-Sotelo J, Morrey BF. Surgical techniques for reconstruction of chronic insufficiency of the triceps. Rotation flap using anconeus and tendo achillis allograft. J Bone Joint Surg Br 2002;84(8): 1116–20.

52. Macken AA, Lans J, Miyamura S, et al. Soft-tissue coverage for wound complications following total elbow arthroplasty. Clin Shoulder Elb 2021;24(4): 245–52.

53. Okamoto S, Tada K, Ai H, et al. Flexor carpi ulnaris muscle flap for soft tissue reconstruction after total elbow arthroplasty. Case Rep Surg 2014;2014: 798506.

54. Hacquebord JH, Hanel DP, Friedrich JB. The pedicled latissimus dorsi flap provides effective coverage for large and complex soft tissue injuries around the elbow. Hand (N Y). 2018 Sep;13(5): 586–92.

55. Goldberg SH, Cohen MS, Young M, et al. Thermal tissue damage caused by ultrasonic cement removal from the humerus. J Bone Joint Surg Am 2005;87(3):583–91.

56. Eyre-Brook AI, Gandhi MJ, Gopinath P, et al. Revision total elbow arthroplasty: Is it safe to perform a single-stage revision for presumed aseptic loosening based on clinical assessment, normal inflammatory markers, and a negative aspiration? J Shoulder Elbow Surg 2021;30(1):140–5.

57. Dauzere F, Clavert P, Ronde-Oustau C, et al. Is systematic 1-stage exchange a valid attitude in chronic infection of total elbow arthroplasty? Orthop Traumatol Surg Res 2021;107(4):102905.

58. Joo MS, Kim JW, Kim YT. Efficacy of 2-stage revision using a prosthesis of antibiotic-loaded acrylic cement spacer with or without cortical strut allograft in infected total elbow arthroplasty. J Shoulder Elbow Surg 2021;30(12):2875–85.

59. Williams KE, MacLean S, Jupiter J. An articulating antibiotic cement spacer for first-stage reconstruction for infected total elbow arthroplasty. Tech Hand Up Extrem Surg 2017;21(2):41–7.

60. Gerow DE, Tan EH, Bamberger HB. Cue ball arthroplasty with humeroradial total elbow arthroplasty (TEA) revision: an approach to managing infection and severe ulnar bone loss in TEA. J Shoulder Elb Arthroplast 2020;4. 2471549220961592.

61. Kwak JM, Kholinne E, Sun Y, et al. Clinical results of revision total elbow arthroplasty: comparison of infected and non-infected total elbow arthroplasty. Int Orthop 2019;43(6):1421–7.

62. Streubel PN, Simone JP, Morrey BF, et al. Infection in total elbow arthroplasty with stable components: outcomes of a staged surgical protocol with retention of the components. Bone Joint Lett J 2016;98-B(7):976–83.

63. Foruria AM, Sanchez-Sotelo J, Oh LS, et al. The surgical treatment of periprosthetic elbow fractures around the ulnar stem following semiconstrained total elbow arthroplasty. J Bone Joint Surg Am 2011; 93:1399e407.

64. Kamineni S, Morrey BF. Proximal ulnar reconstruction with strut allograft in revision total arthroplasty. J Bone Joint Surg Am 2004;86:1223e9.

65. Renfree KJ, Dell PC, Kozin SH, et al. Total elbow arthroplasty with massive composite allografts. J Shoulder Elbow Surg 2004;13:313–21.

66. Lee DH. Impaction allograft bone-grafting for revision total elbow arthroplasty. A case report. J Bone Joint Surg Am 1999;81(7):1008–12.

67. Loebenberg MI, Adams R, O'Driscoll SW, et al. Impaction grafting in revision total elbow arthroplasty. J Bone Joint Surg Am 2005;87(1):99–106.

68. Rhee YG, Cho NS, Parke CS. Impaction grafting in revision total elbow arthroplasty for aseptic loosening and bone loss: surgical technique. JBJS Essent Surg Tech 2013;3(3):e17.

69. Bellevue KD, Lorenzana DJ, Klifto CS, et al. Revision total elbow arthroplasty with the ulnar component implanted into the radius for management of large ulna defects. J Shoulder Elbow Surg 2021;30(4): 913–7.

70. Fevang BT, Lie SA, Havelin LI, et al. Results after 562 total elbow replacements: a report from the Norwegian Arthroplasty Register. J Shoulder Elbow Surg 2009;18(3):449–56.

71. Geurts EJ, Viveen J, van Riet RP, et al. Outcomes after revision total elbow arthroplasty: a systematic review. J Shoulder Elbow Surg 2019;28(2):381–6.

Wrist Arthritis and Arthrodesis
Preserving Function, Minimizing Problems

Anthony LoGiudice, MD[a], Hisham Awan, MD[b],*

KEYWORDS

- Wrist arthritis • Wrist fusion • Wrist arthroplasty

KEY POINTS

- Wrist arthritis can involve several different joints and is caused by numerous underlying conditions.
- Evaluation and imaging focused on identifying the joints generating pain can help guide management.
- The goal of surgical treatment of the arthritic wrist is to minimize pain while preserving motion and optimizing function.
- For SLAC and SNAC wrist, proximal row carpectomy and scaphoid excision and midcarpal arthrodesis are well established procedures with comparable results.
- Total wrist arthrodesis is the most commonly used salvage procedure for pancarpal arthrosis, but improvements in total wrist arthroplasty design have expanded the indications for this evolving technique.

INTRODUCTION

Wrist arthritis is a common condition that is frequently encountered by hand surgeons and results from several different etiologies. The presentation and symptoms can vary, and numerous surgical and nonsurgical treatment options are available for these patients. This article reviews the causes and patterns of wrist arthritis and discusses treatment strategies aimed at preserving function and minimizing complications.

ANATOMY AND KINEMATICS

The wrist joint includes the distal radius and ulna, and the proximal and distal carpal rows. Extrinsic and intrinsic ligaments stabilize the articulations within the wrist. Intrinsic ligaments run between carpal bones. These include the scapholunate ligament (SL) and lunotriquetral ligament. Extrinsic ligaments originate outside the carpus but insert onto the carpal bones. The palmar ligaments[1] (**Fig. 1**) have an arc shape and include the radioscaphocapitate, long radiolunate, and short radiolunate on the radial side and the ulnocapitate and ulnotriquetral ligaments on the ulnar side. On the dorsal side (**Fig. 2**), the important extrinsic ligament is the dorsal radiocarpal ligament. The dorsal intercarpal ligament is technically an intrinsic ligament because it resides solely within the carpus, but it is often considered an extrinsic ligament because it spans three carpal bones.

The scaphoid is thought of as a link between the proximal and distal rows. During radial deviation and flexion, the scaphoid is pushed into flexion by the distal carpal row. Because of the intercarpal ligament attachments, the lunate and triquetrum are also brought into flexion. The opposite happens when the wrist is extended or ulnarly deviated and this extension of the scaphoid is the basis of the scaphoid view radiograph. Injury to the intercarpal ligaments can lead to carpal

[a] Department of Orthopaedic Surgery, Medical College of Wisconsin, 8701 Watertown Plank Road, Milwaukee, WI 53226, USA; [b] Ohio State University Hand and Upper Extremity Center, 915 Olentangy River Road, Suite 3200, Columbus, OH 43212, USA
* Corresponding author.
E-mail address: Hisham.awan@osumc.edu

Hand Clin 39 (2023) 353–365
https://doi.org/10.1016/j.hcl.2023.04.001
0749-0712/23/© 2023 Published by Elsevier Inc.

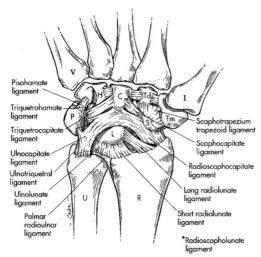

Fig. 1. Palmar wrist ligaments. (Reprinted with permission from Buijze GA, Lozano-Calderon SA, Strackee SD, Blankevoort L, Jupiter JB. Osseous and ligamentous scaphoid anatomy: Part I. A systematic literature review highlighting controversies. J Hand Surg Am. 2011;36:1926-1935.)

instability and secondary attenuation of the extrinsic ligaments is responsible for the characteristic changes in chronic SL injuries, which ultimately lead to an scapholunate advanced collapse (SLAC) wrist.[2]

CAUSES OF WRIST ARTHRITIS

Wrist arthritis can involve several different joints and is caused by numerous underlying conditions. Wrist arthritis can be idiopathic (scaphotrapeziotrapezoidal [STT] or pisotriquetral arthritis) but more often results from avascular necrosis

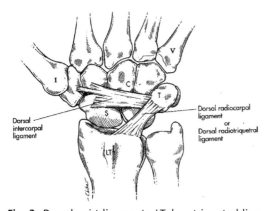

Fig. 2. Dorsal wrist ligaments. LT, lunotriquetral ligament; RSC, radioscaphocapitate; RSL, radioscapholunate. (Reprinted with permission from Buijze GA, Lozano-Calderon SA, Strackee SD, Blankevoort L, Jupiter JB. Osseous and ligamentous scaphoid anatomy: Part I. A systematic literature review highlighting controversies. J Hand Surg Am. 2011;36:1926-1935.)

(Kienböck, Preiser), posttraumatic conditions (SLAC/scaphoid nonunion advanced collapse [SNAC] or radius malunion), congenital or developmental abnormalities (Madelung), or inflammatory causes (gout, rheumatoid arthritis [RA]). The pattern of arthritis and the joints involved are related to the cause. For instance, SLAC and SNAC wrist result in a characteristic progression of arthritis starting at the radioscaphoid joint and progressing into the midcarpal joint.[3] The distal radioulnar joint can also be involved in arthritis of the wrist, but this article focuses on the radiocarpal, intercarpal, and midcarpal joints. **Box 1** lists some common causes of wrist arthritis.

Idiopathic

The wrist is not frequently involved in idiopathic osteoarthritis, but there are a few joints that become arthritic and cause patients to consult a hand surgeon. On the radial side of the wrist, the STT joint can become arthritic and is commonly associated with basal joint arthrosis or dorsal intercalated segment instability (DISI) deformity. The treatment of STT arthritis is dependent on the concurrent pathology with options that include distal scaphoid excision, trapeziectomy with partial trapezoid excision, or STT arthrodesis.[4] On the ulnar side, the pisotriquetral articulation (**Fig. 3**) is often the culprit leading to volar ulnar wrist pain. Pisiform excision has been shown to be a reliable and effective treatment when conservative treatment is ineffective.[5]

Traumatic

Wrist arthritis is commonly seen as a sequela from prior trauma and often results in a characteristic pattern and progression of arthritis. Some common causes are distal radius fractures/malunions, scaphoid nonunion, and SL injuries.

Scapholunate advanced collapse and scaphoid nonunion advanced collapse wrist

SL injuries can lead to the development of arthritis when not adequately treated. Because of the anatomy and kinematics of the wrist, alterations in the anatomy can lead to arthritic changes. SL injuries lead to disruption of secondary stabilizers and results in flexion and some protonation of the scaphoid. In addition, the lunate falls into extension and this results in the characteristic DISI deformity. The radioscaphoid articulation does not tolerate alterations in the joint contact forces and the degenerative changes in SLAC wrist start here and progress in stages (**Figs. 4** and **5**).[3] The degenerative changes begin at the radial styloid (stage 1), then the proximal radioscaphoid joint (stage 2),

Box 1
Causes of wrist arthritis

I. Idiopathic
   a. STT
   b. Pisotriquetral
II. Traumatic
   a. SLAC wrist
   b. SNAC wrist
   c. Secondary to distal radius fracture/malunion
III. Inflammatory
   a. RA
   b. Gout/pseudogout
   c. Psoriatic arthritis
   d. Other inflammatory arthropathies
IV. Infectious
   a. Septic arthritis
   b. Osteomyelitis
V. Kienböck disease/Preiser disease
   a. Madelung disease

followed by the capitolunate joint (stage 3), and finally pancarpal arthrosis (stage 4). Because of the spherical shape of the lunate, the radiolunate joint is more accommodating of extension of the lunate and this joint is often preserved until very late stages of SLAC wrist. Scaphoid nonunion can also lead to progressive degenerative changes in a similar fashion (**Fig. 6**), although the proximal scaphoid articulation is more likely spared in this setting. Knowing the pattern of arthritic involvement has important treatment implications because some treatment options may be contraindicated when various joints are involved.

Radius fractures/malunions

Intra-articular fractures of the radius can result in arthritic changes secondary to joint incongruity. Knirk and Jupiter[6] showed that greater than 2 mm of intra-articular stepoff can lead to a higher risk of posttraumatic arthritis leading to subsequent pain and loss of function.

Malunions without intra-articular stepoff may also lead to progressive arthrosis because of alteration of carpal kinematics. The most common scenario is a dorsally angulated malunion of the radius. This can lead to degeneration at the radiocarpal joint from the lunate loading the dorsal rim of the radius, or at the midcarpal joint secondary to an adaptive DISI deformity (**Figs. 7** and **8**).[7]

Inflammatory Conditions

The most common inflammatory arthritis is RA, and it affects roughly 1% of individuals in the United States. It is an inflammatory autoimmune condition characterized by joint synovitis, articular cartilage degradation, and ligament attenuation. The wrist is a common location affected by RA; 50% of patients are affected within the first 2 years and 90% of patients after 10 years of disease onset.[8]

In patients with RA, synovitis attacks the ligamentous components of the wrist, including the triangular fibrocartilage complex and volar and dorsal ligaments. Because of these pathologic changes, the proximal row supinates and translates palmarly and ulnarly. Treatment is based on the pattern of joint destruction and severity of symptoms. There is a wide spectrum in presentation. In some cases, the arthritis is limited to the radiolunate joint, and in some cases there is severe pancarpal arthrosis (**Fig. 9**). Rheumatoid involvement can also lead to associated pathologies, particularly tenosynovitis and tendon ruptures.

Gout is also known to cause arthritis of the wrist because of crystal deposition within the articular surfaces or by causing attenuation of the SL ligament, which can cause a pattern of arthritis similar to an SNAC wrist, but with more pronounced periarticular erosions.

Other Conditions

Some other potential causes of wrist arthritis are Kienböck disease; infection (septic arthritis, osteomyelitis); and systemic disorders, such as sarcoid arthropathy or other systemic diseases. As described by Lichtman in **Table 1**, Kienböck disease progresses through various stages starting with mild disease at stage I to advanced degenerative changes at stage IV.[9]

EVALUATION
History and Physical

Evaluation of all arthritic conditions of the wrist should start with a history and physical examination. The patient should be asked about any personal or family history of inflammatory arthritis, any prior injury to that wrist, and any associated medical conditions. The history should be followed by a focused physical examination that identifies which joints are generating pain, because arthritis of the wrist is not always symptomatic. The presence of erythema or swelling and constitutional symptoms could indicate an inflammatory or infectious cause. In the presence of diffuse

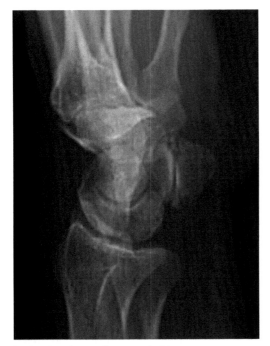

Fig. 3. Pisotriquetral osteoarthritis.

degenerative changes, it is important to palpate individual joints to ascertain which joints are most symptomatic. Provocative maneuvers, such as the Watson scaphoid shift test or lunotriquetral ligament shear or ballottement tests, can also aid in diagnosis.[10,11] In addition to palpation, selective lidocaine injections can also assist in determining which joints are symptomatic.

Laboratory Studies

Bloodwork can also be ordered when considering inflammatory arthropathy or infection as the underlying cause for the arthritis. An erythrocyte sedimentation rate and C-reactive protein levels

are often obtained when these conditions are suspected, but they are not specific. In addition, rheumatoid factor and anti-cyclic citrullinated peptide antibodies can help make the diagnosis of RA. Finally, a uric acid level can aid in the diagnosis of gout but is often not elevated in an acute gout flare.

Joint Fluid Analysis

Aspiration of involved joints is helpful, particularly when infection or crystalline arthropathy is suspected, and it can help distinguish between the conditions. This is especially important, because both conditions can present with acute swelling and erythema, and making the correct diagnosis is paramount because infection likely requires surgical debridement, whereas crystalline arthropathy is treated with supportive medical management.

Imaging

Standard radiographs of the wrist can identify the pattern of arthritic changes. Special views, such as a supinated oblique view, can more accurately identify pathology, such as pisotriquetral arthritis. Advanced imaging is typically not necessary in the work-up of wrist arthritis but occasionally computed tomography scans and MRI can provide further information to help in diagnosing the cause of a patient's wrist pain, or to help with surgical planning.

MANAGEMENT OPTIONS
Conservative Management

A plethora of options and pathways exist in conservative management for arthritis of the wrist. On initial flare up, selective periods of immobilization with a splint or cast is considered along with

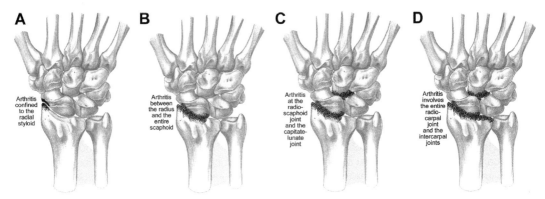

Fig. 4. Stages of progression in SLAC wrist. (*A*) Stage I, arthritis confined to radial styloid. (*B*) Stage II, arthritis progresses to the entire scaphoid. (*C*) Stage III, arthritis progresses to the capitolunate articulation. (*D*) Stage IV, pancarpal arthritis. (With the kind permission of Dr. Imbriglia.)

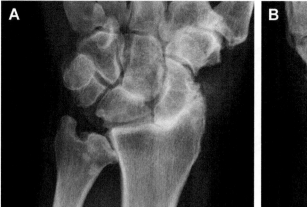
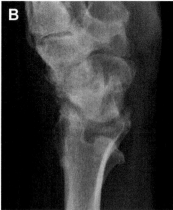

Fig. 5. Anteroposterior (A) and lateral (B) radiographs of a patient with stage III SLAC wrist and DISI deformity. Note the relative sparing of the radiolunate joint.

activity modifications to avoid repetitive use or heavy lifting. Caution should be exercised with extended immobilization that could cause more rapid onset of stiffness in an arthritic wrist. A balance of gentle motion between periods of brief immobilization may be pursued, as per the patient's tolerance.

There is strong evidence to suggest that common prefabricated splints are more efficacious that custom orthoses for wrist arthritis.[12] Further adjuncts may include ice and heat, depending on the acuity of symptoms. Medications are a common pillar in conservative management, which include oral nonsteroidal anti-inflammatory drugs or acetaminophen. Patients can benefit from direct analgesic and anti-inflammatory effects, although complications are associated with renal, liver, or gastrointestinal disease.[13,14]

Intra-articular steroid injections are commonly used, although with transient or limited effect at times, depending on the particular joint or severity. Injection of other medications, such as platelet rich plasma and hyaluronic acid, are also being performed in some centers, but currently the most common practice for hand surgeons remains corticosteroid injection.

Topical medications may include a litany of different active ingredients from capsaicin to salicylates, diclofenac, menthol, eucalyptus oil, and camphor. These have a milder effect that may only last a few hours, but also have a low side effect profile. Some evidence points to early relief with topicals for the first 2 weeks with a limited effect noted thereafter, compared with placebo.[15] Lastly, prescription medications may be indicated for severe disease, particularly with inflammatory (gout/pseudogout) or autoimmune disease (RA, lupus). These are often managed by a primary care physician or rheumatologist who can monitor for various symptomatic or metabolic side effects.

Surgical Treatment

The goal of surgical treatment of the arthritic wrist is to minimize pain while preserving motion and optimizing function. Traditional surgical options for a painful arthritic wrist relied on total or subtotal fusions across the radiocarpal joint. The undesired associated loss of motion has pushed these to be end-salvage options and several other motion-preserving treatments have emerged. Once conservative treatment has been considered unsuccessful, many surgical options exist. These include debridement, denervation, proximal row carpectomy (PRC), and a variety of fusions. Lastly there is still an emerging role for total wrist

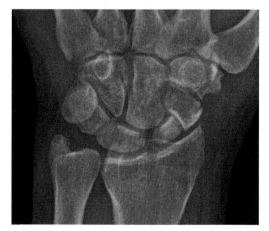

Fig. 6. Radiograph of a patient with chronic scaphoid nonunion resulting in stage I SNAC wrist.

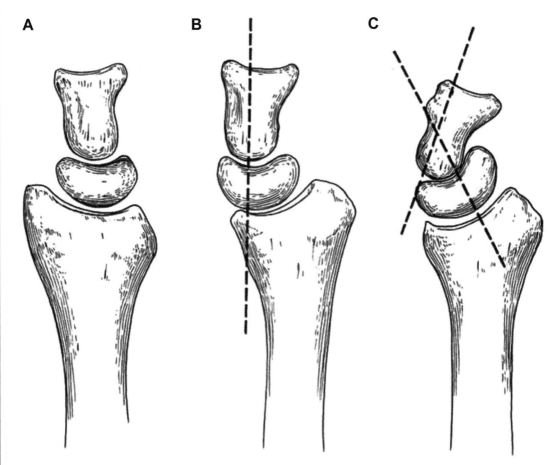

Fig. 7. Patterns of instability with dorsal radius malunions. Normal anatomy (*A*) and two patterns of instability caused by dorsal malunion of the distal radius: dorsal radiocarpal subluxation with maintenance of midcarpal alignment (*B*) and adaptive midcarpal DISI deformity (*C*). (Reprinted with permission from Bushnell BD, Bynum DK. Malunion of the distal radius. J Am Acad Orthop Surg. 2007;15:27-40.)

arthroplasty (TWA) that continues to evolve with improved implant design.

Arthroscopy

Persistent symptoms of wrist pain and synovitis that fail to respond to conservative measures may benefit from arthroscopic debridement. This treatment offers the benefit of limited postoperative restrictions and time for return to activities while also sparing motion. Arthroscopic debridement for undifferentiated monoarticular arthritis may be controversial in large joints, such as the knee, but in the wrist there is a role that is diagnostic and therapeutic.[16] Kim and colleagues[17] found that arthroscopic synovectomy of wrist arthritis showed significant improvement in pain relief and range of motion and Mayo wrist scores in 9 of 20 patients. Patients with persistent symptoms demonstrated signs of inflammatory disease and were successfully treated with disease-modifying antirheumatic drugs. Preoperative work-up of persistent synovitis that cannot easily be attributed to a repetitive trauma or event should include a battery of inflammatory markers to screen for autoimmune diseases, such as RA, lupus, psoriatic arthritis, ankylosing spondylitis, and so forth.

Denervation

Whether degenerative changes are mild or severe, wrist denervation can play a role with minimal morbidity to function or motion. Long since it was first described by Wilhelm in 1958, wrist denervation has seen multiple iterations and modifications including Dellon's partial denervation involving the posterior interosseus nerve and the inclusion of the anterior interosseus nerve through a single incision by Berger in 1998.[18–20] Only in the past few years has this gained momentum to be included as a routine option for treating wrist

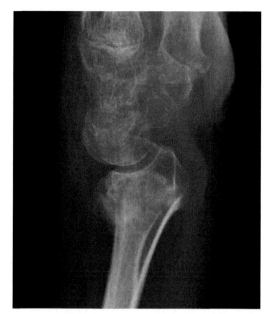

Fig. 8. Lateral radiograph of distal radius malunion resulting in carpal malalignment.

pain. The technical demands of total wrist denervation, however, have led more surgeons to adopt a partial wrist denervation approach. With a dorsal midline incision with straight forward dissection, excision of the anterior interosseus nerve and posterior interosseus nerve has been shown to have consistently good short- to medium-term outcomes.[21–23]

Despite the outcome, this has not been found to preclude or complicate any subsequent salvage procedures undertaken at a later date. The role for denervation offers a quick recovery, limited postoperative restrictions, and no functional or

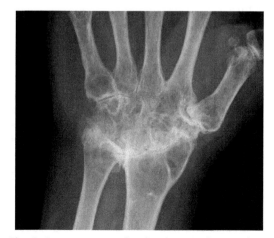

Fig. 9. Severe pancarpal arthrosis secondary to rheumatoid arthritis.

adaptive changes required for rehabilitation. A recent review compiling nine studies and 292 patients who underwent partial wrist denervation showed a reoperation rate of 24% at 18 months but there was a lack of long-term follow-up to compared with more extensive total wrist denervation studies, such as the 10-year follow-up by Schweitzer and colleagues reporting subjective pain improvement in two-thirds of 71 patients.[24,25] A Mayo Clinic study from 2018 had comparable outcomes with partial wrist denervation, reporting 69 of 100 patients requiring no further treatments at 6.75 years, with the remaining 31 patients experiencing symptom relief until 2 years before requiring another procedure.[26] This can represent years of relief to reach retirement, save for needed time off for a more extensive salvage procedure, or vocational retraining to avoid need for further surgery. If patients are indicated for a salvage procedure (described later) earlier in their course, most often have some partial denervation included to maximize outcomes of pain relief and take advantage of the same approach.[27]

There is only one study published in 2018 that looked at denervation combined with arthroscopic synovectomy along with radial styloidectomy for SLAC 2-3 wrist patients with good Disabilities of the Arm, Shoulder, and Hand (DASH) and return to work outcomes; however, there are no control or cohort groups for comparison. Further research is required to delineate how these motion-sparing procedures can be optimally implemented.

Partial arthrodesis

Surgical treatment of radiocarpal arthritis patterns is dictated by the involved joints. Posttraumatic arthritis caused by intra-articular distal radius fractures may involve degenerative disease at the radioscaphoid and/or radiolunate fossas. Isolated radiolunate fusions have been described with good results for focal symptomatic disease after trauma, and in patients with focal disease secondary to RA or in persistent global instability.[28–31] This preserves dart throwers motion through the midcarpal joint and, in the case of RA or instability, prevents ulnar translocation of the carpus. The most common technique involves dorsal preparation of the joint with headless screw fixation, although plate, k-wire, or staple fixation methods have also been described. The SL ligament should be inspected and confirmed intact, or additional fusion across the radioscaphoid joint is recommended to prevent progression of arthritis as the scaphoid falls into flexion.

More extensive destruction of the distal radius after intra-articular fracture can otherwise be treated with radioscapholunate (RSL) fusion.[32–35]

Table 1 Modified Lichtman classification for Kienböck disease	
Stage I	Normal radiographs or linear fracture Abnormal but nonspecific bone scan Diagnostic MRI appearance
Stage II	Lunate sclerosis One or more fracture lines with possible early collapse
Stage III	Lunate collapse
IIIA	Normal carpal alignment and height
IIIB	Fixed scaphoid rotation[a] Carpal height decreased Capitate migrates proximally
Stage IV	Severe lunate collapse with intra-articular degenerative changes at the midcarpal joint, radiocarpal joint, or both

[a] Radioscaphoid angle $\geq 60°$.

Reprinted with permission from Rhee PC, Jones DB, Moran SL, Shin AY. The effect of lunate morphology in Kienböck disease. J Hand Surg Am. 2015 Apr;40(4):738-44.

These fusions were originally met with several complications, however. Range of motion (ROM) was observed to decrease by 33% to 40%, whereas nonunion occurred up to 27% of attempts.[36,37] Progression of midcarpal arthritis caused by the scaphoid bridging to two carpal rows also was reported between 35% and 53% of patients.[38]

To address this issue, excision of the distal pole of the scaphoid improved the rates of union, pain scores, and ROM by preserving the midcarpal row motion.[39–41] Further cadaveric studies have demonstrated that excision of the triquetrum along with RSL fusion and distal scaphoid excision could achieve motion similar to or better than baseline, including flexion, extension, and deviation arc,[42] but follow-up cadaveric models also demonstrated concerns for midcarpal instability.[43] There are only limited case studies thus far comparing the outcomes of RSL fusion with distal scaphoid excision with or without triquetrum excision and as such insufficient evidence to determine superiority of triquetrum excision with RSL and distal scaphoid excision and whether it demonstrates clinical instability in patients.[44]

Proximal row carpectomy versus four-corner fusion

The most common motion-sparing surgeries elected over the decades of treating wrist arthritis are PRC and scaphoid excision with four-corner fusion (4CF). PRC offers the simplest motion-sparing salvage option by not requiring any fusion mass to heal, thus making it an ideal option for situations of bone loss, patients who use nicotine, or those who are immunocompromised. This pattern is suitable for arthritis patterns with preserved capitolunate and radiolunate joints, providing durable results in motion and grip.[45] Through a dorsal approach, careful excision of the scaphoid, lunate, and triquetrum allow the capitate to migrate and rest in the lunate fossa of the radius. After elevating the capsule, direct observation of the capitolunate and radiolunate joints should confirm the integrity of the chondral surfaces. Use of elevators, such as McGlamry, or similar curved broad tools aid in isolating the proximal row atraumatically. A radial styloidectomy is often included to avoid impingement at the trapezium with deviation.[46] Once the proximal row is excised, visualization and repair/imbrication of the volar radioscaphocapitate ligament has been shown to prevent ulnar translation if damaged during excision.[47]

When the capitolunate joint is degenerative but the radiolunate remains intact, a scaphoid excision with midcarpal fusion may be performed. Traditionally the lunate, capitate, hamate, and triquetrum would be fused together to form a single carpal mass.[48] This required a reasonable amount of bone preparation and fixation is pursued with pinning, headless screws, dorsal plate, or staples. Earlier studies believed this to be a more anatomic solution than a PRC because it preserved the radiolunate joint and carpal height, thus achieving greater grip strength and prolonged time to subsequent arthritis at the remaining proximal joint. Several systematic reviews,[49,50] however, showed no clear difference in grip strength or mobility after 4CF or PRC, with 70% to 75% of grip retained versus the contralateral side, and roughly 60% of normal joint motion preserved. However, there was a trend toward improved motion with the PRC. Patients reported pain relief after PRC and 4CF at nearly identical rates (84% vs 85%, respectively). Complications were notable for patients undergoing PRC developing further osteoarthritis at the radiolunate joint radiographically.[50] Saltzman and coworkers[49] demonstrated twice the complication rate with 4CF, citing nonunion at 6%, dorsal impingement at 3%, and other hardware-related problems. Rahgozar and colleagues[51] showed nearly four times rate of conversion to total wrist fusion (TWF) after partial fusion versus PRC. Currently the two procedures are performed at similar rates, most often dictated by the pattern of arthritis and patient history including nicotine use, effect of prolonged rehabilitation, patient age, and cost.

Both of these procedures have seen modifications to address unexpected variants or as simplifications. Capitolunate fusions have emerged as an alternative to 4CF, offering similar outcomes in motion and grip strength with shorter operative times, lower costs because of less hardware, and lower nonunion rates, albeit with an elevated incidence of reoperation for hardware removal because of screw migration.[52,53] Other limited intercarpal fusions may serve a particularly unique pattern but ultimately are grouped based on whether or not it remains within the proximal row of if it arrests motion through the midcarpal joint. Union rates vary depending on the particular fusion attempted but generally outcomes reflect the preservation of dart throwers motions as seen in comparisons of PRC versus 4CF.

PRC offers a shorter recovery, lower complication rate, and excellent ROM and functional outcomes, but a damaged radiolunate joint caused by early osteoarthritis can pose a risk to such reliable outcomes. Interposition of the dorsal wrist capsular tissue is performed to provide a resurfacing layer for a degenerative lunate fossa or proximal capitate. A matched cohort looked at 25 patients with capitate or lunate fossa degenerative changes and performed PRC with capsule interposition and then compared them with 50 patients undergoing PRC alone with intact lunate fossa and capitate chondral surfaces. At nearly 6 years average follow-up there were no differences between the two groups regarding the improved grip strength, ROM arc, QuickDASH, and Patient-Rated Wrist Evaluation scores.[54] A recent meta-analysis of retrospective, prospective, cross-sectional, and randomized controlled studies delved into data comparing the outcomes for 4CF and PRC.[55] No significant difference in outcomes could be found across all studies; however, there was a consistent risk of bias observed in each study. Ultimately the authors favored PRC because of its lower hardware-related complication, relative simplicity, and comparable long-term outcomes.[55]

Capitate resurfacing offers a final salvage for a failed PRC or Kienböck for which other limited arthrodeses are not favored. It addresses capitate osteoarthritis while also improving carpal height and conforming to the lunate fossa more completely.[53] There are no studies demonstrating long-term outcomes with the previously established pyrocarbon implants, and recent cobalt chrome/titanium implants have only demonstrated similar efficacy at 1 year. Capitate resurfacing does allow one further possibility to preserve motion with a PRC.

Total wrist fusion versus arthroplasty

Total wrist arthrodesis remains the ultimate salvage option for pancarpal arthritis, whether indicated initially, such as in patients with RA because of poor soft tissue stability, or as a revision to prior surgeries.[56] Popularized by Mannerfelt and Malmsten,[57] wrist arthrodesis has seen several iterations and methodologies over the years to deliver a stable radiocarpal fusion that is durable and relieving of pain. Similar to their original method, Millender and Nalebuff[58] described using a smooth Steinmann pin (rather than a Rush pin) placed retrograde through the third metacarpal and into the radial shaft to achieve fusion in patients with RA. As methods and materials have advanced, so too have outcomes. Hastings and coworkers[59] reviewed outcomes in the 1990s demonstrating high rates of fusion (98%) when using dorsal plating, but with persistently high complication rates (51%), including high rates of tendon adhesions and tenosynovitis, and one extensor rupture. Green and Henderson[60] combined a PRC with the arthrodesis, decreasing the number of fusion sites and making use of the proximal row as bone graft. They achieved high union rates with only 2 of 110 patients experiencing nonunion, but they did perform 12 plate removals with tenolysis for adhesions and contractures, attributed to their high-profile plates that extended significantly down the metacarpal shaft. Further plate developments incorporating lower profile and precontoured designs, along with locking screw technology, seem to lower hardware complication rates, but larger reviews have yet to be gathered. A recent review in 104 wrists in patients with RA reported a 98% fusion rate using a modified Clayton-Mannerfelt technique, with no hardware removals required.[61]

There is lingering controversy about the use of TWA as an alternative treatment of those patients who previously only had TWF as an option. Several generations of TWA have emerged over the years, with high rates of early complications and need for reoperation caused by instability or osteolysis/loosening.[62] Long described as an alternative to fusion in patients with RA with early devastating outcomes from underlying disease, TWA was considered only for those lowest-demand patients given the high rates of loosening and failure. Implant survival rates were 50% to 60% at 5 years and the goal of achieving success on par with large joint arthroplasty seemed to be farfetched.[63–65] As biologic medications for RA and other inflammatory arthritides have matured, the prior population of patients have dwindled and outcomes have focused on patients with posttraumatic arthritis, namely those with sequelae of a distal radius fracture, SLAC or SNAC wrist.

A 2018 metanalysis of 43 studies of TWF and TWA outcomes demonstrated incremental improvements in survivorship, stability, and functional outcomes for TWA, with higher complication rates seen in the TWA outcomes.[5] Newer fourth-generation implants had lower complication rates up to only 2.9%, reflecting similar rates as with TWF.[66] Similar but elevated rates were recently noted in a meta-analysis of 343 cases of TWF and 618 cases of TWA in patients with RA (17% vs 19%, respectively).[67] Pain relief and grip strength were improved in both groups, without adequate data to measure DASH and Patient-Rated Wrist Evaluation scores. Of note, follow-up only averaged 5.5 years in the arthroplasty group, leaving long-term effects unappreciated. This echoed a prior review by Cavaliere and Chung[68] that found similar satisfaction rates between TWA and TWF (91% vs 93%, respectively). The trend of literature reflects that TWA methods are closing in on the long-term reliability of TWF; however, many outcomes are in patients with RA with limited salvage options beyond TWF. The young, active patient or laborer remains a challenging population for TWA treatment, much like is seen in other large joint arthroplasty studies.[69,70] Although indications expand to younger and more active populations, TWA remains a choice among only a select group of hand surgeons comfortable with the technical challenges of primary and revision surgeries.

Revision of TWA has several difficulties noted, including osteolysis and loose components, fracture, and adjacent joint arthritis.[62,71] As a result, TWF, the most common revision treatment, has a higher rate of complications, notably nonunion.[62] Early attempts at implementing iliac crest graft had failed to correct nonunion rates to equal primary TWF attempts, because of the global bone loss appreciated on explant.[72,73] However, follow-up techniques using larger struts fashioned from femoral head allograft seem to offer an acceptable salvage with high rates of fusion (87% to 100%).[74–76] Adapting this technique from Carlson and Simmons,[76] Adams and coworkers[75] demonstrated union at a mean of 4 months in 19 of 20 patients by using an allograft femoral head that was contoured to re-establish carpal height while accommodating a dorsal fusion plate.

SUMMARY

Wrist arthritis is a common condition that has numerous causes and a myriad of different presentations. Because of the number of joints in the wrist, it is important to isolate the ones generating pain. Several management options exist, and the treatment should be individualized based on several factors including the patient's age, comorbidities, occupation, duration of symptoms, and failed treatment modalities. Treatment should be aimed at minimizing pain and preserving motion and function. Less-invasive options, such as arthroscopy and denervation, are appealing because of the shorter recovery time and preservation of motion, but the duration of effectiveness can vary greatly between patients. Scaphoid excision midcarpal arthrodesis and PRC are well established procedures that have shown excellent results in patients with SLAC and SNAC wrist, with comparable outcomes. Finally, patients who have failed these smaller procedures or those with pancarpal arthrosis are treated effectively with total wrist arthrodesis or even TWA in lower-demand patients.

CONFLICTS OF INTEREST

The authors report no conflicts of interest and received no funding for this study.

REFERENCES

1. Buijze GA, Lozano-Calderon SA, Strackee SD, et al. Osseous and ligamentous scaphoid anatomy: Part I. A systematic literature review highlighting controversies. J Hand Surg Am 2011;36:1926–35.
2. Laulan J, Marteau E, Bacle G. Wrist osteoarthritis. Orthop Traumatol Surg Res 2015;101:S1–9.
3. Weiss KE, Rodner CM. Osteoarthritis of the wrist. J Hand Surg Am 2007;32:725–46.
4. Catalano LW 3rd, Ryan DJ, Barron OA, et al. Surgical management of scaphotrapeziotrapezoid arthritis. J Am Acad Orthop Surg 2020;28:221–8.
5. O'Shaughnessy MA, Lewallen LW, Moran SL, et al. Dreaded ulnar wrist pain: long-term results of pisiformectomy for painful pisotriquetral arthrosis. J Surg Orthop Adv 2019;28:196–200.
6. Knirk JL, Jupiter JB. Intra-articular fractures of the distal end of the radius in young adults. J Bone Joint Surg Am 1986;68:647–59.
7. Bushnell BD, Bynum DK. Malunion of the distal radius. J Am Acad Orthop Surg 2007;15:27–40.
8. Awan HM, Waljee J. Rheumatoid arthritis and other inflammatory arthropathies. In: Weiss APC, editor. ASSH Textbook of hand and upper extremity surgery. Chicago: ASSH; 2019. p. XXX.
9. Rhee PC, Jones DB, Moran SL, et al. The effect of lunate morphology in Kienböck disease. J Hand Surg Am 2015;40(4):738–44.

10. Elhassan B, Shin AY, Alexander Y. Management of wrist arthritis secondary to advance Kienbock disease. Tech Orthop 2009;24:27–31.

11. von Unger S, Thumm N, Rodner CM. Work-up of the arthritic wrist. Tech Orthop 2009;24:2–7.

12. Becker SJE, Bot AGJ, Curley SE, et al. A prospective randomized comparison of neoprene vs thermoplast hand-based thumb spica splinting for trapeziometacarpal arthrosis. Osteoarthritis Cartilage 2013;21(5):668–75.

13. Wongrakpanich S, Wongrakpanich A, Melhado K, et al. A comprehensive review of non-steroidal anti-inflammatory drug use in the elderly. Aging Dis 2018;9(1):143.

14. Chang RW, Tompkins DM, Cohn SM. Are NSAIDs safe? Assessing the risk-benefit profile of nonsteroidal anti-inflammatory drug use in postoperative pain management. Am Surg 2021;87(6):872–9.

15. Lin J, Zhang W, Jones A, et al. Efficacy of topical non-steroidal anti-inflammatory drugs in the treatment of osteoarthritis: meta-analysis of randomised controlled trials. BMJ 2004;329(7461):324.

16. Laupattarakasem W, Laopaiboon M, Laupattarakasem P, et al. Arthroscopic debridement for knee osteoarthritis. Cochrane Database Syst Rev 2008;1. https://doi.org/10.1002/14651858.CD005118.PUB2/EPDF/ABSTRACT.

17. Kim SM, Park MJ, Kang HJ, et al. The role of arthroscopic synovectomy in patients with undifferentiated chronic monoarthritis of the wrist. J Bone Joint Surg Br 2012;94(3):353–8.

18. Berger RA. Partial denervation of the wrist: a new approach. Tech Hand Upper Extrem Surg 1998;2(1):25–35.

19. Dellon AL, Mackinnon SE, Daneshvar A. Terminal branch of anterior interosseous nerve as source of wrist pain. J Hand Surg Br 1984;9(3):316–22.

20. Wilhelm A. Zur Innervation der Gelenke der oberen Extremität. Z Anat Entwicklungsgeschichte 1958;120(5):331–71.

21. Dellon AL. Partial dorsal wrist denervation: Resection of the distal posterior interosseous nerve. J Hand Surg Am 1985;10(4):527–33.

22. Hofmeister EP, Moran SL, Shin AY. Anterior and posterior interosseous neurectomy for the treatment of chronic dynamic instability of the wrist. Hand (N Y) 2006;1(2):63.

23. Weinstein LP, Berger RA. Analgesic benefit, functional outcome, and patient satisfaction after partial wrist denervation. J Hand Surg Am 2002;27(5):833–9.

24. Kadhum M, Riley N, Furniss D. Is partial wrist denervation beneficial in chronic wrist pain? A systematic review. J Plast Reconstr Aesthet Surg 2020;73(10):1790–800.

25. Schweizer A, von Känel O, Kammer E, et al. Long-term follow-up evaluation of denervation of the wrist. J Hand Surg Am 2006 Apr;31(4):559–64.

26. O'Shaughnessy MA, Wagner ER, Berger RA, et al. Buying time: long-term results of wrist denervation and time to repeat surgery. Hand (N Y) 2019;14(5):602.

27. van Hernen JJ, Lans J, Garg R, et al. Factors associated with reoperation and conversion to wrist fusion after proximal row carpectomy or 4-corner arthrodesis. J Hand Surg Am 2020;45(2):85–94.e2.

28. Ryu J, Cooney WP, Askew LJ, et al. Functional ranges of motion of the wrist joint. J Hand Surg Am 1991;16(3):409–19.

29. McGuire D, Bain G. Radioscapholunate fusions. J Wrist Surg 2012;1(2):135–40.

30. Linscheid RL, Dobyns JH. Radiolunate arthrodesis. J Hand Surg Am 1985;10(6 Pt 1):821–9.

31. Saffar P. Radio-lunate arthrodesis for distal radial intraarticular malunion. J Hand Surg Br 1996;21(1):14–20.

32. Moritomo H, Apergis EP, Herzberg G, et al. 2007 IFSSH committee report of wrist biomechanics committee: biomechanics of the so-called dart-throwing motion of the wrist. J Hand Surg Am 2007;32(9):1447–53.

33. Brigstocke GHO, Hearnden A, Holt C, et al. In-vivo confirmation of the use of the dart thrower's motion during activities of daily living. J Hand Surg Eur 2014;39(4):373–8.

34. Edirisinghe Y, Troupis JM, Patel M, et al. Dynamic motion analysis of dart throwers motion visualized through computerized tomography and calculation of the axis of rotation. J Hand Surg Eur 2014;39(4):364–72.

35. Bain G, Sood A, Yeo C. RSL fusion with excision of distal scaphoid and triquetrum: a cadaveric study. J Wrist Surg 2014;03(01):037–41.

36. Nagy L, Büchler U. Long-term results of radioscapholunate fusion following fractures of the distal radius. J Hand Surg Br 1997;22(6):705–10.

37. Yeoh D, Tourret L. Total wrist arthroplasty: a systematic review of the evidence from the last 5 years. J Hand Surg Eur 2015;40(5):458–68.

38. McCombe D, Ireland DCR, McNab I. Distal scaphoid excision after radioscaphoid arthrodesis. J Hand Surg Am 2001;26(5):877–82.

39. Garcia-Elias M, Lluch A, Ferreres A, et al. Treatment of radiocarpal degenerative osteoarthritis by radioscapholunate arthrodesis and distal scaphoidectomy. J Hand Surg Am 2005;30(1):8–15.

40. Mühldorfer-Fodor M, Ha HP, Hohendorff B, et al. Results after radioscapholunate arthrodesis with or without resection of the distal scaphoid pole. J Hand Surg Am 2012;37(11):2233–9.

41. Crisco JJ, Coburn JC, Moore DC, et al. In vivo radiocarpal kinematics and the dart thrower's motion. J Bone Joint Surg Am 2005;87(12):2729–40.

42. Pervaiz K, Bowers WH, Isaacs JE, et al. Range of motion effects of distal pole scaphoid excision and

triquetral excision after radioscapholunate fusion: a cadaver study. J Hand Surg Am 2009;34(5):832–7.

43. Suzuki D, Omokawa S, Iida A, et al. Biomechanical effects of radioscapholunate fusion with distal scaphoidectomy and triquetrum excision on dart-throwing and wrist circumduction motions. J Hand Surg Am 2021;46(1):71.e1–7.

44. Degeorge B, Dagneaux L, Montoya-Faivre D, et al. Radioscapholunate fusion for posttraumatic osteoarthritis with consecutive excision of the distal scaphoid and the triquetrum: a comparative study. Hand Surg Rehabil 2020;39(5):375–82.

45. Ali MH, Rizzo M, Shin AY, et al. Long-term outcomes of proximal row carpectomy: a minimum of 15-year follow-up. *Hand* (NY) 2012;7(1):72–8.

46. van Rijt WG, Delnoy RE, Bonhof-Jansen EEDJ, et al. The role of routine radial styloidectomy in proximal row carpectomy: a retrospective review of 120 patients. J Hand Surg Eur 2022;47(7):705–10.

47. Wagner ER, Barras LA, Harstad C, et al. Proximal row carpectomy in young patients. JBJS Essent Surg Tech 2021;11(1):428–63.

48. Watson HK, Ballet FL. The SLAC wrist: scapholunate advanced collapse pattern of degenerative arthritis. J Hand Surg Am 1984;9(3):358–65.

49. Saltzman BM, Frank JM, Slikker W, et al. Clinical outcomes of proximal row carpectomy versus four-corner arthrodesis for post-traumatic wrist arthropathy: a systematic review. J Hand Surg Eur 2015;40(5):450–7.

50. Mulford JS, Ceulemans LJ, Nam D, et al. Proximal row carpectomy vs four corner fusion for scapholunate (SLAC) or scaphoid nonunion advanced collapse (SNAC) wrists: a systematic review of outcomes. J Hand Surg Eur 2009;34(2):256–63.

51. Rahgozar P, Zhong L, Chung KC. A comparative analysis of resource utilization between proximal row carpectomy and partial wrist fusion: a population study. J Hand Surg Am 2017;42(10):773–80.

52. Ferreres A, Garcia-Elias M, Plaza R. Long-term results of lunocapitate arthrodesis with scaphoid excision for SLAC and SNAC wrists. J Hand Surg Eur 2009;34(5):603–8.

53. Dunn JC, Polmear MM, Scanaliato JP, et al. Capitolunate arthrodesis: a systematic review. J Hand Surg Am 2020;45(4):365.e1–10.

54. Gaspar MP, Kane PM, Shin EK. Management of complications of wrist arthroplasty and wrist fusion. Hand Clin 2015;31(2):277–92.

55. Ahmadi AR, Duraku LS, van der Oest MJW, et al. The never-ending battle between proximal row carpectomy and four corner arthrodesis: a systematic review and meta-analysis for the final verdict. J Plast Reconstr Aesthet Surg 2022;75(2):711–21.

56. Wei DH, Feldon P. Total wrist arthrodesis: indications and clinical outcomes. J Am Acad Orthop Surg 2017;25(1):3–11.

57. Mannerfelt L, Malmsten M. Arthrodesis of the wrist in rheumatoid arthritis. A technique without external fixation. Scand J Plast Reconstr Surg 1971;5(2):124–30.

58. Millender LH, Nalebuff EA. Arthrodesis of the rheumatoid wrist: an evaluation of sixty patients and a description of a different surgical technique. J Bone Joint Surg Am 1973;55(5). https://journals.lww.com/jbjsjournal/Fulltext/1973/55050/Arthrodesis_of_the_Rheumatoid_Wrist__AN_EVALUATION.11.aspx.

59. Hastings H, Weiss APC, Quenzer D, et al. Arthrodesis of the wrist for post-traumatic disorders. J Bone Joint Surg Am 1996;78(6):897–902.

60. Green DP, Henderson CJ. Modified AO arthrodesis of the wrist (with proximal row carpectomy). J Hand Surg Am 2013;38(2):388–91.

61. Kluge S, Schindele S, Henkel T, et al. The modified Clayton-Mannerfelt arthrodesis of the wrist in rheumatoid arthritis: operative technique and report on 93 cases. J Hand Surg Am 2013;38(5):999–1005.

62. Berber O, Garagnani L, Gidwani S. Systematic review of total wrist arthroplasty and arthrodesis in wrist arthritis. J Wrist Surg 2018;07(05):424–40.

63. Logan JS, Warwick D. The treatment of arthritis of the wrist. Bone and Joint Journal 2015;97-B(10):1303–8.

64. Ward CM, Kuhl T, Adams BD. Five to ten-year outcomes of the universal total wrist arthroplasty in patients with rheumatoid arthritis. J Bone Joint Surg Am 2011;93(10):914–9.

65. Chevrollier J, Strugarek-leCoanet C, Dap F, et al. Results of a unicentric series of 15 wrist prosthesis implantations at a 5.2 year follow-up. Acta Orthop Belg 2016;82(1):31–42.

66. Fischer P, Sagerfors M, Jakobsson H, et al. Total wrist arthroplasty: a 10-year follow-up. J Hand Surg Am 2020 Aug;45(8):780.e1–10.

67. Zhu XM, Perera E, Gohal C, et al. A systematic review of outcomes of wrist arthrodesis and wrist arthroplasty in patients with rheumatoid arthritis. J Hand Surg Eur 2021;46(3):297–303.

68. Cavaliere CM, Chung KC. A systematic review of total wrist arthroplasty compared with total wrist arthrodesis for rheumatoid arthritis. Plast Reconstr Surg 2008;122(3):813–25.

69. Kuijpers MFL, Hannink G, van Steenbergen LN, et al. Outcome of revision hip arthroplasty in patients younger than 55 years: an analysis of 1,037 revisions in the Dutch Arthroplasty Register. Acta Orthop 2020;91(2):165.

70. Walker-Santiago R, Tegethoff JD, Ralston WM, et al. Revision total knee arthroplasty in young patients: higher early reoperation and rerevision. J Arthroplasty 2021;36(2):653–6.

71. Wagner ER, Srnec JJ, Fort MW, et al. Outcomes of revision total wrist arthroplasty. J Am Acad Orthop Surg Glob Res Rev 2021;5(3). https://doi.org/10.5435/JAAOSGlobal-D-21-00035.

72. Rizzo M, Ackerman DB, Rodrigues RL, et al. Wrist arthrodesis as a salvage procedure for failed implant arthroplasty. J Hand Surg Eur 2011;36(1): 29–33.

73. Beer TA, Turner RH. Wrist arthrodesis for failed wrist implant arthroplasty. J Hand Surg Am 1997;22(4): 685–93.

74. Zijlker HJA, Fakkert RK, Beumer A, et al. Comparative outcomes of total wrist arthrodesis for salvage of failed total wrist arthroplasty and primary wrist arthrodesis. J Hand Surg Eur 2022;47(3):302.

75. Adams BD, Kleinhenz BP, Guan JJ. Wrist arthrodesis for failed total wrist arthroplasty. J Hand Surg 2016;41(6):673–9.

76. Carlson JR, Simmons BP. Wrist arthrodesis after failed wrist implant arthroplasty. J Hand Surg 1998; 23(5):893–8.

Management of Complex Hand and Wrist Ligament Injuries

Hannah C. Langdell, MD[a], Gloria X. Zhang, BS[b], Tyler S. Pidgeon, MD[b], David S. Ruch, MD[a], Christopher S. Klifto, MD[b], Suhail K. Mithani, MD[a,b,*]

KEYWORDS

- Ligament injury • Ulnar collateral ligament • Radial collateral ligament • Hand • Wrist • Thumb
- Scapholunate • Skier's thumb

KEY POINTS

- Treatment of thumb collateral ligament injuries depends on instability grading. Nondisplaced or minimally displaced avulsion fractures can be treated with conservative measures.
- Finger collateral ligament injuries remain underreported but typically can be managed conservatively. Options for repair and reconstruction using tendon grafts can be considered for chronic injuries.
- Treatment of scapholunate interosseous ligament (SLIL) injuries depends on the degree of scapholunate instability, portion of the SLIL torn, chronicity of the injury, and reducibility of the deformity.

INTRODUCTION

Ligamentous injuries are commonly seen in the hand and wrist. Timely recognition of the injury and adequate repair or reconstruction are critical in restoring joint stability and mobility. In the United States, upper extremity injuries represented more than 3,468,996 emergency department visits in 2009, whereas injuries to the fingers and wrist represented 38.4% and 15.3% of the population, respectively.[1] Incidence of upper extremity ligamentous injuries remains underreported but estimates range from 17.87 per 100,000 persons for forearm and hand extensor tendons, 9.89 per 100,000 for mallet fingers, and 3.42 per 100,000 for ulnar collateral ligament (UCL) injuries, with a greater prevalence in men than in women.[2,3] The scapholunate interosseous ligament (SLIL) is a commonly injured wrist ligament.[4] Although the incidence of this injury is unknown, in a cadaveric study, up to 35% of the wrists had at least a partial SLIL tear.[5] Other common ligamentous injuries

include thumb ulnar and radial collateral ligament tears,[3] which can result in instability of the metacarpophalangeal joint (MCPJ). The thumb UCL injury is particularly common with an incidence of 50 per 100,000.[6]

Injuries to the thumb MCPJ and SLIL are common in young, active adults.[4] This population represents a challenge for repairs and reconstructions as young individuals tend to place a high biomechanical demand on the thumb and wrist joint. These are complex injuries that often are undiagnosed at the time of the initial visit. Furthermore, there is controversy regarding the most appropriate management algorithm. Surgeons must consider a wide range of nonoperative and operative techniques that will allow for the greatest degree of satisfactory range of motion and strength. Incomplete resolution of symptoms from thumb UCL/radial collateral ligament (RCL) tears may lead to decreased thumb pinch and grasp strength while SLIL injuries may lead to carpal instability and severe osteoarthritis.

[a] Division of Plastic and Reconstructive Surgery, Duke University Medical Center, Durham, NC, USA;
[b] Department of Orthopedic Surgery, Duke University Medical Center, Durham, NC, USA
* Corresponding author. North Carolina Orthopaedic Clinic, 3609 Southwest Durham Drive, Durham, NC 27707.
E-mail address: suhail.mithani@duke.edu

Hand Clin 39 (2023) 367–377
https://doi.org/10.1016/j.hcl.2023.03.002
0749-0712/23/

The purpose of this review is to provide an overview of the MCPJ, SLIL, and non-SLIL carpal ligament anatomy, diagnosis, imaging, treatment consideration and options, as well as surgical techniques encompassing repair, reconstruction, and fusion.

THUMB METACARPOPHALANGEAL JOINT LIGAMENTOUS INJURIES
Anatomy and Etiology

In addition to the volar plate and dorsal capsule, the UCL and RCL are important static stabilizers of the thumb MCPJ. Both the UCL and RCL consist of a proper and accessory collateral ligament. The proper collateral ligament runs in a dorsal to volar trajectory from the metacarpal head to the base of the proximal phalanx. The accessory collateral ligament inserts on the volar aspect of the proximal phalanx and volar plate and is volar to the proper collateral ligament. The UCL is critical for grip strength, pinch, and stability of the MCPJ. Additionally, both the UCL and RCL help provide dorsal support to the MCPJ.

Mechanisms of thumb UCL injuries typically involve forced abduction, rotation, or hyperextension.[7] Thus, UCL injuries are commonly called skier's thumb because skiers often place their thumbs at risk for forced radial deviation. The distal insertion of the UCL at the proximal phalanx is the most common region for injuries but tears can involve the dorsal capsule, palmar plate, and adductor aponeurosis.[7,8] Typical fracture patterns include avulsion of the ulnar base of proximal phalanx, which have a reported frequency of 20% to 30%.[9] An additional 64% to 87% of complete UCL injuries are associated with Stener lesions,[10] which occur when the UCL dislocates over the aponeurosis of the adductor pollicis, often with a bone fragment from its distal insertion attached. The interposition of the adductor between the torn collateral ligament and its insertion can prevent healing and is therefore associated with a poorer prognosis without surgical intervention. In contrast to UCL injuries, RCL injuries may occur in variable locations with reports in the proximal area encompassing 55% of patients, distal area 29%, and midsubstance 16%.[11]

Diagnosis and Imaging

On clinical examination, patients with acute collateral ligament injuries may present with pain, swelling, ecchymosis, and decreased range of motion. Patients with acute injuries will likely have pain to palpation over the ulnar or radial aspect of the MCPJ. The clinician should attempt to palpate a Stener lesion in suspected UCL injuries, although inability to palpate the lesion does not preclude its presence. In more chronic injuries, patients may complain of decreased grip strength or weakened grasp. A complete tear can be diagnosed on stressed radiographs if the proximal phalanx of the thumb is angulated 30° to 35° with the MCPJ fully extended, which tests the accessory collateral ligament, or at 30° of flexion, which tests the proper collateral ligament.[12] Alternatively, a diagnosis of collateral ligament tear can be made if there is no firm end point or angulation of greater than 15° compared with the contralateral side. Concomitant injury to the dorsal capsule and volar plate may result in radiographic evidence of volar radial subluxation of the proximal phalanx due to the pull of the abductor pollicis brevis muscle. Given that stressing the MCPJ in an acute injury is often painful and can lead to guarding or muscle spasm, it is possible to have a false-negative examination. Performing the examination under local anesthesia has been shown to increase the accuracy of the clinical diagnosis from 28% to 98% in a study of 47 patients.[13]

Although radiographs are the initial imaging of choice when collateral ligament injuries are suspected, advanced imaging may be needed to confirm the diagnosis if the clinical examination is uncertain or to distinguish between nondisplaced and displaced injuries.[7] Use of ultrasound or MRI has been used to help identify UCL and RCL injuries. A prospective trial of ultrasound versus MRI found that both had a sensitivity of 65%.[14] In the presence of a Stener lesion, MRI was found to have a sensitivity of 73%, whereas ultrasound had a sensitivity of 36%.[14] However, other reports in the literature show ultrasound to be an accurate tool in identifying displaced UCL tears with an overall sensitivity of 76% and specificity of 81%.[15] A systematic review found that when compared with ultrasound, MRI had a higher specificity for displaced UCL tears (92%) and greater specificity for diagnosis of UCL tears (100%).[16] Thus, both ultrasound and MRI are reliable tools for ruling out UCL tears but MRI is superior to ultrasound when differentiating displaced versus nondisplaced UCL tears.[16]

Classification

Thumb UCL and RCL injuries can be divided into 3 grades.[17] Grade I is defined as an incomplete ligament tear with tenderness along the collateral ligament without laxity to stress. Grade II is defined by a greater number of torn fibers but remains an incomplete tear. On clinical examination, the pain and swelling are more significant, and patients will have laxity under stress but with a discernible end point. A Grade III tear is defined as a complete tear of the ligament, with significant pain, swelling, and increased laxity without an end point.

Approach to Management

Treatment of collateral ligament injuries depends on instability grading. For stable collateral ligament tears (Grade I and II) that are nondisplaced, or minimally displaced avulsion fractures, conservative treatment with functional bracing, casting, or splinting are typically used for 4 to 6 weeks.[18] Grip and pinch strengthening exercises may begin after 6 weeks.[12] Nonsteroidal anti-inflammatory drugs and steroid injections should be used with caution because they may suppress the prostaglandin-based inflammatory cascade that promotes ligament healing. Similarly, steroid injections have been shown to be effective with pain in the acute period of 6 to 8 weeks but may cause collagen breakdown at the injection site and ultimately hinder ligament healing. Conservative treatment has been shown to be effective in injuries without significant laxity or disability. However, patients that fail conservative treatment report persistent pain, decreased pinch strength, limited range of motion, continued instability, and early arthrosis.[19]

There are many surgical options for Grade III UCL injures depending on the chronicity of the injury. Indications for surgical intervention include the presence of gross instability with joint subluxation, Stener lesions, or displaced avulsion fractures.[20] Techniques to repair the UCL include pullout suture over button with or without Kirschner wire (K-wire) immobilization, suture anchors, soft tissue periosteal suture, and arthroscopic Stener reduction with K-wire fixation.[21] One study reported that the use of suture anchors had shorter surgical times, fewer soft-tissue complications, and overall lower cost compared with a pullout suture.[22] Additionally, UCL repair to the adductor or the periosteum has been described.[23] A newer option to augment the repair is the use of suture tape. Biomechanical studies have shown a higher load to failure when using suture tape augmentation compared with UCL repair alone.[24] Furthermore, in a study of 17 competitive athletes with acute UCL injuries treated with primary repair via suture tape augmentation, all returned to their previous level of play, and no postoperative complications were reported.[25]

In chronic UCL injuries in which the ligament is attenuated and not able to be repaired, autograft tendon is often used. Typically, the palmaris longus is used as the graft material but other materials such as half of the flexor carpi radialis or the fourth toe extensor can be used.[9] Glickel and colleagues performed reconstruction with a palmaris longus graft by using a bone tunnel in the metacarpal and the proximal phalanx.[26] Breek and colleagues report the use of a free tendon graft in 70 patients to repair collateral ligament injuries.[27] They report excellent patient satisfaction and normal grip strength in 48 patients. Approximately a third of patients had decreased flexion and extension but none of the patients reported any significant disability. Additionally, a previous systematic review of 293 thumb UCL injuries showed that both acute repair and delayed reconstruction have excellent functional outcomes and similar rates of complications and failures.[21]

Operative management is often considered for Grade III RCL injuries as various authors have argued that the unopposed ulnar deviation of the proximal phalanx from the adductor pollicis or extensor pollicis longus will cause the RCL to heal in an incompetent manner.[28] Lack of treatment in the acute period may lead to complications such as chronic pain, swelling, joint instability, and lack of preoperative function. Repair of the RCL in the acute period has thus been suggested to allow for greater anatomic healing and stability to the MCPJ. RCL repair is similar to UCL repair in that both pullout sutures and suture anchors are used. Techniques for RCL reconstruction in the setting of chronic injuries include repair to the bone on the radial side, distal advancement of the abductor pollicis brevis tendon, tendon graft reconstruction, and repair of the abductor aponeurosis.[29] Other methods of reconstruction described in the literature include the reconstruction of the volar capsule and radial collateral ligament by using the extensor pollicis brevis tendon.[30] Although the use of pinning is not typically performed in UCL repairs unless the reduction using soft tissue repair is inadequate or there is an avulsion fragment needing fixation, in RCL injuries, there have been some reports of pinning the MCPJ particularly when there is volar subluxation.[31] Overall, when assessing the results of repair versus reconstruction for Grade III tears of the RCL, Catalano and colleagues found no statistically significant difference in MCP or interphalangeal joint motion, grip or pinch strength, and MCPJ stability between the 2 groups.[32]

FINGER LIGAMENT INJURIES
Anatomy and Etiology

Injuries to the finger MCPJ collateral ligaments are rare compared with thumb injuries and are underreported in the literature. Ligamentous injuries in the hand have been estimated at an incidence of 1 in 1000 hand injuries with 61% in the thumb and the remaining 39% occurring within the fingers.[33] The most common mechanism of injury to the collateral ligament of the fingers occurs when a laterally directed force is directed to a finger with some degree of flexion.[33] Radial and UCL injuries occur in equal distributions within the fingers; however, radial collateral injuries are more common in the ring and small fingers while ulnar collateral injuries have been more commonly reported in the index finger.[34] The RCL of the index finger is thicker and wider compared with the index UCL and plays a large role in resisting ulnarly directed forces, whereas the UCL contributes more toward extension and flexion.[35] As the collateral ligaments serve as the primary stabilizers allowing for abduction and adduction,[36] untreated injuries may result in decreased pinch strength and joint instability.

Diagnosis and Imaging

Diagnosis of finger collateral injuries is primarily clinical; however, the use of arthrograms has been advocated for diagnosis and surgical planning.[37] Clinically, patients may present with tenderness at the base of the finger with laxity of the MCPJ. Radiographs may show osteochondral avulsion of the proximal phalanx or metacarpal head.[38] Because the collateral ligaments help provide stability to the MCPJ, physical examination maneuvers include lateral stress testing of the first phalanx on the metacarpal bone while the hand is in full flexion.

Classification

Previously reported classification systems for collateral ligament injuries to the PIP joint and the thumb MCPJ RCL have also been used in describing collateral injuries to the fingers.[39] Classification is divided into 3 grades. Grade I is defined as tenderness over the joint but with no significant laxity when compared with the contralateral side. Grade II injuries are described a greater laxity compared with the contralateral side but with a defined end point. Grade III injuries are defined as having no defined end point in terms of laxity.

Approach to Management

Although collateral ligamentous injuries to the fingers are relatively rare, the presence of joint instability and gross pain are advocated as markers for surgical repair or reconstruction. Nonoperative treatment remains understudied. However, one author proposed an algorithm in which Grade I injuries with no laxity can be managed using buddy taping and splinting.[39] Grade II injuries may similarly be managed nonoperatively with 3 weeks of immobilization followed by 3 weeks of splinting with the potential for surgical intervention. The authors advocate that for Grade III injuries, early repair of the ligament is recommended using methods such as suture anchors. Outcomes with early repair have been favorable,[34,37,40] with one study reporting 10 patients with full MCP collateral ligament ruptures in the fingers regaining full mobility within 10.7 weeks with no complications at the 2-year mark.[41] However, chronic injuries (4–6 weeks) to the collateral ligaments have shown variable results with repair or reconstruction,[37,42] with some reports of MPJ fusion needed for persistent pain and stiffness. Reconstruction options including tendon repair have been reported using the flexor digitorum superficialis tendon or palmaris longus with good results but literature on outcomes remains low.[43–45]

SCAPHOLUNATE INTEROSSEOUS LIGAMENT INJURIES
Anatomy and Etiology

The SLIL complex has both extrinsic and intrinsic components and provides stability to the carpal bones of the wrist. The intrinsic component, the SLIL itself, is a C-shaped ligament that has 3 distinct segments: the dorsal, volar, and proximal ligaments.[46] The dorsal component is primarily composed of strong transverse fibers in parallel that provides most of tensile strength and resistance to rotation. Similarly, the volar component is comparable in length and width to the dorsal component but is half the thickness and is composed of oblique fibers that help with rotation in the sagittal plane. The proximal component differs from both the dorsal and volar components because it is primarily composed of anisotropic fibrocartilage and has very little strength or blood supply; thus, it is common to see degenerative tears.[4] The extrinsic ligaments of the wrist are composed of the volar radioscaphocapitate ligament, long radiolunate ligament (LRL), and the short radiolunate ligament.[47]

Injuries to the SLIL can result in dynamic SLIL dissociation (gaps), carpal collapse, and scapholunate advanced collapse of the wrist (commonly known as SLAC wrist). However, many injuries to the SLIL are undiagnosed at time of injury because it takes 3 to 12 months after a traumatic event for instability and dissociation to be seen on routine radiographs.[48] Thus, mechanisms of SLIL injury remain largely unknown. The most cited mechanism of SLIL rupture is a fall onto the hypothenar eminence while the wrist is simultaneously in extension, ulnar deviation, and midcarpal supination.[49] In this position, the capitate may intrude into the scapholunate articulation. Thus, a high degree of suspicion is required to diagnose SLIL injuries after falls on an outstretched wrist. Reports in the literature show that 5% of all wrist sprains have an associated SLIL tear and can often be associated with distal radius fractures, scaphoid fractures, and other ligamentous injuries.[50–52]

The role of the scapholunate interosseous, dorsal intercarpal, and radiolunate ligaments has been explored in wrist biomechanical studies. Although SLIL rupture is the most common, SLIL injuries can be further compounded by injuries to the dorsal intercarpal (DIC) ligament and LRL. One study found that injury to the SLIL alone did not result in changes to wrist range of motion (ROM) while injury to the SLIL, DIC ligament, and LRL caused significant changes in radial deviation, radial extension, and ulnar flexion.[53] Similarly, a prospective in vivo study found that in 85 cases of wrist pain with SL instability, a lesion to the SLIL was associated with lesions to the LRL, radioscaphocapitate, scaphotrapezial, and dorsal intercarpal ligaments.[54] Thus, injuries to the extrinsic ligaments are often associated with intrinsic ligamentous injuries and contribute to carpal instability.[55]

Diagnosis and Imaging

For SLIL injuries, patients may present on clinical examination with symptoms of pain, snapping, clicking, or grinding when loading the affected wrist. Tenderness to palpation may localize to the dorsal aspect of the SLIL distal to Lister tubercle. Examination may show decreased grip strength and range of motion. A positive Watson's scaphoid test may also be a sign of a complete SL tear.[48] In this maneuver, the examiner applies dorsally directed pressure on the scaphoid tubercle and ranges the wrist from ulnar deviation to radial deviation. Application of dorsal pressure will subluxate the scaphoid onto the radius if the SLIL is torn, resulting in a painful clunk. However, rates of false positives are high, and clinical examination should be followed with imaging.

Imaging in suspected SLIL tears can be helpful in timely recognition of these injuries. Radiographs with PA, lateral, AP clenched fist, and scaphoid views can potentially show signs of scapholunate instability and dissociation but small differences in wrist positions may change radiographic measurements. Additionally, there is significant variability in what defines an abnormal scapholunate interval. One study found that when set at 2.5 mm, the

sensitivity for identifying an SLIL lesion was 60% while specificity was 75%.[56] Other methods of visualization include MRI and diagnostic arthroscopy. Wrist MRI has been shown to have a sensitivity of 59% to 79% and specificity ranging from 32% to 88%.[57] Using magnetic resonance arthrography had even greater diagnostic accuracy for the detection of partial tears, with an accuracy of 91.7%.[58] Diagnostic arthroscopy can also be used in the diagnosis of acute and chronic SLIL tears and has the advantage of being a diagnostic and treatment tool.

Classification

The degree of severity for SLIL injuries can be classified using the Geissler methodology, which divides ligament injuries into 4 grades based on arthroscopic findings.[47] Grade I is defined as the presence of attenuation and or hemorrhage of the interosseous ligament observed from the radiocarpal space. There is no incongruence of carpal alignment in the midcarpal space. Grade II is similarly defined as the presence of attenuation and or hemorrhage of the interosseous ligament observed from the radiocarpal space but with incongruence or step-off in the midcarpal space. A small gap less than 2 mm between the carpal bones may also be present. Grade III is defined as incongruence and or step-off present in both the radiocarpal and midcarpal space. There is a gap of greater than 2 mm between the carpal bone. Grade IV is similarly defined as incongruence and or step-off present in both the radiocarpal and midcarpal space but with gross instability. An arthroscope of 2.7 mm can be passed through the gap in the carpal bones.

The Geissler classification is often combined with a series of questions proposed by Garcia-Elias, which aims to grade SLIL injury severity and treatment options.[59] Garcia-Elias propose 5 prognostic factors to consider when evaluating SLIL injuries: (1) the integrity of the dorsal SL ligament, (2) the healing potential of the disrupted ligaments, (3) the status of the secondary scaphoid stabilizers, (4) the reducibility of the carpal malalignment, and (5) the cartilage status. The answers to these can then be used to divide scapholunate injuries into 6 grades with stage 1 being partial SLIL injury, stage 2 as complete disruption with repairable ligament, stage 3 as complete disruption with irreparable ligament but normal alignment, stage 4 as complete disruption with irreparable ligament and reducible rotary subluxation of the scaphoid, stage 5 as complete disruption with irreducible malalignment and intact cartilage, and stage 6 as chronic SLIL disruption with cartilage loss (SLAC).

Approach to Management

Treatment of SLIL injuries depends on the degree of scapholunate instability, chronicity of the injury, and reducibility of the deformity. The appropriate treatment algorithm remains controversial because there is debate as to whether certain surgical interventions improve long-term functional outcomes or prevent the rate of progression of osteoarthritis.[46] Nonsurgical intervention with cast immobilization is recommended immediately after an acute injury; however, patients with symptomatic, complete SLIL injuries should be offered surgical management.[46]

Overall, there is an underreporting of partial SLIL injuries but small cohorts of studies have reported the use of arthroscopic debridement for symptom resolution. Ruch and Poehling reported a series of 14 patients with isolated partial scapholunate and lunotriquetral ligament injuries and showed that 11 patients had complete resolution of symptoms and were able to return to work by postoperative week 7.[60] There was no statistically significant reduction in either grip or pinch strength. Similarly, Weiss and colleagues examined the role of arthroscopic debridement alone for both complete and incomplete intercarpal ligament tears of the wrist and showed that 85% of wrists with partial SLIL tears had complete symptom resolution.[61] Grip strength similarly improved by 23% postoperatively.

Arthroscopic debridement was found to have similarly favorable outcomes in children and adolescents with partial SLIL tears (Geissler Grade II and III) that had failed nonoperative treatment. The authors reported an improvement in Mayo wrist scores from 66.3 to 91.6 at 43 months of follow-up.[62] Children with Grade III tears eventually required reoperation. Nonetheless, in the management of partial SLIL tears, arthroscopic debridement is an appropriate option because it results in high rates of symptomatic relief in Geissler I and II injuries.

Acute injuries to the SLIL are defined as occurring within 2 to 3 weeks from injury[4] and most commonly involve avulsion of the ligament off the scaphoid. With timely surgery, the ligament is typically amenable to direct repair with suture anchors. To perform a repair, the SLIL interval should be easily reducible with 0.045 K-wires. Bickert and colleagues used a technique involving suture anchors and showed that of the 12 patients that underwent SLIL repair, 8 patients had excellent or good functional outcomes.[63] They determined that 10 of the 12 patients had stable SL ligaments by examining normal rotation behavior at the scaphoid and lunate with stable angles and intervals.

An SLIL repair may be augmented with a capsulodesis procedure. Capsulodesis procedures aim to anchor the scaphoid to prevent abnormal flexion but do not address abnormalities with lunate extension of the scapholunate gap. In the Blatt capsulodesis, a flap of dorsal capsule and dorsal radiocarpal ligament are sutured to the distal pole of the scaphoid. Although this maneuver does help prevent scaphoid flexion, there is a decrease in wrist ROM.[64] Minami and colleagues describe the use of a modified dorsal capsulodesis combined with ligamentous repair of scapholunate dissociation.[65] The authors found that compared with SLIL repair alone, there was a better maintenance of the SL angle (average of 49°) with the addition of a dorsal capsulodesis. However, Pomerance found that in a cohort of 17 patients with 66 months follow-up, there was deterioration of clinical and function outcomes in patients who had high physical demand placed on the wrist on a daily basis.[66] Additionally, there was persistent instability radiographically. Thus, the author suggests that direct repair with additional dorsal capsulodesis may be an insufficient repair option for patients who place high demands on the wrists.[66] The Mayo capsulodesis builds on the Blatt technique and tries to reduce the tether crossing the radiocarpal joint. In this technique, a strip of dorsal intercarpal ligament that originates from the trapezoid is sutured to the distal scaphoid.[67] Szabo described a case report using direct repair with dorsal intercarpal ligament capsulodesis for a patient with open transstyloid perilunate fracture dislocation.[68] The patient was able to maintain an SL angle of 49° and a 2-mm scapholunate gap with good functional results 1 year postoperatively.[68] After repair, the carpal bones can be stabilized with K-wires for 8 to 12 weeks or with an intercarpal screw for 6 to 9 months. Overall, primary repair of the SLIL with capsulodesis has shown variable results with up to 78% of patients having radiographic evidence of arthritis at 8-year follow-up.[69]

There are various reconstruction options for sub-acute or chronic SLIL tears in which there is an irreparable ligament but a reducible deformity. At this point, the secondary scaphoid stabilizers are intact and may provide additional support to prevent rotational subluxation. Weiss and colleagues describe the design of a bone-reticulum-bone-graft to reconstruct a complete tear of the SLIL.[70] They report a series of 13 patients with 100% satisfaction and return to former work activities. In the group with dynamic instability, 12 patients had resolution of pain and 2 had pain with heavy activities. Grip strength improved by an average of 46%. In the group with static instability, 2 patients had resolution of pain, 1 with heavy activity, and 2 with constant pain. Grip strength improved by 30%. The use of a bone-retinaculum-bone graft was thus a suitable option for patients with dynamic stability but showed inconsistent results within the static instability group. Other reconstruction options include the use of a dorsal-medial navicular first cuneiform ligament graft from the foot as well as distal radius bone-retinaculum-bone-constructs.[71] Improvement in short-term symptom relief is noted but has shown persistent radiographic irregularities over time. Arthroscopic debridement with pinning has also been described in patients with Geissler Grade III and IV tears. However, the results have been suboptimal to date and have been reported only in small cohorts of patients. The authors described a cohort with 11 patients where 3 patients required revision procedures due to failure and 8 patients reported good to excellent Mayo scores.[72] However, none of the patients showed deterioration to static instability, and there was no evidence of dorsal intercalated segment instability.

Tendon weaving procedures, such as the Brunelli tenodesis,[73] are another reliable option in cases of chronic ligamentous injures with an irreparable ligament. Tendon-weaving procedures aim to decrease motion across the scaphoid. Brunelli and colleagues describe a technique in which the tendon of the flexor carpi radialis is threaded in a tunnel in the distal scaphoid and then attached to the distal radius and lunate.[73] A modification to the Brunelli technique has been reported by performing a triligament tenodesis using the flexor carpi radialis tendon and passing it through the scaphoid to recreate the dorsal radiotriquetral ligament, scaphotrapeziotrapezoid joint, and SLILs.[59] Overall, tendon-weaving techniques using the Brunelli method have shown improvement in functional outcomes and pain relief in the short term but inferior function compared with the contralateral side. Furthermore, radiographic outcomes show evidence of deterioration over time.[74] A tendon-weaving procedure using the extensor carpi radialis brevis has also been described in which the tendon is passed through the scaphoid, lunate, capitate, and distal radius.[75]

There are many other methods that have been used to reconstruct the SLIL. In the RASL (reduction and association of the scaphoid and lunate) procedure, a compression screw is placed across the scaphoid and lunate in order to create a fibrous nonunion. Although the procedure has been shown to improve patients' pain, several studies report unfavorable outcomes such as decreased ROM, hardware loosening, and the development of arthritic changes.[76,77]

The palmaris longus tendon graft has been used to reconstruct the ligament with suture anchors and has shown acceptable results in terms of patient satisfaction, return to work, and ROM at 4-year follow-up.[78] Finally, the use of an internal brace to reconstruct the dorsal SLIL is gaining in popularity and can be augmented with tendon grafts.[79]

Treatment of irreducible injuries can pose difficulties. In Grade 5 lesions in which the cartilage is still intact, it may be possible to aggressively release the soft tissue and mobilize scar tissue around the scaphoid and lunate enough to reduce the deformity.[4] However, few results have been published about this stage of injury and careful preoperative counseling is needed before attempting a reduction. Surgeons may consider proceeding to salvage procedures similar to the treatment of Grade 6 injuries. In cases of chronic injuries in which there is degenerative cartilage or if there is progression of arthritis after repair or reconstruction, salvage procedures are commonly needed. Treatments for SLAC wrist include neurectomies, partial row carpectomy (PRC), scaphoidectomy with 4-corner fusion, and total wrist arthrodesis depending on the extent of arthritis. Total wrist denervation involves dividing a total of 10 nerve branches including the anterior interosseous nerve (AIN), the posterior interosseous nerve (PIN), the superficial sensory branch of the radial nerve, as well as branches of the median and ulnar nerves while partial wrist denervation involves dividing the AIN and PIN.[80] Both have been successful in treating wrist pain and may be combined with other salvage procedures.[81] PRC and scaphoidectomy with 4-corner fusion are the 2 main operations for SLAC wrist. Both require an intact radiolunate articulation, and a PRC traditionally requires a normal head of the capitate. In general, both surgeries result in a wrist flexion-extension arc of approximately 70° to 80° and grip strength of 70% to 75% compared with the contralateral hand.[48] Thus, both options should be considered in SLAC wrist with a preference for PRC in patients at risk for nonunion such as smokers.[82] Other salvage operations or adjunctive procedures include radial styloidectomy with scaphocapitate arthrodesis, scaphoidectomy with capitolunate arthrodesis, PRC with osteochondral resurfacing in cases of capitate arthrosis, and PRC with capsular interposition with or without leveling of the proximal end of the capitate.[82]

SUMMARY

Ligamentous injuries in the hand and wrist present a significant challenge to patients and clinicians.

Optimal treatment relies on a combination prompt diagnosis of the injury and a patient-centered discussion of the various nonoperative and surgical options. More robust long-term outcome data for UCL/RCL and SLIL injuries are needed to evaluate treatment decision-making strategies and algorithms.

CLINICS CARE POINTS

- Since ligamentous injuries are often missed, clinicians must maintain a high index of suspension and utilize stress radiographs and MRI to confirm the diagnosis and guide treatment.
- Use of suture tape can be considered to augment the primary repair of acute, complete thumb UCL injuries.
- Chronic UCL and RCL injuries can be treated with tendon graft reconstruction with excellent functional outcomes.
- Performing a dorsal capsulodesis after repair of the SLL with suture anchors may help prevent scaphoid flexion, but direct repair should only be attempted if the SLL interval is easily reducible.
- In cases of an irreparable SLL but a reducible deformity, tendon weaving procedures, compression screws, or tendon grafts can reliably treat patients' pain with but mixed with long-term results.

DISCLOSURES

Dr S.K. Mithani reports the following relationships and activities: Integra LifeScience (Paid presenter or speaker), and Tissium (Paid consultant). Dr D.S. Ruch reports the following relationships and activities: Acumed, LLC (IP royalties, paid presenter or speaker), and American Society for Surgery of the Hand (Board or committee member). Dr C.S. Klifto reports the following relationships and activities: Acumed, LLC (Paid consultant), GE Healthcare (Stock or stock options), Johnson & Johnson (Stock or stock options), Merck (Stock or stock options), Pfizer (Stock or stock options), Restore3d (Paid consultant), and Smith & Nephew (Paid consultant).

REFERENCES

1. Ootes D, Lambers KT, Ring DC. The Epidemiology of Upper Extremity Injuries Presenting to the Emergency Department in the United States. HAND 2011;7(1):18–22.

2. Taylor KF, Lanzi JT, Cage JM, et al. Radial Collateral Ligament Injuries of the Thumb Metacarpophalangeal Joint: Epidemiology in a Military Population. J Hand Surg 2013;38(3):532–6.

3. Clayton RAE, Court-Brown CM. The epidemiology of musculoskeletal tendinous and ligamentous injuries. Injury 2008;39(12):1338–44.

4. Pappou IP, Basel J, Deal DN. Scapholunate ligament injuries: a review of current concepts. Hand (N Y). 2013;8(2):146–56.

5. Lee DH, Dickson KF, Bradley EL. The incidence of wrist interosseous ligament and triangular fibrocartilage articular disc disruptions: a cadaveric study. J Hand Surg Am 2004;29(4):676–84.

6. Jones MH, England SJ, Muwanga CL, et al. The use of ultrasound in the diagnosis of injuries of the ulnar collateral ligament of the thumb. J Hand Surg Br 2000;25(1):29–32.

7. Stener B. Skeletal injuries associated with rupture of the ulnar collateral ligament of the metacarpophalangeal joint of the thumb. A clinical and anatomical study. Acta Chir Scand 1963;125:583–6.

8. Kaplan EB. The pathology and treatment of radial subluxation of the thumb with ulnar displacement of the head of the first metacarpal. J Bone Joint Surg Am 1961;43-a:541–6.

9. Tsiouri C, Hayton MJ, Baratz M. Injury to the ulnar collateral ligament of the thumb. Hand (N Y). 2009; 4(1):12–8.

10. Mahajan M, Rhemrev SJ. Rupture of the ulnar collateral ligament of the thumb - a review. Int J Emerg Med 2013;6(1):31.

11. Coyle MP Jr. Grade III radial collateral ligament injuries of the thumb metacarpophalangeal joint: treatment by soft tissue advancement and bony reattachment. J Hand Surg Am 2003;28(1):14–20.

12. Tang P. Collateral Ligament Injuries of the Thumb Metacarpophalangeal Joint. JAAOS - Journal of the American Academy of Orthopaedic Surgeons. 2011;19(5).

13. Cooper JG, Johnstone AJ, Hider P, et al. Local anaesthetic infiltration increases the accuracy of assessment of ulnar collateral ligament injuries. Emerg Med Australas 2005;17(2):132–6.

14. Hamborg-Petersen E, Torfing T, Viberg B. The value of magnetic resonance imaging and ultrasound in diagnosing displaced rupture of the thumb ulnar collateral ligament. J Hand Surg 2020;45(10):1098–100.

15. Papandrea RF, Fowler T. Injury at the thumb UCL: is there a Stener lesion? J Hand Surg Am 2008;33(10): 1882–4.

16. Rashidi A, Haj-Mirzaian A, Dalili D, et al. Evidence-based use of clinical examination, ultrasonography, and MRI for diagnosing ulnar collateral ligament tears of the metacarpophalangeal joint of the thumb: systematic review and meta-analysis. Eur Radiol 2021;31(8):5699–712.

17. Rozmaryn LM. The Collateral Ligament of the Digits of the Hand: Anatomy, Physiology, Biomechanics, Injury, and Treatment. J Hand Surg Am 2017; 42(11):904–15.

18. Pichora DR, McMurtry RY, Bell MJ. Gamekeepers thumb: a prospective study of functional bracing. J Hand Surg Am 1989;14(3):567–73.

19. Dinowitz M, Trumble T, Hanel D, et al. Failure of cast immobilization for thumb ulnar collateral ligament avulsion fractures. J Hand Surg Am 1997;22(6): 1057–63.

20. Chuter GS, Muwanga CL, Irwin LR. Ulnar collateral ligament injuries of the thumb: 10 years of surgical experience. Injury 2009;40(6):652–6.

21. Samora JB, Harris JD, Griesser MJ, et al. Outcomes after injury to the thumb ulnar collateral ligament–a systematic review. Clin J Sport Med 2013;23(4): 247–54.

22. Landsman JC, Seitz WH Jr, Froimson AI, et al. Splint immobilization of gamekeeper's thumb. Orthopedics 1995;18(12):1161–5.

23. Madan SS, Pai DR, Kaur A, et al. Injury to ulnar collateral ligament of thumb. Orthop Surg 2014;6(1):1–7.

24. Shin SS, van Eck CF, Uquillas C. Suture Tape Augmentation of the Thumb Ulnar Collateral Ligament Repair: A Biomechanical Study. J Hand Surg Am 2018;43(9):868.e861–6.

25. Gibbs DB, Shin SS. Return to Play in Athletes After Thumb Ulnar Collateral Ligament Repair With Suture Tape Augmentation. Orthop J Sports Med 2020;8(7). 2325967120935063.

26. Glickel SZ, Malerich M, Pearce SM, et al. Ligament replacement for chronic instability of the ulnar collateral ligament of the metacarpophalangeal joint of the thumb. J Hand Surg Am 1993;18(5):930–41.

27. Breek JC, Tan AM, van Thiel TP, et al. Free tendon grafting to repair the metacarpophalangeal joint of the thumb. Surgical techniques and a review of 70 patients. J Bone Joint Surg Br 1989;71(3):383–7.

28. Edelstein DM, Kardashian G, Lee SK. Radial collateral ligament injuries of the thumb. J Hand Surg Am 2008;33(5):760–70.

29. Camp RA, Weatherwax RJ, Miller EB. Chronic post-traumatic radial instability of the thumb metacarpophalangeal joint. J Hand Surg Am 1980;5(3):221–5.

30. Brewood AF, Menon TJ. Combined reconstruction of volar and radial instability of a thumb metacarpo-phalangeal joint. J Hand Surg Br 1984; 9(3):333–4.

31. Avery DM 3rd, Inkellis ER, Carlson MG. Thumb collateral ligament injuries in the athlete. Curr Rev Musculoskelet Med 2017;10(1):28–37.

32. Catalano LW, Cardon L, Patenaude N, et al. Results of Surgical Treatment of Acute and Chronic Grade II Tears of the Radial Collateral Ligament of the Thumb Metacarpophalangeal Joint. J Hand Surg 2006; 31(1):68–75.

33. Lourie GM, Gaston RG, Freeland AE. Collateral ligament injuries of the metacarpophalangeal joints of the fingers. Hand Clin 2006;22(3):357–64, viii.

34. Ishizuki M, Sugihara T, Wakabayashi Y, et al. Stener-like lesions of collateral ligament ruptures of the metacarpophalangeal joint of the finger. J Orthop Sci 2009;14(2):150–4.

35. Minami A, An KN, Cooney WP 3rd, et al. Ligament stability of the metacarpophalangeal joint: a biomechanical study. J Hand Surg Am 1985;10(2): 255–60.

36. Lee SA, Kim BH, Kim S-J, et al. Current status of ultrasonography of the finger. Ultrasonography 2016; 35(2):110–23.

37. Doyle JR, Atkinson RE. Rupture of the radial collateral ligament of the metacarpo-phalangeal joint of the index finger: a report of three cases. J Hand Surg Br 1989;14(2):248–50.

38. Waxweiler C, Cuylits N, Lumens D, et al. Surgical Fixation of Metacarpophalangeal Collateral Ligament Rupture of the Fingers. Plast Reconstr Surg 2019;143(5):1421–8.

39. Gaston RG, Lourie GM. Radial collateral ligament injury of the index metacarpophalangeal joint: an underreported but important injury. J Hand Surg Am 2006;31(8):1355–61.

40. Dray G, Millender LH, Nalebuff EA. Rupture of the radial collateral ligament of a metacarpophalangeal joint to one of the ulnar three fingers. J Hand Surg Am 1979;4(4):346–50.

41. Delaere OP, Suttor PM, Degolla R, et al. Early surgical treatment for collateral ligament rupture of metacarpophalangeal joints of the fingers. J Hand Surg 2003;28(2):309–15.

42. Riederer S, Nagy L, Büchler U. Chronic posttraumatic radial instability of the metacarpophalangeal joint of the finger. Long-term results of ligament reconstruction. J Hand Surg Br 1998;23(4): 503–6.

43. Carlo J, Dell PC, Matthias R, et al. Collateral Ligament Reconstruction of the Proximal Interphalangeal Joint. J Hand Surg 2016;41(1):129–32.

44. Lee JI, Jeon WJ, Suh DH, et al. Anatomical collateral ligament reconstruction in the hand using intraosseous suture anchors and a free tendon graft. J Hand Surg 2012;37(9):832–8.

45. Mantovani G, Pavan A, Aita MA, et al. Surgical Reconstruction of PIP Joint Collateral Ligament in Chronic Instability in a High Performance Athlete: Case Report and Description of Technique. Tech Hand Up Extrem Surg 2011;15(2):87–91.

46. White NJ, Rollick NC. Injuries of the Scapholunate Interosseous Ligament: An Update. JAAOS - Journal of the American Academy of Orthopaedic Surgeons. 2015;23(11).

47. Geissler WB. Arthroscopic management of scapholunate instability. J Wrist Surg 2013;2(2):129–35.

48. Andersson JK. Treatment of scapholunate ligament injury: Current concepts. EFORT Open Rev 2017; 2(9):382–93.

49. Mayfield JK. Mechanism of carpal injuries. Clin Orthop Relat Res 1980;149:45–54.

50. Chennagiri RJ, Lindau TR. Assessment of scapholunate instability and review of evidence for management in the absence of arthritis. J Hand Surg Eur 2013;38(7):727–38.

51. Jones WA. Beware the sprained wrist. The incidence and diagnosis of scapholunate instability. J Bone Joint Surg Br 1988;70(2):293–7.

52. Reichel LM, Bell BR, Michnick SM, et al. Radial styloid fractures. J Hand Surg Am 2012;37(8): 1726–41.

53. Badida R, Akhbari B, Vutescu E, et al. The role of scapholunate interosseous, dorsal intercarpal, and radiolunate ligaments in wrist biomechanics. J Biomech 2021;125:110567.

54. Overstraeten L, Camus E. The role of extrinsic ligaments in maintaining carpal stability – A prospective statistical analysis of 85 arthroscopic cases. Hand Surgery and Rehabilitation 2016;35:10–5.

55. Van Overstraeten L, Camus EJ. The role of extrinsic ligaments in maintaining carpal stability – A prospective statistical analysis of 85 arthroscopic cases. Hand Surgery and Rehabilitation 2016; 35(1):10–5.

56. Megerle K, Pöhlmann S, Kloeters O, et al. The significance of conventional radiographic parameters in the diagnosis of scapholunate ligament lesions. Eur Radiol 2011;21(1):176–81.

57. Zanetti M, Saupe N, Nagy L. Role of MR imaging in chronic wrist pain. Eur Radiol 2007;17(4):927–38.

58. Moser T, Dosch JC, Moussaoui A, et al. Wrist ligament tears: evaluation of MRI and combined MDCT and MR arthrography. AJR Am J Roentgenol 2007;188(5):1278–86.

59. Garcia-Elias M, Lluch AL, Stanley JK. Three-ligament tenodesis for the treatment of scapholunate dissociation: indications and surgical technique. J Hand Surg Am 2006;31(1):125–34.

60. Ruch DS, Poehling GG. Arthroscopic management of partial scapholunate and lunotriquetral injuries of the wrist. J Hand Surg Am 1996;21(3):412–7.

61. Weiss AP, Sachar K, Glowacki KA. Arthroscopic debridement alone for intercarpal ligament tears. J Hand Surg Am 1997;22(2):344–9.

62. Earp BE, Waters PM, Wyzykowski RJ. Arthroscopic treatment of partial scapholunate ligament tears in children with chronic wrist pain. J Bone Joint Surg Am 2006;88(11):2448–55.

63. Bickert B, Sauerbier M, Germann G. Scapholunate ligament repair using the Mitek bone anchor. J Hand Surg Br 2000;25(2):188–92.

64. Blatt G. Capsulodesis in reconstructive hand surgery. Dorsal capsulodesis for the unstable scaphoid and volar capsulodesis following excision of the distal ulna. Hand Clin 1987;3(1):81–102.

65. Minami A, Kato H, Iwasaki N. Treatment of scapholunate dissociation: ligamentous repair associated with modified dorsal capsulodesis. Hand Surg 2003;8(1):1–6.

66. Pomerance J. Outcome after repair of the scapholunate interosseous ligament and dorsal capsulodesis for dynamic scapholunate instability due to trauma. J Hand Surg Am 2006;31(8):1380–6.

67. Slater RR Jr, Szabo RM, Bay BK, et al. Dorsal intercarpal ligament capsulodesis for scapholunate dissociation: biomechanical analysis in a cadaver model. J Hand Surg Am 1999;24(2):232–9.

68. Szabo RM. Scapholunate Ligament Repair With Capsulodesis Reinforcement. J Hand Surg 2008; 33(9):1645–54.

69. Megerle K, Bertel D, Germann G, et al. Long-term results of dorsal intercarpal ligament capsulodesis for the treatment of chronic scapholunate instability. J Bone Joint Surg Br 2012;94(12):1660–5.

70. Weiss AP. Scapholunate ligament reconstruction using a bone-retinaculum-bone autograft. J Hand Surg Am 1998;23(2):205–15.

71. Harvey EJ, Berger RA, Osterman AL, et al. Bone-tissue-bone repairs for scapholunate dissociation. J Hand Surg Am 2007;32(2):256–64.

72. Darlis NA, Kaufmann RA, Giannoulis F, et al. Arthroscopic debridement and closed pinning for chronic dynamic scapholunate instability. J Hand Surg Am 2006;31(3):418–24.

73. Brunelli GA, Brunelli GR. A new technique to correct carpal instability with scaphoid rotary subluxation: a preliminary report. J Hand Surg Am 1995;20(3 Pt 2): S82–5.

74. Nienstedt F. Treatment of static scapholunate instability with modified Brunelli tenodesis: results over 10 years. J Hand Surg Am 2013;38(5):887–92.

75. Almquist EE, Bach AW, Sack JT, et al. Four-bone ligament reconstruction for treatment of chronic complete scapholunate separation. J Hand Surg Am 1991;16(2):322–7.

76. Aibinder WR, Izadpanah A, Elhassan BT. Reduction and Association of the Scaphoid and Lunate: A Functional and Radiographical Outcome Study. J Wrist Surg 2019;8(1):37–42.

77. Larson TB, Stern PJ. Reduction and association of the scaphoid and lunate procedure: short-term clinical and radiographic outcomes. J Hand Surg Am 2014;39(11):2168–74.

78. Gandhi MJ, Knight TP, Ratcliffe PJ. Scapholunate ligament reconstruction using the palmaris longus tendon and suture anchor fixation in chronic scapholunate instability. Indian J Orthop 2016;50(6):616–21.

79. Mullikin I, Srinivasan RC, Bagg M. Current Techniques in Scapholunate Ligament Reconstruction. Orthop Clin North Am 2020;51(1):77–86.

80. Hofmeister EP, Moran SL, Shin AY. Anterior and posterior interosseous neurectomy for the treatment of chronic dynamic instability of the wrist. Hand (N Y). 2006;1(2):63–70.
81. Mulford JS, Ceulemans LJ, Nam D, et al. Proximal row carpectomy vs four corner fusion for scapholunate (Slac) or scaphoid nonunion advanced collapse (Snac) wrists: a systematic review of outcomes. J Hand Surg Eur 2009;34(2):256–63.
82. Ben Amotz O, Sammer DM. Salvage Operations for Wrist Ligament Injuries with Secondary Arthrosis. Hand Clin 2015;31(3):495–504.

InternalBrace for Intercarpal Ligament Reconstruction

Brian W. Starr, MD[a,b,*], Kevin C. Chung, MD, MS[c]

KEYWORDS

- Scapholunate • Lunotriquetral • DISI • Intercarpal ligament

KEY POINTS

- Despite innumerable options, no clear consensus exists regarding the treatment of subacute or chronic intercarpal ligament injuries in the setting of predynamic or dynamic instability.
- Intercarpal ligament reconstruction using the Arthrex InternalBrace system and an all-dorsal approach shows immense promise in early outcomes data.
- Preliminary 6-month and 1-year outcomes data demonstrate restoration of grip strength, range of motion, and improvement in patient-reported pain and functional scores.

INTRODUCTION

Scapholunate (SL) and lunotriquetral (LT) instability are common causes of chronic, debilitating wrist pain and functional impairment. Little debate exists regarding the approach to promptly diagnose intercarpal ligamentous injuries. Primary repair, augmented with either capsulodesis or SutureTape, yields satisfactory outcomes if performed within the first several weeks of injury.[1–4] Consensus also exists for injuries on the opposite end of the spectrum. Patients who languish for years with pain and untreated instability inevitably deteriorate to a fixed dorsal intercalated segment instability (DISI) deformity with progressive articular compromise. For these patients, salvage operations, including proximal row carpectomy and limited arthrodesis, offer reliable results. However, in the setting of subacute or chronic injuries with predynamic or dynamic instability, the ideal surgical approach remains unclear. Countless techniques have been proposed for treatment of this subgroup of patients who meet criteria for Garcia-Elias stage 3 and 4. Unfortunately, despite the dedicated work and ongoing innovation of many pioneers of our specialty, consensus on the optimal reconstructive approach remains elusive. Over the years, the senior author (KCC) has performed many of these varying procedures and remains unsatisfied with today's most prominent techniques.

BACKGROUND

Every well-studied technique to date has shortcomings (**Table 1**). Procedures that are solely reliant on tendon-weave techniques, as originally popularized by Brunelli and Brunelli, are inherently prone to laxity and loss of reduction as the tendon attenuates over time.[5] Modifications as discussed by Van Den Abbeele and colleagues, Almquist and colleagues, and Garcia Elias and colleagues are also subject to this intrinsic weakness.[6–8] A recent retrospective review of the 3-ligament tenodesis (3LT) technique noted a startling high percentage—30% (15/50)—of patients required a salvage

---

[a] Section of Plastic Surgery, Cincinnati Children's Hospital Medical Center, 3333 Burnet Avenue MLC 2020, Cincinnati, OH 45229, USA; [b] University of Cincinnati College of Medicine, 3230 Eden Avenue Cincinnati, OH 45267, USA; [c] Section of Plastic Surgery, The University of Michigan Health System, 1500 East Medical Center Drive, 2130 Taubman Center, SPC 5340, Ann Arbor, MI 48109-5340, USA
* Corresponding author.
E-mail address: brian.starr@cchmc.org

Hand Clin 39 (2023) 379–388
https://doi.org/10.1016/j.hcl.2023.02.008

Table 1
Summary of scapholunate reconstruction techniques

Procedure	n/Follow-up	Pain/Disability	ROM[b]	Grip Strength[c]	SL Gap (mm)	SL (deg)	Salvage	Complications
4-Bone, Almquist[6]	36/57 m	92% return to work	52/37	73%	3.3	—	8.3%	Wire loop disruption
Brunelli & Brunelli[5]	11, 6–24 m	100% return to work	—/25	65%	—	—	None	None
3LT, Garcia-Elias[8,9,22]	38/46 m	81% return to work	52/51	65%	—	—	None	AVN scaphoid, CRPS
	50/111 m[a]	PRWE 11[a]	55/57[a]	73%[a]	3.4[a]	80[a]	30% at 33 m	
RASL[13]	8/38 m	PRWE 26	55/44	77%	4.5	59	None	Radiographic failure, screw loosening, partial destruction of scaphoid/lunate
Arthroscopic-assisted volar/dorsal[13]	17/48 m	VAS 1.8	60/52	84%	2.9	—	None	AVN scaphoid, 4/17 with DISI
SLAM[15,21]	13/11 m	VAS 1.7	56/45	62%	2.1	59	7.7%	AVN scaphoid, AVN lunate
ANAFAB[16]	10/>24 m	VAS 1.0	60/50[d]	94%	3	"Close to or within normal"	None	DRUJ subluxation
All-dorsal Internal Brace[e]	*7/6 m*	*PRWE 37*	*51/41*	*80%*	*2.5*	*50*	*None*	*—*
	3/12 m	*PRWE 11*	*60/56*	*88%*	*2.2*	*57*		

Abbreviations: AVN, avascular necrosis; CRPS, complex regional pain syndrome; deg, degrees; DRUJ, distal radioulnar joint; LTF, lost to follow-up; m, months; PRWE, patient-rated wrist evaluation.
[a] Excluding 30% salvage and 38% LTF.
[b] Extension/flexion (in degrees).
[c] Percentage of contralateral, uninjured extremity.
[d] Median.
[e] Performed by senior author (KCC).

operation at a mean of 34 months post-op.[9] Nienstedt reported encouraging long-term clinical results using a modified Brunelli technique, with 7 of 8 patients with "good" or "excellent" functional results at 10 years post-op. However, final radiographic measurements were noted to be trending towards preoperative values, with a mean 17 degree increase in SL angle and 0.4 mm widening in SL gap.[10] Rosenwasser's reduction and association of the scaphoid and lunate (RASL) procedure avoids shortcomings associated with soft tissue–based reconstruction; however, this technique has been plagued with hardware complications, as the requisite intercarpal motion weakened this form of reconstruction.[11] Despite recent literature from Koehler and colleagues[12] demonstrating that reliable clinical outcomes depend on precise screw placement, many surgeons have since abandoned this procedure.

In recent years, multiple investigators have advocated combined reconstruction of both volar and dorsal ligaments in an attempt to overcome torsional instability that may result from dorsal-only reconstruction techniques. Ho and colleagues[13] have adopted a novel technique, using an arthroscopic-assisted approach to reconstruct both volar and dorsal ligaments, using palmaris graft. Their 4-year outcomes are encouraging, although it remains to be seen whether other surgeons can replicate these investigators' success and arthroscopic technical prowess that is accomplished by a select few. We remain skeptical regarding the long-term durability of the tendon graft in this technique. Yao and colleagues address this concern in their SL axis method (SLAM), by securing the graft in immediate proximity to the SL interval. The graft is placed along the central axis of rotation, reminiscent of headless compression screw placement for the RASL procedure. Despite early success, our opinion of the technique has been tempered by scattered reports of avascular necrosis of the scaphoid and lunate, which are devastating problems.[14,15] Sandow and Fisher recently reported short-term outcomes in a series of 10 patients treated with their hybrid SutureTape and tendon graft anatomic front and back repair technique. The investigators' initial results show promise, although larger series and longer follow-up are required to determine the ultimate role of this complex technique.[16] Similarly, more data are needed to adequately judge the hybrid SutureTape and graft volar-dorsal (SLITT) technique recently proposed by Kakar and Greene.[17]

Encouraged by reports by Weiss and Harvey, the senior author (KCC) adopted a bone-ligament-bone reconstruction technique between 2013 and 2019.[18,19] In critically evaluating our short-term outcomes with this reconstruction, however, we found that one-third of patients suffered from persistent pain, disability, and suboptimal range of motion postoperatively.[20] In seeking a better alternative, we reflected on the ease-of-use, durability, and reliability of suture tape–based reconstructions (Arthrex InternalBrace [Arthrex Inc., Naples, Florida]) in various applications. The current literature is deficient in well-designed studies applying this technique for intercarpal ligament reconstruction.

Dating back to July, 2019 the senior author (KCC) has performed 20 SL, LT, or combination SL/LT ligament reconstructions with an all-dorsal approach, using the Arthrex InternalBrace system. In critically appraising our surgical technique and initial results, we became convinced of the procedure's merits as a durable option for restoring normal wrist kinematics. In January 2020 we started enrolling patients with predynamic and dynamic instability in an IRB-approved prospective study, aimed at meticulously studying outcomes using the all-dorsal InternalBrace reconstruction technique. If the diagnosis or quality of the articular surfaces is questionable, we perform diagnostic arthroscopy to confirm patients' eligibility for reconstruction (Fig. 1). We use wrist arthroscopy liberally to assess the entire wrist for other pathologies so that we can provide the patient with a coherent treatment plan and to repair all damaged structures. We have been closely following-up these patients and charting functional and radiographic outcomes at 6-week, 3-month, 6-month, 1-year, and 2-year intervals. To date, we have enrolled 16 patients with

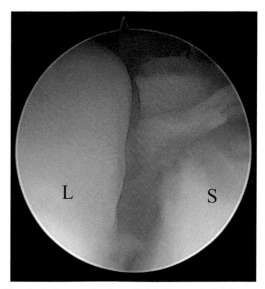

Fig. 1. Arthroscopic view of Geissler grade 3 injury as viewed through the midcarpal portal.

encouraging early results. We will publish our pro-spective outcomes data after at least a 1-year follow-up for this cohort.

TECHNIQUE

We approach the wrist via a dorsal longitudinal incision centered over the SL interval. The incision is designed to incorporate prior 3 to 4 and midcarpal arthroscopy portal scars (**Fig. 2**). We take a standard approach to the carpus, between the third and fourth dorsal compartments. The extensor pollicis longus tendon is left within its sheath. The fourth dorsal compartment is incised, and the posterior interosseous nerve is located at the radial base of the compartment and excised (**Fig. 3**). We perform a longitudinal capsulotomy and sharply elevate capsular flaps to provide wide exposure of the proximal row (**Fig. 4**). The extensor carpi radialis brevis (ECRB) tendon is identified, proximal to its insertion on the base of the third metacarpal. A 2-mm slip of ECRB tendon graft is harvested from distal to proximal, for a distance of approximately 10 cm to provide a biological construct to augment the suture tape

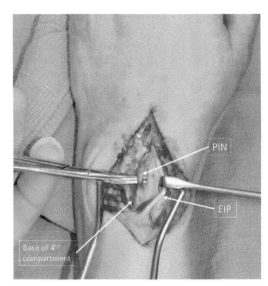

Fig. 3. The fourth dorsal compartment is incised, and the posterior interosseous nerve (PIN) is located at the radial base of the compartment and excised.

for longevity of the reconstruction stability (**Fig. 5**).

Next, the lunate is reduced out of DISI deformity with the aid of a 0.062″ joystick K-wire. With the lunate reduced as aggressively as possible, we use the Linscheid technique, transfixing the lunate with a second 0.062″ K-wire driven from the dorsal distal radius to the dorsal lunate to keep the lunate in perfect aligned for the reconstruction. In our experience, it is impossible to overreduce the

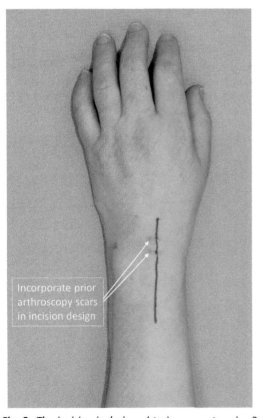

Fig. 2. The incision is designed to incorporate prior 3 to 4 and midcarpal arthroscopy portal scars.

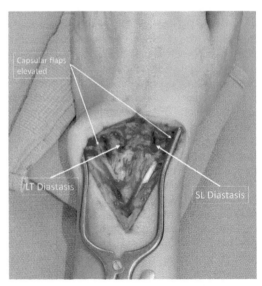

Fig. 4. Longitudinal capsulotomy is performed and capsular flaps elevated to provide wide exposure of the proximal row.

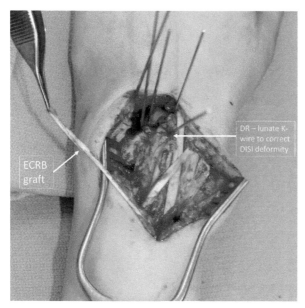 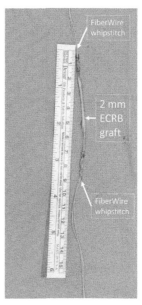

Fig. 5. A 2-mm slip of ECRB tendon graft is harvested from distal to proximal, for a distance of approximately 10 cm to provide a biological construct to augment the suture tape for longevity of the reconstruction stability.

lunate. Next, depending on the specific injury pattern, the 1.35 mm guidewires are inserted into the central lunate, proximal pole of the scaphoid, and central triquetrum as indicated. The wires are inserted to a depth as marked on the laser line, and proper placement is confirmed on fluoroscopy. The lunate, scaphoid proximal pole, and triquetrum (as indicated) are drilled with the 3.5-mm (gold) cannulated drill bit. To drill, place the blue drill guide over the intended guidewire and drill concentrically until reaching the 1-cm depth-stop (**Fig. 6**). The 3.5-mm drill hole accommodates the SutureTape and 2-mm tendon graft (**Fig. 7**). If tendon graft is not used, the 3.0-mm cannulated drill (silver) is selected instead. However, we always add the tendon graft for the theoretical advantage of biologic reconstruction. Once the 3.5-mm drill holes have been made, the SutureTape and tendon graft are loaded onto the forked eyelet of the SwiveLock SL anchor (**Fig. 8**). The

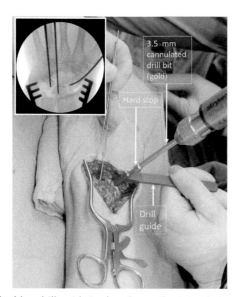 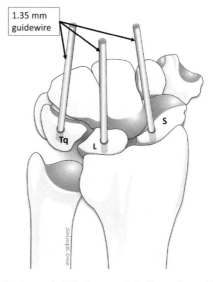

Fig. 6. The blue drill guide is placed over the intended guidewire and drilled concentrically until reaching the 1-cm depth-stop.

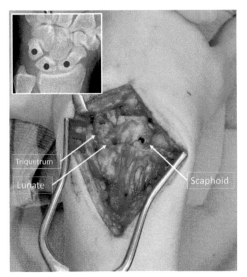
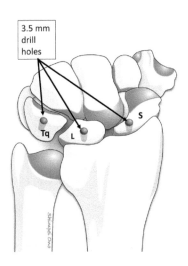

Fig. 7. The 3.5-mm drill hole accommodates the SutureTape and 2-mm tendon graft.

SutureTape is loaded with equal length on either side. The graft is loaded on the eyelet 2 to 3 mm from one end—loading of the graft is facilitated by the previously placed FiberLoop whipstitch. The anchor, graft, and SutureTape complex are inserted into the proximal pole of the scaphoid first. The graft and SutureTape are then loaded on a new SwiveLock SL anchor and inserted into the lunate (**Fig. 9**). If LT ligament is also being reconstructed, both limbs of the SutureTape are loaded; if only the SL ligament is being reconstructed, one limb of the SutureTape may be trimmed at the proximal pole of the scaphoid. Joysticks inserted into the scaphoid and lunate are often needed to reduce the diastasis, before securing the graft and SutureTape. To reconstruct the LT ligament, the graft and a single limb of the SutureTape are again gathered on a new SwiveLock SL anchor and inserted into the triquetrum. As a final step to help maintain scaphoid extension and resist progressive flexion deformity that can weaken the SL ligament reconstruction, the remaining limb of the SutureTape is directed from the lunate to the dorsal distal pole of the

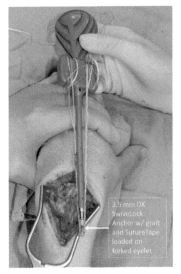
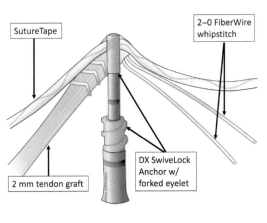

Fig. 8. Once the 3.5-mm drill holes have been made, the SutureTape and tendon graft are loaded onto the forked eyelet of the SwiveLock SL anchor.

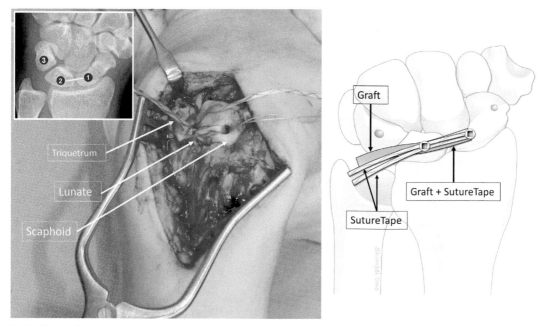

Fig. 9. The graft and SutureTape are then loaded on a new SwiveLock SL anchor and inserted into the lunate.

scaphoid. For this, a 1.35-mm guidewire is inserted into the distal pole of the scaphoid. The drill guide is placed over the guidewire, and the 3.0-mm cannulated drill bit (silver) is used to drill the distal pole (**Fig. 10**). The remaining SutureTape is loaded on a 3.0-mm SwiveLock SL anchor and inserted into the distal pole, under moderate tension. The final construct is seen in **Fig. 11**.

Technical tips of this operation are as follows: (1) be sure the guidewires are placed center of the axis of the bones and verify by fluoroscopy to avoid eccentric drilling that can fracture the

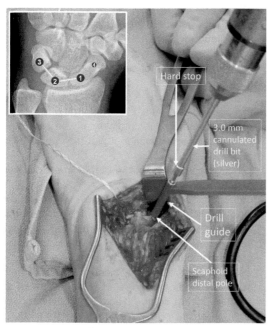

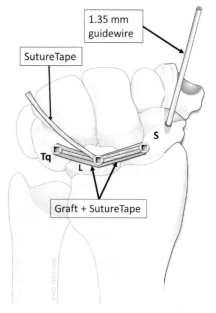

Fig. 10. The drill guide is placed over the guidewire, and the 3.0-mm cannulated drill bit (silver) is used to drill the scaphoid distal pole.

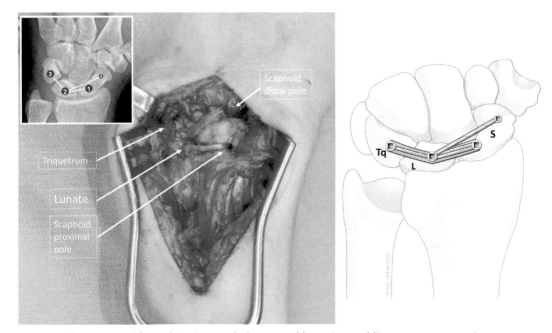

Fig. 11. Final construct with combination scapholunate and lunotriquetral ligament reconstruction.

delicate carpal bones. (2) Push the SwiveLock in the precise direction of the drill hole and feel entire seating of the lock before turning the hand drill guide, otherwise the lock will not be fully engaged and will be proud over the carpal bone. (3) For dynamic instability, we do not need to fix the carpal bones with K-wires because the carpus will be well aligned. We keep the wrist immobilized for 6 weeks before initiating patient-directed active motion exercises. At no point do we prescribe passive exercises by the therapist, in order to avoid overzealous recovery of wrist motion that may weaken the reconstruction. A successful wrist ligament reconstruction is to achieve painless wrist motion at whatever motion arc the patient can achieve. (4) With reducible static deformity and no articular wear, we will use intercarpal wires to mainly wrist alignment until the ligament reconstruction has healed at 6 weeks. In this scenario, we cut the pins under the skin to avoid devastating pin-site infections and retrieve the pins at a second procedure.

OUTCOMES

We are pleased to report early success with this technique, in a small cohort of patients at short-term follow-up (see **Table 1**). We are still actively enrolling patients in our prospective study and aim to follow our existing patients for many more months. At present, we have at least 6 months of follow-up on 7 patients with unilateral SL or LT instability. At their 6-month postoperative appointment, these patients demonstrated a mean extension/flexion arc of 51 and 41 degrees, respectively. Grip strength was measured to be 80% of the contralateral, uninjured extremity. Disability as scored on the patient-rated wrist evaluation (PRWE) remained elevated at 37/100. Three patients with unilateral injuries have at least 1 year of follow-up data. These data demonstrate ongoing recovery beyond the 6-month mark. At 1 year, patients demonstrated a mean extension/flexion arc of 60 and 56 degrees, respectively, and grip strength was measured to be 88% of the contralateral, uninjured extremity. These patients also noted substantial improvement in their overall pain and functional status, with a PRWE of 11/100.

In comparison to existing techniques, our early results demonstrate equal-or-better functional outcomes (see **Table 1**). Many recent studies lack consistent measurement of pain and functional status using patient-reported, validated surveys such as the PRWE. In the absence of consistent outcome surveys across studies, we instead must rely on objective measurements such as range of motion and grip strength for immediate, direct comparison. Our preliminary findings for wrist range of motion using the all-dorsal InternalBrace technique—92° total arc of motion at 6 months and 116° total arc of motion at

12 months—are as good or better than other techniques. Similarly, grip strength recovery at just 6 months (80% of contralateral) is superior, in comparison to other approaches such as the Garcia-Elias 3LT (65%) and SLAM (62%).[8,21] A rarely acknowledged shortcoming of many recent techniques is the steep learning curve. We contend that the all-dorsal technique described herein is straightforward and easy to learn. In contrast to time-intensive, complex procedures that require bone tunnels and multiple exposures, our tourniquet time for this technique is routinely less than 1 hour.

SUMMARY

The list of techniques described for treatment of subacute and chronic intercarpal injuries is near-endless. Despite the array of options, historical outcomes have been suboptimal, and consensus on the ideal technique remains elusive. In our experience, intercarpal ligament reconstruction using the Arthrex InternalBrace system and an all-dorsal approach shows immense promise. Early data demonstrate restoration of grip strength, range of motion, and substantial improvement in patient-reported pain and functional scores. The all-dorsal technique is straightforward, efficient, and easy to teach. More data and longer follow-up are certainly required, but we are cautiously optimistic that this technique may one day become the standard.

CLINICS CARE POINTS

- Preliminary 6-month and 1-year outcome data using an all-dorsal approach with the InternalBrace system demonstrate restoration of grip strength, range of motion, and improvement in patient-reported pain and functional scores.

- The all-dorsal InternalBrace technique is straightforward and efficient and does not require multiple incisions, bone tunnels, or elaborate tendon weaves.

- For dynamic instability, we do not need to fix the carpal bones with K-wires because the carpus will be well aligned. We keep the wrist immobilized for 6 weeks before initiating patient-directed active motion exercises.

- With reducible static deformity and no articular wear, we will use intercarpal wires mainly for wrist alignment until the ligament reconstruction has healed at 6 weeks.

ACKNOWLEDGMENTS

Special thanks to Shimpei Ono, MD, PhD for the beautiful illustrations.

DISCLOSURES

Dr K.C. Chung receives funding from the National Institutes of Health, book royalties from Wolters Kluwer and Elsevier, and a research grant from Sonex to study carpal tunnel outcomes. The authors have no financial relationship to Arthrex and have received no funding for research related to intercarpal ligament reconstruction using the InternalBrace system.

REFERENCES

1. Beredjiklian PK, Dugas J, Gerwin M. Primary repair of the scapholunate ligament. Tech Hand Up Extrem Surg 1998;2(4):269–73.
2. Thompson RG, Dustin JA, Roper DK, et al. Suture tape augmentation for scapholunate ligament repair: a biomechanical study. J Hand Surg Am 2021;46(1):36–42.
3. Minami A, Kato H, Iwasaki N. Treatment of scapholunate dissociation: Ligamentous repair associated with modified dorsal capsulodesis. Hand Surg 2003;8(1):1–6.
4. Zarkadas PC, Gropper PT, White NJ, et al. A survey of the surgical management of acute and chronic scapholunate instability. J Hand Surg 2004;29(5):848–57.
5. Brunelli GA, Brunelli GR. A new surgical technique for carpal instability with scapho-lunar dislocation. (eleven cases). Ann Chir Main Memb Super 1995;14(4–5):207–13.
6. Almquist EE, Bach AW, Sack JT, et al. Four-bone ligament reconstruction for treatment of chronic complete scapholunate separation. J Hand Surg 1991;16(2):322.
7. Van Den Abbeele KL, Loh YC, Stanley JK, et al. Early results of a modified brunelli procedure for scapholunate instability. J Hand Surg Br 1998;23(2):258–61.
8. Garcia-Elias M, Lluch AL, Stanley JK. Three-ligament tenodesis for the treatment of scapholunate dissociation: Indications and surgical technique. J Hand Surg Am 2006;31(1):125–34.
9. Goeminne S, Borgers A, van Beek N, et al. Long-term follow-up of the three-ligament tenodesis for scapholunate ligament lesions: 9-year results. Hand Surg Rehabil 2021;40(4):448–52.
10. Nienstedt F. Treatment of static scapholunate instability with modified brunelli tenodesis: results over 10 years. J Hand Surg Am 2013;38(5):887–92.

11. Rosenwasser MP, Miyasajsa KC, Strauch RJ. The RASL procedure: Reduction and association of the scaphoid and lunate using the herbert screw. Tech Hand Up Extrem Surg 1997;1(4):263–72.

12. Koehler SM, Beck CM, Nasser P, et al. The effect of screw trajectory for the reduction and association of the scaphoid and lunate (RASL) procedure: A biomechanical analysis. J Hand Surg Eur 2018; 43(6):635–41.

13. Ho PC, Wong CW, Tse WL. Arthroscopic-assisted combined dorsal and volar scapholunate ligament reconstruction with tendon graft for chronic SL instability. J Wrist Surg 2015;4(4):252–63.

14. Chan K, Engasser W, Jebson PJL. Avascular necrosis of the lunate following reconstruction of the scapholunate ligament using the scapholunate axis method (SLAM). J Hand Surg Am 2019;44(10):904.e1–4.

15. Mullikin I, Srinivasan RC, Bagg M. Current techniques in scapholunate ligament reconstruction. Orthop Clin North Am 2020;51(1):77–86.

16. Sandow M, Fisher T. Anatomical anterior and posterior reconstruction for scapholunate dissociation: preliminary outcome in ten patients. The Journal of hand surgery, European volume 2020;45(4):389–95.

17. Kakar S, Greene RM. Scapholunate ligament internal brace 360-degree tenodesis (SLITT) procedure. J Wrist Surg 2018;7(4):336–40.

18. Weiss AP. Scapholunate ligament reconstruction using a bone-retinaculum-bone autograft. J Hand Surg Am 1998;23(2):205–15.

19. Harvey EJ, Berger RA, Osterman AL, et al. Bone-tissue-bone repairs for scapholunate dissociation. J Hand Surg Am 2007;32(2):256–64.

20. Ross PR, Gundlach B, Yue M, et al. Outcomes after bone-ligament-bone intercarpal ligament reconstruction. Plast Reconstr Surg 2022;149(4):901–10.

21. Yao J, Zlotolow DA, Lee SK. ScaphoLunate axis method. J Wrist Surg 2016;5(1):59–66.

22. De Smet L, Sciot R, Degreef I. Avascular necrosis of the scaphoid after three-ligament tenodesis for scapholunate dissociation: Case report. J Hand Surg Am 2011;36(4):587–90.

Compression Neuropathies
Revisions and Managing Expectations

Tiam M. Saffari, MD, PhD, MSc, Amy M. Moore, MD, Ryan W. Schmucker, MD*

KEYWORDS

• Compression neuropathy • Revision surgery • Carpal tunnel syndrome • Cubital tunnel syndrome

KEY POINTS

• Making the correct diagnosis in revision nerve cases is key. Clarify by using the: "is it persistent, is it recurrent, or is it new?" approach to evaluating symptoms.
• Preoperative treatment of revision nerve patients must include maximizing therapy, optimizing pain management, and carefully controlling expectations.
• Principles of revision nerve surgery include allowing adequate time for the case, making long incisions, working from known to unknown, avoiding nerve injury, and minimizing tourniquet time.
• For prevention of perineural scarring after revision surgery, surgeons can consider local vascularized tissue transfer or one of a number of commercially available products.

BACKGROUND

Upper extremity nerve compression syndromes, including carpal tunnel syndrome (CTS) and cubital tunnel syndrome (CuTS), are commonly encountered by hand surgeons. When these conditions enter the chronic phase, they can result in damage of the myelin sheath and cause permanent structural changes in the nerve itself.[1,2] Although the anatomic distribution of the symptoms may differ, these syndromes share a similar pathophysiology. Chronic compression neuropathy commences with sensory complaints, progressing from intermittent paresthesia to constant numbness. This was first recognized by an alteration in pressure and vibration thresholds in 1984.[3] Sensory deficits are followed by motor complaints such as weakness and atrophy. These symptoms are directly affected by the degree and duration of compression, respectively.[4]

Surgical decompression can relieve compression symptoms; however, in approximately 25% of the cases, these releases fail. Although a failed decompression is clinically defined as not resolving the pain, paresthesia, and possibly weakness, failure from a patient's perspective could include the absence of a return to normal function.[5] Cubital tunnel release has similar failure rates (2.4%–17%) when compared with carpal tunnel release (CTR, 3%–25%).[5,6] Risk factors contributing to revision CuTS include younger age at presentation, a history of diabetes and a greater static 2-point discrimination.[7] Severe CuTS, involving motor weakness, is not realistically expected to return to normal. Guiding the patient's expectations is the key to patient satisfaction and plays an important role in surgical success. Failure of nerve decompression could be defined as a persistence of, recurrence of or development of new symptoms. Defining the correct diagnosis after a failed nerve decompression will be discussed in this article. Furthermore, the management and revision options for failed upper extremity compression neuropathies will be provided.

BASIC SCIENCE EVIDENCE OF NERVE COMPRESSION

In rabbits, extraneural acute compression of the tibial nerve was found to decrease intraneural microvascular flow and subsequently alter nerve structure and function.[8] Although interference of venular flow was observed with lower pressures

Department of Plastic and Reconstructive Surgery, The Ohio State University Columbus, OH, USA
* Corresponding author. The Ohio State University Wexner Medical Center, 915 Olentangy River Road, Suite 2100, Columbus, OH 43212.
E-mail address: Ryan.Schmucker@osumc.edu

Hand Clin 39 (2023) 389–401
https://doi.org/10.1016/j.hcl.2023.02.009
0749-0712/23/© 2023 Elsevier Inc. All rights reserved.

(20–30 mm Hg), higher pressures (40–50 mm Hg) resulted in arteriolar and intrafascicular capillary flow impairment, explaining the damage by degree of compression.[8] The duration of compression has also been tested in animal models; it has been found that short-term compression at low pressures increases endoneurial pressures and subsequently causes persistent intraneural edema,[9] whereas long-term compression results in inflammation and fibrin deposits followed by proliferation of endoneurial fibroblasts and capillary endothelial cells.[10] Demyelination and Schwann cell necrosis were also found after long-term compression.[10] Differences between early and late decompression have also been investigated. Rats that underwent early decompression (ie, 2 weeks postoperatively) were found to have complete restoration of neural blood flow along with normalization of all electrodiagnostic parameters, compared with a failure of blood flow and electrodiagnostic testing recovery in late decompression (ie, 6 weeks postoperatively).[11,12]

Pathophysiology

The connective tissue matrix (ie, mesoneurium) lays around the epineurium and is critical to gliding of the nerve during movement of the extremity.[4,13] The median nerve may glide 7.3 mm during full flexion and extension of the elbow and has an excursion of 14.5 mm just proximal to the carpal tunnel, respectively.[14] For the ulnar nerve, these excursions are 9.8 mm at the elbow and 13.8 mm just proximal to Guyon canal, respectively.[14] In case of trauma and subsequent edema in the endoneurial space, the pressure in the nerve fascicles may increase, resulting in inhibition of nerve gliding. Swelling further compromises the microvascular blood supply and could lead to focal ischemia of the nerve and scarring of the mesoneurium,[15] leading to more traction injury during motion. Other causes of swelling include renal failure, diabetes, thyroid disease, alcoholism, and pregnancy. Most cases of swelling, however, are idiopathic.[16] The spectrum of histopathologic changes that occur with the progression of nerve compression is illustrated in **Fig. 1**. Nerve compression syndromes occur at sites where the nerve passes through relatively fixed anatomic structures, or tunnels, which are unable to accommodate swelling. In 1973, Upton and McComas introduced the controversial concept of a "double-crush phenomenon."[17] After distal nerve compression, changes proximal to the nerve cell bodies and impaired axoplasmic flow have been observed. Similarly, it is suggested that proximal levels of compression could predispose distal

sites to be more sensitive to compression.[17] It is hypothesized that when one level of a nerve trunk is compressed, the rest of the nerve is more likely to undergo a pathologic change, explaining the double crush concept.[17,18] Other possible explanations include the interruption of lymphatic or venous drainage at the proximal site, or proximal endoneurial edema, resulting in disrupted intraneural blood flow distally.[19,20]

PREOPERATIVE REVISION NERVE SURGERY PRINCIPLES
Diagnosis: Is It Persistent, Is It Recurrent, or Is It New?

Although it can often be difficult to confirm whether the nerve compression is recurrent or persistent, the correct diagnosis is of the utmost importance. The evaluation of patients after failed surgery begins with a thorough history of previous treatments and evaluation of the change in character, intensity, and chronicity of the symptoms.[21] Unchanged numbness and/or dysesthesia may indicate persistent symptoms, whereas return of preoperative symptoms after a period of relief would suggest recurrent symptoms. Recurrent compression is most often defined as a return of symptoms more than 3 months after surgery and suggests postoperative scarring, traction, or new compression points. The distinction between persistent and recurrent symptoms is often not clear and complicates directing toward the optimal recommended treatment, with no relief of symptoms in 20% and 35% of patients after a second carpal tunnel[22,23] and cubital tunnel release, respectively.[24] Incomplete release may be relieved by repeat decompression; however, revision surgery is more complicated due to the scarring that is inherent to the first operation and can put the nerve at risk if not careful.[25]

A change in the character of the symptoms can indicate a new cause. New symptoms may be caused by incomplete release, devascularization of the nerve, or iatrogenic nerve injuries in up to 15% of cases.[26] Patients may also describe new symptoms that could be related to postoperative neuromas.[21,25] An overview of the clinical categorization of secondary CTS and CuTS is provided in **Table 1**.[21,25,27,28] Possible missed diagnoses in the setting of CTS include cervical radiculopathy, spinal cord lesions, proximal median nerve compression or other causes of peripheral neuropathy, including diabetes mellitus and thyroid disorders.[29] The presentation of cervical radiculopathy could resemble the distal nerve neuropathies and the correct location of compression, via physical examination and electrodiagnostic

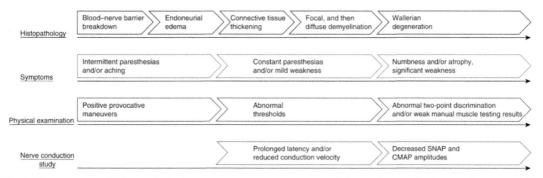

Fig. 1. The spectrum of histopathologic changes, signs, symptoms, and electrodiagnostic changes that occur with progression of nerve compression. CMAP, Compound muscle action potential; SNAP, sensory nerve action potential. (*Adapted from* Mackinnon SE, Novak CB. Compression neuropathies. In: Wolfe SW, Hotchkiss RN, Pederson, WC, et al, eds. Green's Operative Hand Surgery . 7th ed. Philadelphia: Elsevier; 2017, with permission.)

studies, needs to be identified before treatment. In some cases, the nerve is entrapped in multiple areas (ie, double crush syndrome), [30] which could complicate diagnosis and treatment. It is imperative that proximal entrapment syndromes affecting the median and ulnar nerves, including thoracic outlet syndrome, pectoralis minor syndrome, and cervical radiculopathy are ruled out.

Revision surgery of CuTS has been recommended by Lowe and Mackinnon when motor conduction velocities are less than 20 m/s. [21] Recent evidence suggests that compound muscle action potential (CMAP) amplitude can be used to predict the severity of CuTS. Power and colleagues recommended that a reduced first dorsal interosseous amplitude predicts weakness in grip and key pinch strength, however, isolated slowing of conduction velocity across the elbow does not.[31] Although the CMAP amplitude is a sensitive indicator of the severity of CuTS, we prefer to base the decision for additional surgery on a clinical picture of sensory complaints and/or motor function deterioration. Gruber and colleagues suggested the use of ultrasonography in persistent symptoms after ulnar nerve transposition and found kinked fascial compression in 6 out of 8 patients.[32] Conservative therapy, such as rehabilitation focused on nerve glides and muscle rebalancing, has been suggested for patients with mild symptoms, with the goal to decrease the frequency of symptoms and further progress the disease.[33,34] Although activity modification and splinting play a successful role in the primary setting of nerve compression, these modalities are not nearly as effective after failed nerve decompression.[21,28,35–38]

Preoperative Treatment

The most difficult part of evaluating patients after a failed nerve decompression, is deciding when to

not operate. First and foremost, patient expectations must be carefully assessed and deemed to be reasonable before proceeding with any reoperation. If patient and surgeon expectations are not well aligned, surgery should be deferred. In situations of 3 or more repeat decompressions without success, further decompression is unlikely to be successful because the complication of nerve devascularization (causing complete nerve palsy) or nerve injury is dramatically increased.

Clinicians can provide individually tailored education and pain management plans to the patient through a shared decision-making approach, discussing treatment options, expectations, and documenting pain treatment goals. Individually tailored education preoperatively is proven to result in beneficial effects including less preoperative anxiety, fewer requests for sedative medications and reduced postoperative opioid consumption.[39–41] Moreover, documenting pain patterns preoperatively could be used to compare postoperative severity and distribution of symptoms and aid in defining the correct diagnosis (ie, recurrent, persistent, new pain).[42] Carroll and colleagues suggest that preventing postsurgical chronic pain is the responsibility of the surgeon and that medications could be started preoperatively to manage the pain postoperatively. [43] An overview of the pharmacotherapeutic recommendations for reducing the risk of chronic postoperative pain is provided in **Table 2**.[43]

INTRAOPERATIVE PRINCIPLES OF REVISION NERVE SURGERY
Allow Adequate Time

Once a diagnosis is made, patient expectations are extensively discussed, preoperative therapy is completed, and medical management is optimized. As revision nerve cases have increased

Table 1
Clinical categorization of secondary carpal tunnel syndrome and cubital tunnel syndrome

	Category	Symptoms	Causes
Carpal Tunnel Syndrome	Persistent	Paresthesia and weakness Patient complaint: symptoms same or worse after intervention	• Incorrect primary diagnosis • Incomplete release • Concomitant disease • Missed proximal compression site, for example, lacertus fibrosus, pronator teres, or fibrous arch of the flexor digitorum superficialis • Tenosynovitis
	Recurrent	Paresthesia and weakness Patient complaint: symptoms improved for period of time, then returned	• Postoperative scarring • Chronically proliferative tenosynovitis • Distal radius fracture with or without malunion • New compression points
	New	New pain Patient complaint: symptoms different from preoperatively, worsened symptoms	• Neuroma of palmar cutaneous branch of median nerve • Incomplete release causing new point of compression (proximal or distal) • Iatrogenic nerve injury
CuTS	Persistent	Paresthesia and weakness Patient complaint: symptoms same or worse after intervention	• Incorrect diagnosis • Incomplete release • Concomitant disease: Guyon canal distally, thoracic outlet syndrome, or pectoralis minor proximally • Medial instability of the elbow or extension contracture of the elbow joint
	Recurrent	Paresthesia and weakness Patient complaint: symptoms improved for period of time, then returned	• Postoperative scarring • Traction • New compression point • (Re)subluxation of nerve back into epicondylar groove after transposition • Development of elbow osteoarthritis with new osteophytes
	New	New pain Patient complaint: symptoms different from preoperatively, worsened symptoms	• Neuroma of medial antebrachial cutaneous nerve • Iatrogenic nerve injury • Incomplete release causing new point of compression (proximal or distal)

complexity due to scarring, one must ensure that sufficient operating time is scheduled. Leaving plenty of time to operate will allow for thoughtful intraoperative decision-making and the ability to do what is necessary depending on the multitude of difference scenarios one can encounter during revision nerve cases. An unexpected nerve transection or neuroma-in-continuity when a recurrent nerve compression was suspected can drastically change the operative plan and the amount of time required to complete the operation. Overbooking these cases (ie, allowing more time than you anticipate) will provide the time necessary for unexpected intraoperative findings.

Increase Length of Incisions

The first principle that is key to revision nerve surgery is to extend the previous incision proximally and distally. The goal is to identify the nerve safely

Table 2
Preoperative pharmacotherapeutic recommendations to reduce the risk of postoperative chronic pain

Agent	Dose	Benefits	Important Considerations
Gabapentin	1200 mg 2 h preincision and 400–600 mg 3 times daily postoperatively for 14 d	• Promotes opioid cessation and prevents chronic opioid use[43] • Effective in neuropathic pain syndromes	Caution in patients with: • Advanced age • Reduced lung function Dose adjustment in patients with renal impairment
Pregabalin	300 mg 2 h preincision and 150 mg 2 times daily postoperatively for 14 d		
Ketamine	Preincision intravenous bolus of 0.5 mg/kg followed by intravenous infusion 0.25 mg/kg/h	• Low-dose ketamine provides immediate postoperative analgesia • Opioid-sparing effects	Not to be used in patients with: • Liver disease • Significant risk for liver disease (eg, alcoholism)
Venlafaxine	37.5 mg 1 d before surgery and continuing for 10–14 d postoperatively	• Significantly reduces opioid use compared with placebo and gabapentin[44]	Not suggested for patients that are taking (other) antidepressants

outside of the zone of scar. Although it may seem obvious, thick white scar tissue and nerve are very difficult to distinguish even while operating under tourniquet control. Thus, identifying the nerve in healthy tissue where anatomic landmarks are still intact is crucial for the success of the operation.

Work from Known to Unknown

Using the increased operative field by making longer incisions, as discussed above, allows for the identification of the nerve out of a scarred field. Dissection is carried most commonly from known to unknown, or healthy toward scarred tissue. Native unscarred planes allow for clean separation of the nerve from surrounding structures with preservation of vascular structures and motor or sensory branches in the area. When neuromas are suspected, it is useful to mark the sites of pain, that is, an acute Tinel sign, on the skin with an arrow before entering the operating room (**Fig. 2**). These markings can help you identify areas of nerve injury, such as inadvertently injured branches of the medial antebrachial cutaneous (MABC) nerve branches in CuTS.

Avoid Nerve Injury

Occasionally the scarred area of the nerve is so thick that the identification of the nerve itself or individual fascicles is nearly impossible. Decompression with or without nerve reconstruction in these cases is still necessary. The surgeon should not be surprised to find oneself entering the nerve even with the utmost careful and tedious dissection. Knowing the anatomy and topography of

the nerve at the level of injury, careful preoperative examination of the patient, and use of hand-held electrical stimulation (ES) all aid in these difficult dissections in order to preserve, and potentially improve, the function that is present.

Minimize Tourniquet Use to Allow for Hand-Held Electrical Stimulation

The use of tourniquet can be helpful for visualization as scarred fields are often bloody and can distort anatomy. If testing of nerve function is desired, the surgeon should seek to isolate the nerve in the healthy tissue bed proximal to the previously operative site expeditiously at the start of

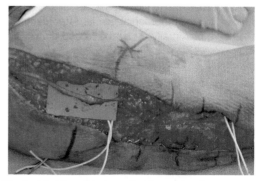

Fig. 2. Marking the sites of pain on the skin preoperatively when neuromas are expected. A MABC neuroma could occur after cubital tunnel release and presents with severe electrical shooting pain into the MABC distribution. In this photo, we can see that the site of pain (marked on the skin) correlates to the position of the neuroma found. (*Courtesy of* Amy Moore, MD, FACS, Columbus, OH.)

the operation. After 30 to 45 minutes of tourniquet use, direct hand-held ES of the nerve will start to get weak and eventually disappear, which eliminates this often helpful strategy to avoid nerve injury during the revision surgery. Awareness of tourniquet neuropraxia allows the surgeon to prioritize the critical dissection. The use of ES to potentially aid nerve regeneration will be discussed later in the article.

COMMON INTERVENTIONS FOR REVISION NERVE RELEASES
Revision Carpal Tunnel Release

Postoperative scarring is the most significant cause of recurrent CTS. Contributory factors include poor hemostasis and hematoma formation during the primary surgery, prolonged immobilization, or inadequate therapy. Excessive or inappropriate manipulation of the median nerve during the initial surgery may enhance intraneural or perineural scarring and adherence of the nerve to surrounding structures. The astute nerve surgeon can avoid persistent symptoms by careful preoperative examination to rule out proximal compression by checking for a Tinel sign and compression test over the median nerve in the proximal volar forearm. In the setting of a previous endoscopic CTR with either persistent or recurrent symptoms, the surgical technique proceeds as an open release.

Revision carpal tunnel surgery starts by identifying and marking the patient's previous surgical scar as well as the sites of the patient's most prominent Tinel sign. This aids in identifying the area of maximal compression before surgery. If central, the incision is made 8 to 10 mm ulnar to the previous scar. The incision is extended proximally across the wrist crease to allow for the release of the antebrachial fascia. After identifying the nerve proximally, it can be traced distally and will most often be found tethered under the radial leaflet of the transverse carpal ligament surrounded by dense scar tissue. If there are any concerns for concomitant ulnar nerve compression as a contributor to continued symptoms, Guyon canal can be decompressed through the same incision. We then prefer to neurolyse the median nerve circumferentially to ensure that no further compression remains. Care must be taken to do this neurolysis bluntly because the thenar motor branch is often difficult to identify in a scarred bed. A bulky dressing is applied, and an early movement is initiated by our hand therapists who also focus on desensitization and nerve gliding exercises in the first postoperative week.

An external neurolysis should be performed in cases where the epineurium has attached fibrous bands with maintenance of fascicular architecture. Hunter found that in these cases, rerelease resulted in restoration of the nerve gliding with good success.[44] In a prospective randomized controlled trial, no benefit of additional internal neurolysis could be found,[23] making this procedure controversial in revision carpal tunnel surgery.[25] The authors prefer a thorough external neurolysis at the time of revision CTR with meticulous removal of the often thick surrounding scar tissue that can envelope the nerve. Although some reports provide good results with neurolysis alone, many favor providing vascularized tissue or nerve wraps to the nerve bed after rerelease to prevent the scarring process. Small case series suggest that perineural autologous fat grafting could provide significant improvement in symptom severity and function severity scores after 1 to 2 years. [45,46] The effectiveness of free nonvascularized fat grafting should be thoroughly investigated because preclinical evidence suggests that a large proportion of adipocytes in a nonvascularized fat graft are unlikely to survive even when the graft

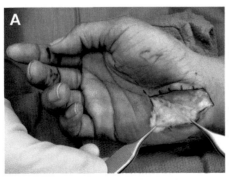
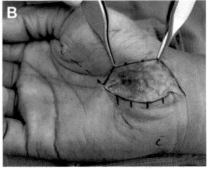

Fig. 3. A hypothenar fat pad flap could be used as a protective barrier in a case of recurrent CTS. (*A*) The hypothenar fat pad is dissected from the overlying skin of the palm, preserving its vascular supply from the ulnar artery. (*B*) The hypothenar fat pad has been placed over the median nerve and loosely secured to the radial leaflet of the transverse carpal ligament. (*Courtesy of* Sonu Jain, MD, Columbus, OH.)

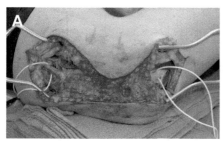
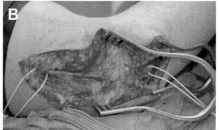

Fig. 4. Revision ulnar nerve decompression. A scarred ulnar nerve bed is depicted. The large incision will allow you to work from the known (ie, distal and proximal ends) to the unknown (ie, the scarred area). (*Courtesy of Amy Moore, MD, FACS, Columbus, OH.*)

is placed in a good recipient bed.[47] Flap coverage options at the level of the wrist could be grouped into local (synovial flap, lumbrical muscle flap, hypothenar fat flap, palmaris brevis flap), regional (radial forearm adipofascial flap, distal ulnar adipofascial flap), and distant flaps (pedicled groin flap, free tissue transfer).[25] Here, we will discuss the most commonly used flap for recurrent CTS, the hypothenar fat pad flap.

Hypothenar Fat Pad Flap

The hypothenar fat pad flap, first described in 1985 by Cramer[48] and subsequently modified by Strickland and Mathoulin,[49,50] is a technically simple procedure that interposes a barrier between the median nerve and the transverse carpal ligament, preventing median nerve readherence and scarring. This vascularized pedicle flap is based on the vasculature of the ulnar artery to the hypothenar fat. It is raised by subcutaneous dissection from the hypothenar eminence on the ulnar border of the carpal tunnel incision (**Fig. 3**A). The ulnar leaflet of the transverse carpal ligament can be removed to achieve mobilization of the flap and further dissection is carried out until Guyon canal is released and the ulnar artery and nerve are visualized and protected. The flap is mobilized to cover the median nerve, and securely inset by suturing

the free edge of the flap to the deep side of the radial leaf of the transverse carpal ligament while avoiding injury to the thenar motor branch of the median nerve (**Fig. 3**B). Retrospective studies found a significant decrease in pain scores by 74% and a distal latency decrease by 15%.[51] In a prospective study of 20 patients, relief of pain was found in 18 patients that received the hypothenar fat pad flap.[52] Complication rates of this flap are found to be low.[49,52–56] Regardless, this flap is not fully accepted to be the ideal method to treat recurrent CTS because concerns remain regarding the insufficient padding and inadequate size[57–59] or the tendency of the flap to undergo fibrosis and form scar tissue.[60]

Revision Cubital Tunnel Release

Revision surgery is often associated with increased technical difficulty due to significant scarring of the nerve to surround soft tissue (**Fig. 4**). On dissection, a scarred nerve bed may be seen, stressing the importance of creating long incisions and working from known (ie, distally and proximally to the scarred tissue area, see **Fig. 4**A) to the unknown (ie, scarred area). On identification of the nerve outside of the scarred area, careful and safe dissection can be carried out in

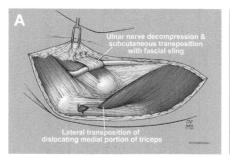
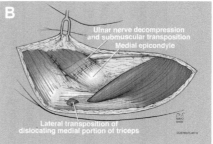

Fig. 5. An overview of ulnar nerve decompression and subcutaneous versus submuscular transposition. Figure A depicts the subcutaneous transposition and Figure B depicts a submuscular transposition of the ulnar nerve. (Used with permission of Mayo Foundation for Medical Education and Research, all rights reserved.)

Table 3
Comparison of nerve barrier options based on ideal characteristics for a barrier to epineural scarring

Ideal Characteristics	Adipofascial or Muscle Flap	Vein Wrapping	HA-CMC Membrane (Seprafilm)	Bovine Collagen (Neurawrap, Neuramend)	Porcine Small Intestine Submucosa (Axoguard)	Human Amnion Matrix (Arthrex, Amniox)
Biocompatible	Yes, Nonabsorbable	Yes, Nonabsorbable	No reports of rejection Absorbs by 7 d	No reports of rejection Absorbs by 4–8 mo	No reports of rejection Absorbs by 3 mo	Absorbs by 3 mo
Semipermeable	Yes	Yes	Yes	Yes	Yes	Yes
Nonconstricting	No reported cases of cicatrix formation after use	No reported cases of cicatrix formation after use	No reported cases of cicatrix formation after use	No reported cases of cicatrix formation after use	No reported cases of cicatrix formation after use	No reported cases of cicatrix formation after use
Promote nerve gliding	Yes	Yes, demonstrated in animal model	Unknown	Unknown	Unknown	Unknown
Minimal/no donor site morbidity	Depends on flap harvested (minimal for local fat pad flap)	Yes, (typically edema)	No donor site morbidity	No donor site morbidity	No donor site morbidity	No donor site morbidity
Minimal cost or supply restraints	Increased surgery time	Increased surgery time	Subject to implant cost and availability	Subject to implant cost and availability	Subject to implant cost and availability	Subject to implant cost and availability

Adapted from Dy, C.J., B. Aunins, and D.M. Brogan, Barriers to Epineural Scarring: Role in Treatment of Traumatic Nerve Injury and Chronic Compressive Neuropathy. J Hand Surg Am, 2018. 43(4): p. 360-367; with permission.

the scarred field to achieve complete decompression (see **Fig. 4**B).

The revision surgery performed is determined by the initial technique. If an in situ decompression was performed, then the decision to transpose anteriorly is the most common approach. However, if submuscular transposition was performed, then transposing the nerve into the superficial soft tissue is performed. Anterior transposition of the ulnar nerve is performed when subluxation occurs, and includes 2 techniques: subcutaneous (**Fig. 5**A) and submuscular transposition, respectively (**Fig. 5**B). Subcutaneous transposition is associated with few relative contraindications and provides the nerve with a smooth gliding surface; however, in some patients, it may result in a visible, palpable, and irritable ulnar nerve due to the lack of much overlying soft tissue to serve as cushioning. Another option is submuscular transposition, which was first described by Learmonth in 1942 and involved elevation of the flexor-pronator muscle and positioning of the nerve deep below.[61] A systematic review and meta-analysis by Liu and colleagues suggest that anterior subcutaneous and submuscular transposition are equally effective in patients with ulnar neuropathy at the elbow.[62] Currently, the authors prefer to avoid taking down the entire flexor pronator origin and instead position the nerve in a muscle trough beneath a fascial sling created after Z-lengthening similar to what has been described by Dy and Mackinnon,[63] known as intramuscular transposition.

PREVENTION OF PERINEURAL SCARRING AFTER REVISION SURGERY

After revision nerve decompression and/or transposition, the prevention of repeat scar formation and adherence of the nerve to the surrounding tissue is paramount. At this point, there may be significant scar tissue around the nerve bed which can cause painful re-entrapment of the nerve. Despite early nerve glide exercises and range of motion, the nerve can still become encased in scar all over again. Scar formation prevents nerve gliding, can apply traction and cause ischemia to the nerve, resulting in recurrent or new symptoms over time. Many treatment modalities and products have been investigated to prevent epineural scarring and adhesions; an overview is provided in **Table 3**. The ideal nerve wrap should be absorbable, provide a gliding surface for the nerve, and prevent scar formation around the nerve while also preventing axonal escape. It is important to not place these wraps tightly around the nerves. Postoperative nerve edema can lead to ischemia

of the nerve and further symptoms if not careful. Furthermore, these wraps should have very little chance of inducing inflammation, have adequate porosity to allow for diffusion of nutrients, and minimal donor site morbidity.[64]

Use of autologous tissue such as adipofascial flaps and vein wrapping has also been described. Adipofascial flaps provide healthy vascularized tissue to prevent scar formation around the nerve.[65,66] These flaps could be free or pedicled and dependent on the location to harvest the flap. Autologous vein wrapping has been studied in the setting of nerve decompression and shown promising results as the vein intima provides a gliding surface for the nerve.[67,68] Donor site morbidity, difficulty of application, and possible incorrect application causing further ischemia can be hazards of this technique.[67,68]

Commercially available materials used for nerve wraps include type 1 collagen, porcine small intestine submucosa (mixture of type 1 and 3 and collagen), hyaluronic acid-based wraps, and human amniotic membrane. The degradation time of these products highly differs and can be as long as 48 months, whereas most have a short degradation time of a few months.[69] There is evidence that each of these wraps can provide a barrier to perineural scarring.[68,70–73] The author's preference is the use of human amniotic membrane-derived products for a few key reasons. First, amnion wraps are thin and pliable and do not require any sutures to hold them in place. This makes them applicable to allow for postoperative swelling of the nerve, which inevitably occurs after surgical decompression. Wraps that are inadvertently applied too tightly can become constrictive and cause a new area of compression. Second, amnion tissue seems to cause minimal inflammation, resorbs after 3 months, and contains anti-inflammatory cytokines and growth factors that can aid in preventing significant perineural scarring. For these reasons, we currently prefer amnion as our barrier of choice for the prevention of postoperative scarring after revision nerve decompression (**Fig. 6**).

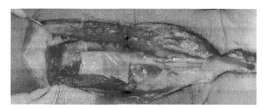

Fig. 6. The use of an amnion wrap. Depicted is the use of an amnion wrap around the median nerve after decompression. (*Courtesy of* Ryan Schmucker, MD, Columbus, OH.)

Failed nerve decompression

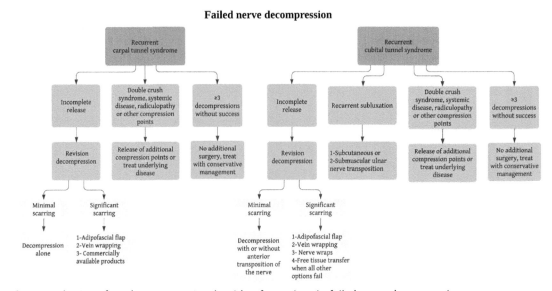

Fig. 7. Author's preferred treatment. An algorithm for options in failed nerve decompression.

A schematic algorithm of revision surgery options for recurrent CTS and CuTS is provided in **Fig. 7**.

FUTURE DIRECTIONS

Due to the severity of nerve compression that is encountered in many patients with longstanding nerve compression, therapies aimed at accelerating axonal regeneration have been investigated. ES shows great promise in this arena. The technique of ES relies on brief low-frequency (20 mHz or less) stimulation applied directly after nerve repair for a variable duration of time. Both animal and human studies have found that ES enhances functional recovery in both motor and sensory nerves.[74–78] The biologic basis of ES was discovered by the finding that applying tetrodotoxin, which blocks proximal electrical impulses, to the proximal nerve negated the benefits of ES on regenerating nerves.[79] ES exerts its influence through the retrograde conduction of action potentials to the neuronal cell bodies in the central nervous system. This upregulates neurotrophic factors and genes that are expressed in the neuron and crucial to accelerating nerve regeneration. In turn, this leads to increased axonal regeneration along with remyelination of regenerating axons.[74,78–82]

In the clinical realm, recent prospective randomized controlled studies have shown the benefit of ES on nerve regeneration in the setting of chronic median and ulnar nerve compression.[83,84] Power and colleagues recently assessed the effects of 1 hour of postsurgical ES after ulnar nerve decompression in patients with severe cubital tunnel. In a total of 31 patients, 11 patients received surgery alone and 20 received surgery with ES. If was found that motor unit number estimation, key pinch strength, and other functional and physiologic outcomes all increased significantly in the ES group compared with controls.[84] Currently, studies have been investigating the optimal delivery, duration of stimulation needed and timing of the application (intraoperative vs postoperative) in different nerve injury models to evaluate therapeutic benefit.[85] It is expected that ES will play a major role in the clinical treatment of severe compression neuropathies in the very near future.

SUMMARY

Defining the correct diagnosis after a failed nerve decompression (ie, persistent, recurrent, or new symptoms) is of the utmost importance and guides further surgical planning. We prefer to base the decision for additional surgery on a clinical picture of sensory complaints and/or motor function deterioration combined with careful consideration of previous surgical procedures. If patient and surgeon expectations are not well aligned, reoperation should be deferred. Revision surgery principles include (1) long incisions, (2) allowing sufficient operative time, and (3) working from known to unknown. Although incomplete release may be treated by repeat decompression alone, the options for a nerve in a scarred bed are more complicated and include transposition of the nerve anteriorly or superficially, the use of adipofascial flaps, vein wrapping, commercially available nerve wraps, or free tissue transfer when all other options fail.

CLINICS CARE POINTS

- Define if the symptoms are persistent, recurrent, or new
- If patient and surgeon expectations are not well aligned, reoperation should be deferred
- Revision surgery principles include (1) long incisions, (2) allowing sufficient operative time, and (3) work from known to unknown
- ES is expected to play a major role in clinical treatment of severe compression neuropathies in the very near future

DISCLOSURES

Commercial and financial: The authors are participating in a clinical trial that investigates the use of electrical stimulation (Checkpoint Surgical Inc) during cubital tunnel decompression.

REFERENCES

1. Gupta R, Steward O. Chronic nerve compression induces concurrent apoptosis and proliferation of Schwann cells. J Comp Neurol 2003;461(2):174–86.
2. Mackinnon SE, Dellon AL, Hudson AR, et al. Chronic human nerve compression–a histological assessment. Neuropathol Appl Neurobiol 1986;12(6):547–65.
3. Szabo RM, Gelberman RH. Peripheral nerve compression: etiology, critical pressure threshold, and clinical assessment. Orthopedics 1984;7(9):1461–6.
4. Mackinnon SE. Pathophysiology of nerve compression. Hand Clin 2002;18(2):231–41.
5. Burahee AS, Sanders AD, Power DM. The management of failed cubital tunnel decompression. EFORT Open Rev 2021;6(9):735–42.
6. Neuhaus V, Christoforou D, Cheriyan T, et al. Evaluation and treatment of failed carpal tunnel release. Orthop Clin North Am 2012;43(4):439–47.
7. Izadpanah A, Maldonado AA, Bishop AT, et al. Risk factors for revision cubital tunnel surgery(☆). J Plast Reconstr Aesthet Surg 2020;73(5):959–64.
8. Rydevik B, Lundborg G, Bagge U. Effects of graded compression on intraneural blood blow. An in vivo study on rabbit tibial nerve. J Hand Surg Am 1981;6(1):3–12.
9. Rydevik B, Lundborg G. Permeability of intraneural microvessels and perineurium following acute, graded experimental nerve compression. Scand J Plast Reconstr Surg 1977;11(3):179–87.
10. Powell HC, Myers RR. Pathology of experimental nerve compression. Lab Invest 1986;55(1):91–100.
11. Jung J, Hahn P, Choi B, et al. Early Surgical Decompression Restores Neurovascular Blood Flow and Ischemic Parameters in an in Vivo Animal Model of Nerve Compression Injury. J Bone Joint Surg Am 2014;96(11):897–906.
12. Hollie A, Power AMM. In: Skirven TM, editor. Rehabilitation of the hand and upper extremity, Chapter 48 Basic science of nerve compression. Philadelphia, PA: Elsevier Mosby; 2011.
13. Koop LK, Tadi P. Neuroanatomy, sensory nerves. Treasure Island (FL): StatPearls; 2022.
14. Wilgis EF, Murphy R. The significance of longitudinal excursion in peripheral nerves. Hand Clin 1986;2(4):761–6.
15. Rempel D, Dahlin L, Lundborg G. Pathophysiology of nerve compression syndromes: response of peripheral nerves to loading. J Bone Joint Surg Am 1999;81(11):1600–10.
16. Brunton LM. Hand, Upper Extremity, and Microvascular Surgery. In: Miller M, Thompson SR, Hart JA, et al, editors. Review of Orthopaedics. 2012. p. 517–87.
17. Upton AR, McComas AJ. The double crush in nerve entrapment syndromes. Lancet 1973;2(7825):359–62.
18. Dahlin LB, Lundborg G. The neurone and its response to peripheral nerve compression. J Hand Surg Br 1990;15(1):5–10.
19. Russell BS. Carpal tunnel syndrome and the "double crush" hypothesis: a review and implications for chiropractic. Chiropr Osteopat 2008;16:2.
20. Phan A, Shah S, Hammert W, et al. Double Crush Syndrome of the Upper Extremity. JBJS Rev 2021;9(12):e21.00082.
21. Lowe J, Mackinnon S. Management of Secondary Cubital Tunnel Syndrome. Plast Reconstr Surg 2004;113:E1–16.
22. Raimbeau G. [Recurrent carpal tunnel syndrome]. Chir Main 2008;27(4):134–45.
23. Mackinnon SE, McCabe S, Murray JF, et al. Internal neurolysis fails to improve the results of primary carpal tunnel decompression. J Hand Surg Am 1991;16(2):211–8.
24. Gellman H. Compression of the ulnar nerve at the elbow: cubital tunnel syndrome. Instr Course Lect 2008;57:187–97.
25. Rodrigues RL, Shin AY. Treatment Options for Recurrent Carpal Tunnel Syndrome: Local Flaps. Tech Orthopaedics 2006;21(1):61–74.
26. Lauder A, Mithani S, Leversedge FJ. Management of Recalcitrant Carpal Tunnel Syndrome. J Am Acad Orthop Surg 2019;27(15):551–62.
27. Amadio PC, Beckenbaugh RD. Entrapment of the ulnar nerve by the deep flexor-pronator aponeurosis. J Hand Surg Am 1986;11(1):83–7.
28. Gabel GT, Amadio PC. Reoperation for failed decompression of the ulnar nerve in the region of the elbow. J Bone Joint Surg Am 1990;72(2):213–9.

29. Steyers CM. Recurrent carpal tunnel syndrome. Hand Clin 2002;18(2):339–45.

30. Osterman AL. The double crush syndrome. Orthop Clin North Am 1988;19(1):147–55.

31. Power HA, Sharma K, El-Haj M, et al. Compound Muscle Action Potential Amplitude Predicts the Severity of Cubital Tunnel Syndrome. J Bone Joint Surg Am 2019;101(8):730–8.

32. Gruber H, Baur EM, Plaikner M, et al. The Ulnar Nerve After Surgical Transposition: Can Sonography Define the Reason of Persisting Neuropathy? Rofo 2015;187(11):998–1002.

33. Novak CB. Upper extremity work-related musculoskeletal disorders: a treatment perspective. J Orthop Sports Phys Ther 2004;34(10):628–37.

34. Dellon AL. Review of treatment results for ulnar nerve entrapment at the elbow. J Hand Surg Am 1989;14(4):688–700.

35. Rogers MR, Bergfield TG, Aulicino PL. The failed ulnar nerve transposition. Etiology and treatment. Clin Orthop Relat Res 1991;(269):193–200.

36. Vogel RB, Nossaman BC, Rayan GM. Revision anterior submuscular transposition of the ulnar nerve for failed subcutaneous transposition. Br J Plast Surg 2004;57(4):311–6.

37. Broudy AS, Leffert RD, Smith RJ. Technical problems with ulnar nerve transposition at the elbow: findings and results of reoperation. J Hand Surg Am 1978;3(1):85–9.

38. Caputo AE, Watson HK. Subcutaneous anterior transposition of the ulnar nerve for failed decompression of cubital tunnel syndrome. J Hand Surg Am 2000;25(3):544–51.

39. Horn R, Kramer J. Postoperative pain control. Treasure Island (FL: StatPearls; 2022.

40. Chou R, Gordon DB, de Leon-Casasola OA, et al. Management of Postoperative Pain: A Clinical Practice Guideline From the American Pain Society, the American Society of Regional Anesthesia and Pain Medicine, and the American Society of Anesthesiologists' Committee on Regional Anesthesia, Executive Committee, and Administrative Council. J Pain 2016;17(2):131–57.

41. Agarwal A, Gautam S, Gupta D, et al. Evaluation of a single preoperative dose of pregabalin for attenuation of postoperative pain after laparoscopic cholecystectomy. Br J Anaesth 2008;101(5):700–4.

42. Pripotnev S, Mackinnon SE. Revision of Carpal Tunnel Surgery. J Clin Med 2022;11(5).

43. Carroll I, Hah J, Mackey S, et al. Perioperative interventions to reduce chronic postsurgical pain. J Reconstr Microsurg 2013;29(4):213–22.

44. Hunter JM. Recurrent carpal tunnel syndrome, epineural fibrous fixation, and traction neuropathy. Hand Clin 1991;7(3):491–504.

45. Krzesniak NE, Noszczyk BH. Autologous Fat Transfer in Secondary Carpal Tunnel Release. Plast Reconstr Surg Glob Open 2015;3(5):e401.

46. Gostelie O, et al. Re-Neurolysis and Infiltration of Autologous Lipoaspirate Around the Median Nerve in Secondary Recurrent Carpal Tunnel Syndrome: A Prospective Cohort Study. SSRN Electron J 2020. https://doi.org/10.2139/ssrn.3522582. Electronic Journal.

47. Eto H, Kato H, Suga H, et al. The fate of adipocytes after nonvascularized fat grafting: evidence of early death and replacement of adipocytes. Plast Reconstr Surg 2012;129(5):1081–92.

48. Cramer. Local fat coverage for the median nerve. ASSH Correspondence Newsl 1985;35.

49. Strickland JW, Idler RS, Lourie GM, et al. The hypothenar fat pad flap for management of recalcitrant carpal tunnel syndrome. J Hand Surg Am 1996; 21(5):840–8.

50. Mathoulin C, Bahm J, Roukoz S. Pedicled hypothenar fat flap for median nerve coverage in recalcitrant carpal tunnel syndrome. Hand Surg 2000;5(1):33–40.

51. Payr S, Tiefenboeck TM, Moser V, et al. Surgery of True Recurring Median Carpal Tunnel Syndrome with Synovial Flap by Wulle Plus Integument Enlargement Leads to a High Patient's Satisfaction and Improved Functionality. J Clin Med 2019;8(12).

52. Fusetti C, Garavaglia G, Mathoulin C, et al. A reliable and simple solution for recalcitrant carpal tunnel syndrome: the hypothenar fat pad flap. Am J Orthop (Belle Mead Nj) 2009;38(4):181–6.

53. Plancher KD, Idler RS, Lourie GM, et al. Recalcitrant carpal tunnel. The hypothenar fat pad flap. Hand Clin 1996;12(2):337–49.

54. Chrysopoulo MT, Greenberg JA, Kleinman WB. The hypothenar fat pad transposition flap: a modified surgical technique. Tech Hand Up Extrem Surg 2006;10(3):150–6.

55. Frank U, Giunta R, Krimmer H, et al. [Relocation of the median nerve after scarring along the carpal tunnel with hypothenar fatty tissue flap-plasty]. Handchir Mikrochir Plast Chir 1999;31(5):317–22.

56. Giunta R, Frank U, Lanz U. The hypothenar fat-pad flap for reconstructive repair after scarring of the median nerve at the wrist joint. Chir Main 1998; 17(2):107–12.

57. Craft RO, Duncan SF, Smith AA. Management of recurrent carpal tunnel syndrome with microneurolysis and the hypothenar fat pad flap. Hand (N Y) 2007;2(3):85–9.

58. Stutz NM, Gohritz A, Novotny A, et al. Clinical and electrophysiological comparison of different methods of soft tissue coverage of the median nerve in recurrent carpal tunnel syndrome. Neurosurgery 2008;62(3 Suppl 1):194–9 [discussion: 199–200].

59. Tollestrup T, Berg C, Netscher D. Management of distal traumatic median nerve painful neuromas and of recurrent carpal tunnel syndrome: hypothenar fat pad flap. J Hand Surg Am 2010;35(6): 1010–4.

60. Giunta R, Frank U, Lanz U. Hypothenar fat-pad flap. In: Carpal tunnel syndrome. Springer; 2007. p. 319–23.

61. Leffert RD. Anterior submuscular transposition of the ulnar nerves by the Learmonth technique. J Hand Surg Am 1982;7(2):147–55.

62. Liu CH, Chen CX, Xu J, et al. Anterior Subcutaneous versus Submuscular Transposition of the Ulnar Nerve for Cubital Tunnel Syndrome: A Systematic Review and Meta-Analysis. PLoS One 2015;10(6): e0130843.

63. Dy CJ, Mackinnon SE. Ulnar neuropathy: evaluation and management. Curr Rev Musculoskelet Med 2016;9(2):178–84.

64. Dy CJ, Aunins B, Brogan DM. Barriers to Epineural Scarring: Role in Treatment of Traumatic Nerve Injury and Chronic Compressive Neuropathy. J Hand Surg Am 2018;43(4):360–7.

65. Pace GI, Zale CL, Gendelberg D, et al. Self-Reported Outcomes for Patients Undergoing Revision Carpal Tunnel Surgery With or Without Hypothenar Fat Pad Transposition. Hand (N Y) 2018;13(3): 292–5.

66. Saffari TM, Bedar M, Hundepool CA, et al. The role of vascularization in nerve regeneration of nerve graft. Neural Regen Res 2020;15(9):1573–9.

67. Xu J, Varitimidis SE, Fisher KJ, et al. The effect of wrapping scarred nerves with autogenous vein graft to treat recurrent chronic nerve compression. J Hand Surg Am 2000;25(1):93–103.

68. Kokkalis ZT, Jain S, Sotereanos DG. Vein wrapping at cubital tunnel for ulnar nerve problems. J Shoulder Elbow Surg 2010;19(2 Suppl):91–7.

69. Gaudin R, Knipfer C, Henningsen A, et al. Approaches to Peripheral Nerve Repair: Generations of Biomaterial Conduits Yielding to Replacing Autologous Nerve Grafts in Craniomaxillofacial Surgery. Biomed Res Int 2016;2016:3856262.

70. Soltani AM, Allan BJ, Best MJ, et al. Revision decompression and collagen nerve wrap for recurrent and persistent compression neuropathies of the upper extremity. Ann Plast Surg 2014;72(5): 572–8.

71. Magill CK, Tuffaha SH, Yee A, et al. The short- and long-term effects of Seprafilm on peripheral nerves: a histological and functional study. J Reconstr Microsurg 2009;25(6):345–54.

72. Gaspar MP, Abdelfattah HM, Welch IW, et al. Recurrent cubital tunnel syndrome treated with revision neurolysis and amniotic membrane nerve wrapping. J Shoulder Elbow Surg 2016;25(12):2057–65.

73. Kim SS, Sohn SK, Lee KY, et al. Use of human amniotic membrane wrap in reducing perineural adhesions in a rabbit model of ulnar nerve neurorrhaphy. J Hand Surg Eur 2010;35(3):214–9.

74. Brushart TM, Hoffman PN, Royall RM, et al. Electrical stimulation promotes motoneuron regeneration without increasing its speed or conditioning the neuron. J Neurosci 2002;22(15):6631–8.

75. Geremia NM, Gordon T, Brushart TM, et al. Electrical stimulation promotes sensory neuron regeneration and growth-associated gene expression. Exp Neurol 2007;205(2):347–59.

76. Willand MP, Nguyen MA, Borschel GH, et al. Electrical Stimulation to Promote Peripheral Nerve Regeneration. Neurorehabil Neural Repair 2016;30(5): 490–6.

77. Gordon T. Electrical Stimulation to Enhance Axon Regeneration After Peripheral Nerve Injuries in Animal Models and Humans. Neurotherapeutics 2016; 13(2):295–310.

78. Zuo KJ, Gordon T, Chan KM, et al. Electrical stimulation to enhance peripheral nerve regeneration: Update in molecular investigations and clinical translation. Exp Neurol 2020;332:113397.

79. Al-Majed AA, Neumann CM, Brushart TM, et al. Brief electrical stimulation promotes the speed and accuracy of motor axonal regeneration. J Neurosci 2000; 20(7):2602–8.

80. Al-Majed AA, Tam SL, Gordon T. Electrical stimulation accelerates and enhances expression of regeneration-associated genes in regenerating rat femoral motoneurons. Cell Mol Neurobiol 2004; 24(3):379–402.

81. Gordon T, Udina E, Verge VM, et al. Brief electrical stimulation accelerates axon regeneration in the peripheral nervous system and promotes sensory axon regeneration in the central nervous system. Motor Control 2009;13(4):412–41.

82. Elzinga K, Tyreman N, Ladak A, et al. Brief electrical stimulation improves nerve regeneration after delayed repair in Sprague Dawley rats. Exp Neurol 2015;269:142–53.

83. Gordon T, Amirjani N, Edwards DC, et al. Brief postsurgical electrical stimulation accelerates axon regeneration and muscle reinnervation without affecting the functional measures in carpal tunnel syndrome patients. Exp Neurol 2010;223(1): 192–202.

84. Power HA, Morhart MJ, Olson JL, et al. Postsurgical Electrical Stimulation Enhances Recovery Following Surgery for Severe Cubital Tunnel Syndrome: A Double-Blind Randomized Controlled Trial. Neurosurgery 2020;86(6):769–77.

85. Roh J, Schellhardt L, Keane GC, et al. Short-Duration, Pulsatile, Electrical Stimulation Therapy Accelerates Axon Regeneration and Recovery following Tibial Nerve Injury and Repair in Rats. Plast Reconstr Surg 2022;149(4):681e–90e.

Challenges in Nerve Repair and Reconstruction

James S. Lin, MD[a], Sonu A. Jain, MD[b],*

KEYWORDS

- Peripheral nerve injury • Nerve repair • Nerve reconstruction • Nerve grafting • Nerve transfer

KEY POINTS

- Peripheral nerve injuries remain challenging injuries to manage, as outcomes are often poor despite appropriate surgical intervention.
- Direct end-to-end nerve repair is the standard of care if a minimal tension repair construct can be achieved.
- Nerve autografting is the gold standard for larger nerve defects that preclude primary repair, but donor site morbidity is a notable challenge.
- Nerve transfers are an increasingly popular technique that can be considered for brachial plexus injuries as well as segmental and proximal lesions with a long distance from target motor end plates.
- Molecular and cell-based therapies and pharmacologic agents may play a role to enhance axonal regeneration and improve the outcomes of these challenging injuries in the future.

INTRODUCTION

The treatment of nerve injuries continues to be a challenging issue. Despite appropriate surgical repair or reconstruction, as much as a third of patients may have little to no recovery, and useful results are only obtained in about half of patients.[1,2] There are also considerable economic costs to both the patient and society. The median direct cost to the patient who undergoes brachial plexus surgery has been found to be around $39,000.[3] Even after successful surgical reconstruction, many patients do not return to their previous profession or return to work at all.[4,5] This leads to a mean indirect cost to society of $1.1 million per patient from lost productivity, wages, and disability payments for traumatic brachial plexus injury.[4]

Peripheral nerve injuries are not infrequently encountered. It has been estimated that nearly 3% of all patients treated at a level 1 trauma center had at least one peripheral nerve injury of the extremity. The incidence rises to approximately 5% if plexus and root injuries are also included.[6] These injuries may be challenging to manage, as they have highly variable degrees of severity and potential for recovery. A classification system described by Seddon has often been used.[7] Neurapraxia is the mildest form of injury, where the nerve sustains a stretch or compression injury causing focal demyelination while the axon remains in continuity. The nerve does not undergo distal degeneration, and full spontaneous recovery can typically be expected from days to weeks. Axonotmesis is characterized by the disruption of the continuity of axons, while the epineurium remains intact. Neurotmesis injuries are the most severe, as they describe a physiologic disruption of the entire nerve, and spontaneous recovery is negligible.

Sunderland recognized that axonotmesis injuries can vary substantially depending on the involvement of the surrounding neural structures

Dr Jain has received institutional research funding for the multicenter RANGER study from Axogen, Inc.
a Department of Orthopaedics, The Ohio State University Wexner Medical Center, 241 West 11th Avenue, Suite 6081, Columbus, OH 43201, USA; b Department of Plastic and Reconstructive Surgery, The Ohio State University Wexner Medical Center, 915 Olentangy River Road, 3rd Floor, Suite 3200, Columbus, OH 43212, USA
* Corresponding author.
E-mail address: Sonu.Jain@osumc.edu

hand.theclinics.com

and therefore refined the classification system with 3 additional categories, later modified by Mackinnon with a fourth mixed injury category (**Table 1**).[8] Sunderland Type 1 injuries represent neuropraxia. Type 2 represent axonotmesis with preserved endoneurium, perineurium, and epineurium. Wallerian degeneration occurs distal to the injury. Axonal regeneration is directed by the intact endoneurium at a rate of approximately 1 mm per day or 1 inch per month, and complete recovery can be expected over the course of months.[9,10] Type 3 injuries describes axonotmesis with the disruption of the endoneurium while the perineurium and epineurium are preserved. The added injury to the endoneurium facilitates intrafascicular scar tissue formation that prevent complete contact between regenerating axons and their distal receptors. Since the perineurium and epineurium are preserved, regeneration of the nerve fibers can still occur at approximately 1 mm per day as it is guided by these intact structures. However, recovery will be incomplete and highly variable depending on the extent of scar tissue formation. Type 4 describe axonotmesis with the disruption of the endoneurium and perineurium while only the epineurium is preserved. There is substantial scar tissue formation that prevents regenerating axons from reaching their distal receptors. Minimal recovery can be expected without surgical intervention in these injuries. Type 5 injuries represent neurotmesis. These injuries are typically easier to recognize, as they are often secondary to an open traumatic injury and require surgical management. Type 6 describes nerves with a mixed injury pattern with which may multiple types of interventions and have variable prognosis.[8,9]

While these classification systems can help characterize the structures involved in nerve injuries, surgeons still face notable challenges in diagnosis and treatment. Specifically, it is important to distinguish which injuries will recovery without surgical intervention (Sunderland types 1–3) and those that will not (Sunderland types 4–5). However, many peripheral nerve injuries can be mixed in severity (Sunderland/Mackinnon type 6), where different fascicles sustain different degrees of injury and have different potentials for recovery. Correct subclassification of an axonotmetic injury may also not be possible without histological examination.[10]

EVALUATION

The difficulty in accurate classification of peripheral nerve injuries has led to "watch and wait" strategies in management.[11] However, it has been demonstrated by Mackinnon and other authors that early primary nerve repair where appropriate is associated with improved outcomes compared to delayed surgery.[12] Early decision making is important, as irreversible muscle atrophy and fibrosis can occur in 12 to 18 months, and surgical reconstruction no longer provides benefit.[11,13] Therefore, timely and accurate diagnosis of the peripheral nerve injury is critical. A thorough clinical examination should be a part of the surgeon's evaluation. Any open wounds should be inspected to evaluate the surrounding soft tissues, presence of contamination, and any associated injuries. A complete neurologic examination should assess sensation and motor function of the extremity to determine the presence of deficits as well as intact areas for potential donors if necessary. Motor function is commonly graded by the system developed by the Medical Research Council of Great Britain, and sensation is often classified by the Mackinnon-Dellon scale (**Table 2**).[14,15] Both stationary and moving two-point discrimination should be employed for the evaluation of sensation. A Tinel sign should be able to be elicited at the site of injury, and an advancing Tinel sign can be followed distally at the rate of 1 mm per day as the axon regenerates. If the Tinel sign fails to

Table 1
Seddon and Sunderland Classification System of Peripheral Nerve Injury (including Mackinnon and Dellon modification)

Seddon	Sunderland	
Neuropraxia	Type 1	Focal demyelination. Axon remains intact
Axonotmesis	Type 2	Axonal continuity lost. Endoneurium, perineurium, and epineurium remain intact
	Type 3	Axonal continuity lost. Endoneurium disrupted. Perineurium and epineurium remain intact
	Type 4	Axonal continuity lost. Endoneurium and perineurium disrupted. Epineurium remains intact
Neurotmesis	Type 5	Complete disruption of nerve structures
	Type 6	Mixed injury

Table 2
Medical research Council grading system and Mackinnon-Dellon scale for motor and sensory function

Motor Recovery	
M0	No contraction
M1	Return of perceptible contraction in the proximal muscles
M2	Return of perceptible contraction in the proximal and distal muscles
M3	Return of function in proximal and distal muscles to such a degree that all important muscles are powerful enough to act against gravity
M4	All muscles act against strong resistance, and some independent movements are possible
M5	Complete recovery
Sensory Recovery	
S0	Absent sensation
S1	Recovery of deep cutaneous pain
S1+	Recovery of deep superficial pain
S2	Recovery of superficial pain and some touch
S2+	Same as S2, but with overresponse
S3	Recovery of pain and touch sensibility with the disappearance of overresponse
S3+	Same as S3 with good localization of the stimulus. Imperfect recovery of two-point discrimination
S4	Complete recovery

advance, this may suggest neuroma or fibrosis blocking regeneration.[16]

Electrodiagnostic testing such as electromyography (EMG) and nerve conduction studies can be employed. Needle EMG measures motor unit action potentials to detect changes in recruitment and axonal loss. The presence of fibrillation potentials and positive sharp waves on EMG typically signal that the muscle is denervated. This can be detected approximately 10 to 14 days following injury if the distal nerve end is short, or 21 to 30 days if the distal end is long.[17,18] A nerve conduction study may measure nerve conduction velocity (NCV) by stimulating an electrode placed at the proximal aspect of the nerve and recording the response by an electrode placed distally. If the stimulation occurs distal to the lesion, there may still be a response at the distal recording electrode shortly after injury if Wallerian degeneration has not occurred yet. Therefore, a full evaluation using NCV testing cannot typically be made until

approximately 10 days after injury. Furthermore, these tests cannot reliably differentiate between axonotmesis and neurotmesis – a distinction that is critical in the consideration of surgical versus nonsurgical treatment.[9,19]

Although electrodiagnostic testing may not reveal the precise location of the lesion immediately following injury, imaging studies may help determine the site. For instance, high-resolution ultrasonography has been demonstrated to be a viable tool to assess the location, continuity, and extent of peripheral nerve lesions to the fascicular level.[20] However, a challenge with neurosonography is that visualization may be compromised by the presence of hematoma, seroma, and edema in the acute setting following peripheral nerve injury.[11]

A more recently developed imaging modality is magnetic resonance neurography (MRN), which is magnetic resonance imaging (MRI) modified to target the specific properties of water in nerve tissue, allowing high-resolution visualization of peripheral nerve lesions. This also enables earlier evaluation, as signal increase from Wallerian degeneration can be detected 48 hours following injury by MRN.[21] Moreover, MRN findings specific to the various degrees of nerve injury severity by the Sunderland classification have been described, which is important for surgical considerations.[22] A recent study found that the use of magnetic resonance neurography within the first 90 days for patients with peripheral nerve injuries accelerated decision making by 28 days compared to those who did not receive MRN as part of their evaluation.[11]

SURGICAL TREATMENT

There have been few substantial improvements in the treatment of peripheral nerve injury over the past several decades. In 1873, Huenter described the technique in epineurial nerve repair still used today.[23] In 1945, Sunderland described the principles of microsurgical nerve repair, and in 1964, Kurze and Smith independently employed these principles following the advent of the operating microscope.[24,25] Since then, only minor advancements have been made in surgery for nerve injury. Direct nerve repair, when possible, and autologous nerve grafting, when necessary for larger defects, remain the standard to which other methods are compared. In general, wounds should be thoroughly explored and the extent of injury fully evaluated. Any concomitant skeletal injuries should be addressed in order to achieve an environment of stability and curtail undue tension. A concomitant shortening osteotomy at the time of primary nerve repair can also be considered to achieve a tension-free repair.[26]

Direct Repair

Challenges of direct end-to-end nerve repair include the stringent requirements of the injury that would allow for this technique to be used. Ideally, the injury would be a sharp nerve transection without a crush component, and gapping should be so that minimal tension could be achieved. In addition, the wound must be clean, have adequate vascular supply, and be amenable to soft tissue coverage.[10,27] Following nerve repair, the extremity can be immobilized for a period of 10 to 14 days or longer depending on severity and associated injuries[15] but it is not necessary to do so if the nerve repair does not need to be protected from motion.

Various microsurgical suturing techniques have been described, each with their own advantages and challenges. 8-0 or 9-0 monofilament sutures are typically used.[27] Preferably, the number of suture threads used is as few as possible while maintaining the orientation of the repair.[28] One technique that minimizes sutures required is epineurial neurorrhaphy, where the sutures only pass through the epineurium connecting the nerve stumps together. The needle is passed approximately 1 to 2 mm from the edge of the epineurium on the two nerve ends, using the epineurial vasculature as a guide for aligning the fascicles. The advantage of this technique is that it is less technically demanding than other strategies in addition to requiring fewer sutures. One challenge is that the malalignment of the regenerating fascicles may occur as only the epineurium is sutured[29] particularly when dealing with mixed motor-sensory nerves.

One technique that may improve fascicular alignment is fascicular suturing, where the sutures are passed through the perineural sheaths of individual fascicles. However, this strategy is more technically challenging, and greater dissection is required which leads to greater potential scar formation.[27] A combined repair technique has also been described where both the suture simultaneously passes through both the epineurial and perineurial sheaths. This technique also enables improved fascicular orientation with the disadvantage of being more technically challenging.[28] It should be clearly noted that there is little evidence that more accurate orientation of the regenerating axons afforded by group fascicular repair leads to better functional outcomes than those achieved by the simpler epineurial repair.[30]

Outcomes of primary nerve repairs depend on a variety of factors. In general, better outcomes are associated with early intervention, direct repair rather than grafting, repair of single function nerves, smaller diameter nerves, and distal lesions compared to proximal.[10] However, functional outcomes reported in the literature are difficult to generalize due to the variability of outcome measures, repair techniques, types of lesions, and injury and patient characteristics. Over a 40-year timespan, Mackinnon and Dellon reported very good outcomes (M4, S3+) were obtained in 20% to 40% of patients who underwent direct nerve repair, but very few achieved full recovery.[15] Results may vary considerably. For instance, radial nerve repair has been considered to typically yield favorable results due to its predominantly motor content. In a series of 27 patients who underwent end-to-end repair of the radial nerve following penetrating trauma, wrist extension recovered in 93% of cases, finger extension in 74%, and thumb extension in 52%.[31] In another series, 16 of 18 (89%) patients who underwent primary end-to-end midhumeral radial nerve repair achieved excellent motor recovery (wrist and finger extension of M4 or M5).[32] In contrast, a series of 15 patients who underwent repair for isolated high ulnar nerve lesions were found to have poor intrinsic muscle and sensory recovery.[33]

Furthermore, end-to-side neurorrhaphy can be considered when the proximal end of the injured nerve is not amenable for coaptation. In this technique, the distal end of the injured nerve is sutured to the side of an adjacent nerve, with the goal of reinnervation due to collateral sprouting from the intact axons of the healthy nerve.[34] The success of motor reinnervation with this technique is mixed in the literature.[35,36] One animal study performed end-to-side ulnar to musculocutaneous nerve neurorrhaphy confirmed limited but functional reinnervation does occur.[37]

Fibrin glue

Various methods of augmentation of direct nerve repair have been described. One technique is using fibrin glue to enhance coaptation. A cadaveric study found that the addition of commercially available fibrin sealants to a two 8-0 nylon epineural suture nerve repair increased resistance to gapping, although it did not increase ultimate tensile strength.[38] There has also been evidence supporting the use of fibrin glue as an alternative to suture repair. Animal models have demonstrated the relative ease of use of this technique, and it may also have the advantage of lowering the inflammatory response and fibrosis that one would encounter with sutures.[39,40] A recent randomized clinical trial of 85 patients with injuries of the median and/or ulnar nerves at the wrist and forearm found that repairs performed using autologous fibrin glue were as effective in achieving motor and sensory recovery as those who underwent standard microsurgical epineurial suture repair with the advantage of a shorter operative time.[41]

Conduit wraps

Short conduits can also be wrapped around the nerve ends to augment suture coaptation as a connector-assisted repair. Theoretical benefits of a conduit wrap encapsulating a repair site include the accumulation of positive neurogenic factors, protection from fibroblast influx from surrounding tissue, and decreased likelihood of neuroma formation.[42,43] This conduit-assisted repair technique may also be helpful for inexperienced surgeons, as a cadaveric study found that connector-assistance was associated with improved alignment compared to suture-only or conduit-only repairs.[43] A review of clinical literature concluded that the use of conduit assistance in nerve repair may be associated with improved sensory recovery, reduced operative time, and less pain at the repair site when compared to suture-only repairs.[44] However, it is unclear if this translates to significantly improved clinical outcomes compared to properly performed microsurgical suture repair. Other challenges with this technique include the potential disruption of the suture repair when positioning the connector wrap, the increased cost of materials, and possibility of compression of the regenerating axons at the repair site.[43,45]

Nerve Autografts

Direct nerve repair is often not possible due to nerve defects that would cause excessive tension at a repair site. When intervention is delayed, cleanly transected nerves may also retract and develop neuromas that require excision, creating a defect that precludes primary repair. Nerve mobilization and transposition may be options to decrease tension to allow for the repair of small defects. If too much tension remains, other reconstructive options may be required. Nerve autografts remain the gold standard for the reconstruction of larger nerve defects, as they most closely resemble the architecture and biology of the injured nerve. Various types of autografting have been described, including cable, trunk, interfascicular, and vascularized grafts.[46] Regardless of the technique selected, the length of the prepared graft is generally made 10% to 20% longer than the length of the defect to ensure a tension-free construct.[27] In addition, the interposed graft is reversed in orientation to minimize the dispersion of axons through side nerve branches and therefore maximize axonal regeneration through the graft distally.[23]

Cable grafts

Cable grafts are most commonly used, and this method involves placing multiple small caliber donor grafts in parallel to match the diameter of the injured nerve (**Fig. 1**). This bundle is then placed into the nerve defect and secured with the epineurial suture or fibrin glue. While the cable nerve grafting technique affords advantages in versatility, a limitation is that it requires a well-vascularized bed at the recipient site. Nevertheless, the parallel configuration of the cables does enable greater contact with surrounding tissue and improves the revascularization of the graft.[10]

Trunk grafts

Trunk grafts involve taking a whole segment from a large nerve and interposing it in the gap of the injured nerve. Notable challenges with trunk grafts include poor vascularity and its propensity for internal fibrosis, as the thickness of the graft prevents regenerating axons from reaching the center of the graft before scar formation.

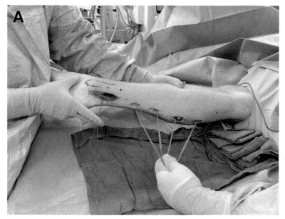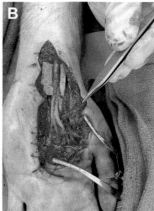

Fig. 1. (*A*) Sural nerve harvest for cable autograft. (*B*) Sural nerve cable autograft for median nerve defect. (*Courtesy of* Sonu Jain MD, Columbus, OH.)

Therefore, these grafts have typically yielded poor functional results.[23]

Interfascicular graft

Interfascicular grafts involve careful dissection of fasciculi or groups of fasciculi at the ends of injured nerves. A donor nerve is similarly separated into strands composed of groups of fasciculi, and these strands are coapted individually to the corresponding ends of the fasciculi or groups of fasciculi of the injured nerve. A proposed advantage of this technique is that the individual strands of graft minimizes tension but maximizes contact area with adjacent tissue and therefore greater chance of survival even in scarred tissue.[47] However, this technique may require greater technical skill and increased operative time due to the meticulous dissection of fascicles needed.[48]

Vascularized graft

The free vascularized nerve graft involves harvesting a donor graft along with its arterial supply.[49] This technique may be considered in instances where the recipient nerve bed has undergone significant fibrosis and therefore unable to provide adequate vascularity to support a nonvascularized nerve graft.[50] The vascularized graft may survive by avoiding the period of ischemia that may lead to the central fibrosis that one may encounter with a trunk graft. Conversely, a challenge of this technique is the greater donor-site morbidity and increased complexity of the procedure, without providing reliably better results than avascular grafts.[28]

Donor graft selection

Donor nerves are typically expendable sensory nerves. The sural nerve is the most commonly sourced autograft due to its relative ease of harvest, a diameter conducive to most cable grafting constructs, and long length of up to 30 to 40 cm that may be obtained for grafting.[51] Other commonly selected grafts include the anterior branch of the medial antebrachial cutaneous neve, lateral femoral cutaneous nerve, and superficial radial sensory nerve.

Donor site morbidity remains a notable challenge for nerve autografting. Although the sural nerve provides a purely sensory function and has relatively low morbidity, the potential effects should be discussed in detail with patients. For sural nerve grafts, sensory loss at the donor is the most commonly reported morbidity at a rate of approximately 87% in the literature.[52] However, partial return of sensation may occur over time, possibly due to collateral sprouting of axons from surrounding sensory nerves.[53] Other commonly reported adverse outcomes include pain and cold sensitivity at rates of 26% and 22%,

respectively. Of note, the extent of sensory loss and pain may be decreased if the proximal sural nerve is spared. Functional impairment has been reported as well, with a rate of approximately 10% in the literature.[52] Furthermore, painful neuromas can occur at the donor site. A systematic review of digital nerves injuries found that 5.7% of patients who underwent autograft repairs developed neuromas, all of which occurred at the medial antebrachial cutaneous (MABC) donor site.[54]

Nerve Allografts

Allografts obviate the need for a nerve harvest, decreasing surgical time and avoiding the potential for donor site morbidity. Historically, a challenge with allografts is rejection due to the immunogenic host response. Animal models have found an increase in T-cell and macrophage proliferation following the implantation of peripheral nerve allografts, likely due to allograft Schwann cells behaving as antigen-presenting cells.[55,56] Many methods have been described to address the immune response. Systemic immunosuppression has been employed in the past, but an obvious disadvantage includes their chemotoxic effects.[57] There has since been a shift in focus toward eliminating the immunogenicity of the allograft via strategies such as host graft irradiation, cold preservation, and chemical processing to create an acellular graft.[58–60]

The use of decellularized cadaveric nerve allografts for patients with either digital or ulnar nerve sensory defects of 5 to 30 mm has been found to have favorable results in recovery of two-point discrimination without infection or rejection[61] (Fig. 2). Data on motor recovery is scarcer. A study employing a rat model with a 10 mm sciatic nerve defect found that those treated with allograft had superior isometric strength compared to those treated with collagen conduit at 16 weeks postoperatively, but autograft was superior to both.[62] Similarly, a rat model with short 14 mm sciatic nerve gaps found greater numbers of myelinated fibers for allografts compared to conduits, although autografts yielded higher axonal counts than both. However, the long gap (28 mm) model in this study demonstrated that only autografts yielded axonal regeneration distal to the graft.[63]

Recently, a database study of patients with mixed motor and sensory nerve injuries underwent processed nerve allografting with a mean graft length of 33 mm (10–70 mm), and meaningful motor recovery (≥M3) was obtained in 73%.[64] In contrast, a study of military servicemembers with mixed motor and sensory nerve injuries who

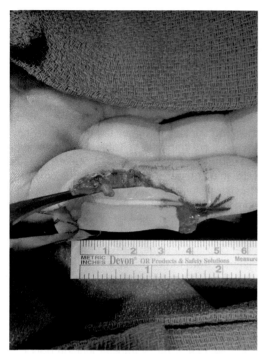

Fig. 2. Processed nerve allograft being used for digital nerve reconstruction. (*Courtesy of* Sonu Jain MD, Columbus, OH.)

underwent processed nerve allograft reconstruction achieved meaningful motor recovery in only 24% of patients.[65] However, the mean nerve defect was 77 mm in this population, often due to a complex mechanism of injury such as a blast or gunshot. Given the paucity and variability of human studies supporting allograft use in motor and mixed motor and sensory nerve reconstruction, their utility in larger diameter and longer gap nerve injuries remains limited.[66]

Nerve Conduits

Nerve conduits are another option for managing nerve defects with gaps of less than 3 cm. Conduits are tubes that can help support nerve regeneration over short distances. The nerve ends placed within the conduit tube, held together with sutures passing through the wall of the tube and capturing the nerve epineurium. In principle, the tube protects the nerve ends and area of regeneration from scar tissue invasion, while neurotropic factors guide the regenerating axons to the distal end of the injured nerve.[67]

Autogenous vein conduits
Many different types of material have been described for conduits. The most commonly employed autogenous source is venous, and vein conduits have been demonstrated to provide satisfactory symptomatic relief and sensory recovery for painful neuromas or segmental nerve injury of 3 cm. Chiu and Strauch's prospective study found that autogenous vein nerve conduits yielded comparable clinical outcomes to sural nerve allografts for the reconstruction of cutaneous sensory nerves, although both were inferior to primary end-to-end repair.[68] There is a theoretical challenge of vein wall collapse, but this has not been demonstrated clinically.[69]

Nonautogenous conduits
Commercially available nonautogenous conduits commonly employed include those made of collagen, polyglycolic acid (PGA), and caprolactone. An animal study comparing these 3 conduits using a rat model with a 10 mm sciatic nerve defect found that caprolactone conduits performed the best, with similar functional outcomes to autograft in terms of recovery of compound muscle action potentials, muscle weight, isometric muscle force, and axonal count.[70] The PGA conduits performed the worst, with complete structural collapse by 12 weeks. In human studies, there are varying amounts of evidence that support the role of these 3 types of commercially available conduits.

Collagen conduits
Collagen conduits are most often comprised of Type-I collagen, a large component of peripheral nerve proteins. The semipermeable framework of collagen conduits allows for controlled diffusion and resorption by approximately 9 months.[69] A series of collagen conduit repairs for digital nerve defects from 10 to 12 mm revealed overall favorable outcomes by two-point discrimination, Semmes-Weinstein monofilament, and Quick Disabilities of the Arm, Shoulder, and Hand (DASH) scores at 2 years.[71] Another series of interpositional collagen conduit repair of digital nerve lesions with a mean 12.5 mm defect found 33% of patients had excellent sensory recovery, 42% good recovery, and 25% had poor or no recovery at 1 year.[72] Until recently, the utility of conduits in large diameter nerves as well as their potential for motor recovery were not well described. Dienstknecht and colleagues report a series of median nerve lesions with gaps of 1 to 2 cm in the distal forearm that undergo collagen conduit repair, achieving good motor function by DASH score and nerve conduction velocity. Klein and colleagues presented a series of radial and ulnar nerve lesions in the forearm with gaps of 8 to 12 mm, also describing overall promising results for sensory and motor recovery.[73]

Polyglycolic acid conduits

Polyglycolic acid (PGA) conduits are considered more flexible and porous, allowing diffusion and resorption by approximately six months.[74] In a level II prospective multicenter trial, Weber and colleagues[75] randomized patients with digital nerve transections with less than 3 cm defects to two groups: 1) reconstruction with a PGA conduit and 2) direct end-to-end primary repair or autograft. Overall, the groups had similar outcomes in terms of two-point discrimination. Further analysis based on gap length found that PGA conduit was superior to primary repair for gaps $\leq$ 4 mm and also superior to autografts for gaps $\geq$ 8 mm. Other studies have compared the PGA conduit to muscle-vein[76] or vein[77] conduits, finding equivalent results. However, one challenge described for PGA conduits is the possibility of extrusion that may require reoperation.[77] In addition, the use of PGA conduits in reconstruction beyond sensory digital nerves has not been well described.

Caprolactone conduits

Poly(DL-lactide-ε-caprolactone), or simply caprolactone, conduits are another type of bioabsorbable synthetic conduit that resorbs in approximately 1 year.[74] A multicenter trial performed by Bertleff and colleagues[78] randomized patients with digital nerve injuries with gaps up to 20 mm into 2 groups: 1) reconstruction with a caprolactone conduit or 2) primary end-to-end repair. These authors found overall favorable and comparable sensory recovery outcomes, although there were more wound-healing complications in the conduit group. Similar to PGA conduits, the utility of caprolactone conduits beyond small sensory nerves has not been well demonstrated.

Recently, Mauch and colleagues[54] performed a systematic review of digital nerve repairs. Articles included 5 examining conduit, 4 allograft, 4 autograft, and 7 studying primary repairs. The review found that allograft and autograft repairs had the highest percentage of patients with normal to near-normal sensory recovery. The studies examining nerve conduit repairs reported higher rates of incomplete sensory recovery. Furthermore, a notable challenge of nerve conduits is the higher rate of reported complications at 10.9%, which included infection, extrusions, amputations, or removal. Therefore, these authors suggested that nerve conduits may be best reserved for uncomplicated cases.[54]

Nerve Transfers

Nerve transfers involve the coaptation of a healthy donor nerve to an injured nerve with the goal of reinnervation and restoration of function. In this technique, a proximal injury is essentially converted to a distal injury, as "nearby" redundant nerve function is transferred to a distal denervated recipient nerve close to its target motor endplates.[79] Nerve transfers share principles with tendon transfers in that the donor nerve is ideally synergistic with the recipient nerve and also redundant in function so minimal morbidity occurs following transfer. Common upper extremity nerve transfers are depicted in **Table 3**. This technique has seen increased usage over the past 2 decades, with many reports of favorable outcomes.[79–81] Nerve transfers can be considered in cases where primary repair or grafting may not be reliable. Specifically, Ray and Mackinnon[79] contend that nerve transfers may be indicated for brachial plexus and other proximal lesions, delayed presentation, long distance from target motor end plates, segmental loss of nerve function, and prior injury with extensive scar formation around vital bony or vascular structures. Furthermore, the proximity of the donor nerve to the target motor endplates enables potentially earlier reinnervation.

Challenges of nerve transfer include donor site morbidity with possible loss of function. Delay of care may also be a challenge, as axonal regeneration and recovery may be limited if significant degeneration of the recipient motor endplates has occurred.[82,83] The optimal timing of nerve transfer remains unclear, but reinnervation of the target muscle by 12 to 18 months following injury is likely ideal.[8] Furthermore, sufficient function of the donor nerve should be confirmed, and an EMG can be obtained if it is questionable. Moreover, there are limited salvage options for cases of failed nerve transfer.

A more recently described technique is the supercharge end-to-side (SETS) nerve transfer. The goal of this technique is to augment, or "supercharge," motor nerve regeneration with a reverse end-to-side coaptation of a normal functioning nerve to the injured nerve. The mechanisms by which donor axons propagate within the recipient nerve and how they affect native axonal regeneration in the recipient nerve remain poorly understood.[84] However, this supercharge technique has seen increasing popularity in anterior interosseous nerve to ulnar motor nerve transfer to enhance intrinsic recovery.[85,86] Over the last decade, indications have been refined, and Mackinnon's team contend that patients most likely to benefit are those with severe cubital tunnel syndrome with substantial intrinsic atrophy, weakness, and attenuated compound muscle action potential amplitude.[87] In addition, evaluation of the intrinsic recipient muscles should include electrodiagnostic testing to confirm significant axonal loss that would benefit from axonal

Table 3
Common upper extremity nerve transfers

Injured Nerve	Impaired Function	Donor Nerve	Recipient Nerve
Motor			
Suprascapular	Shoulder abduction, external rotation	Distal spinal accessory	Suprascapular
Long thoracic	Scapula stabilization, forward abduction	Medial pectoral, thoracodorsal, intercostal	Long thoracic
Axillary	Shoulder abduction	Triceps branch of radial nerve, medial pectoral	Axillary
Musculocutaneous	Elbow flexion	Ulnar nerve fascicle to FCU; median nerve fascicle to FDR, FDS	Brachialis branch; biceps branch
Spinal accessory	Shoulder elevation, abduction	Medial pectoral, C7 redundant fascicle	Spinal accessory
Ulnar	Intrinsic hand	Terminal AIN (branch to pronator quadratus)	Ulnar nerve fascicles to deep motor branch
Median	Thumb opposition	Terminal AIN (branch to pronator quadratus)	Median (recurrent) motor
	Finger flexion	FCU, brachialis	AIN
	Pronation	ECRB, FCU, FDS	Pronator branch
Radial	Wrist and finger extension	FCR, FDS ± PL	ECRB and PIN
Sensory			
Median sensory	Thumb-index key pinch area sensation	Ulnar common sensory branch to 4th web space	Median common sensory branch to 1st web space
	Thumb-index key pinch area sensation	Dorsal sensory branch of the ulnar nerve	Median common sensory branch to 1st web space
Ulnar sensory	Ring and small finger sensation	Median common sensory branch to the 3rd web space	Ulnar common sensory branch to the 4th web space; ulnar digital nerve to the small finger
	Ulnar border of the hand sensation	Lateral antebrachial cutaneous	Dorsal sensory branch of the ulnar nerve

Abbreviations: AIN, anterior interosseous nerve; ECRB, extensor carpi radialis brevis; FCR, flexor carpi radialis; FCU, flexor carpi ulnaris; FDS, flexor digitorum superficialis; PIN, posterior interosseous nerve; PL, palmaris longus.

regeneration and that the denervated motor endplates are still receptive to reinnervation.[87]

FUTURE DIRECTIONS

Some authors have contended that surgical advancements in major nerve repair and reconstruction have plateaued, and that new treatments are needed in improve outcomes.[88] There are still no clinically available pharmacologic agents to aid nerve regeneration.[81] However, many potential avenues such as molecular and cell-based therapy have been proposed.[1] One agent that has profound effects on peripheral nerve regeneration is the immunosuppressant tacrolimus (FK506), which is FDA-approved for the prevention of rejection after solid organ transplantation.[81] In subimmunosuppressive doses, FK506 has neuroprotective and neurotrophic effects that promote neurite elongation and regeneration.[89,90] The potential of adverse systemic effects is a challenge, so there has been interest in developing local delivery methods as well as topical administration.[91,92] Additional agents typically used in other clinical settings that have the potential to enhance neural regeneration include melatonin[93,94] and hyaluronic acid,[95] both of which may also have a role in topical administration.[92]

Neurotrophic factors are critical for maintaining an environment conducive to growth at the distal nerve stump following peripheral nerve repair by facilitating the guidance of axons and accelerating the rate of regeneration. Many neurotrophic factors are secreted by Schwann cells. Stem cells have the potential to differentiate into Schwann cells, and they may be a therapeutic option.[96] A variety of stem cell lineages have been described as acting as Schwann cell precursors, but the optimal source remains unclear.[81,88]

Stabilization of the neuromuscular junction (NMJ) has also been advocated as a potential therapeutic goal, as this may slow the rate of end-organ atrophy following peripheral nerve injury.[88] In the setting of peripheral nerve injury, the NMJ disperses acetylcholine receptor (AChR) clusters at the motor end plates, leading to muscle atrophy. The glycoprotein agrin preserves the integrity of AChR clusters, and increasing local levels of agrin may play a role in preserving NMJ stability and curtailing end-organ atrophy.[97] Matrix melloproteinase-3 (MMP-3) is a serine protease that is increased in concentration following peripheral nerve injury, which degrades agrin at the NMJ. Therefore, inhibition of MMP-3 may also be a therapeutic target, as it would increase levels of agrin and help stabilize the NMJ.[98]

Finally, an area that holds some promise is low-frequency electrical stimulation, which is delivered at the time of surgical repair to help accelerate axonal outgrowth, remyelination, and reinnervation. Further research in this area is ongoing.[99]

SUMMARY

Peripheral nerve injuries can substantially impair a patient's quality of life. Despite appropriate surgical intervention, outcomes often remain poor and functional recovery does not occur in many cases. When possible, direct end-to-end nerve repair is the treatment of choice. The presence of significant retraction or nerve defects causing excessive tension at a repair site often precludes direct repair. Nerve autografts remain the gold standard for the reconstruction of larger nerve gaps, but donor site morbidity remains a notable challenge. Processed nerve allografts and conduits are viable options for reconstruction that avoid donor site morbidity. These two options pose their own challenges, as evidence supporting their use is limited to small-diameter nerve injuries with short defects. Nerve transfers are a relatively new technique that has gained momentum over the past couple of decades. However, functional recovery may be limited if the degeneration of the recipient motor endplates has already occurred. Future directions include molecular and cell-based therapies and pharmacologic agents to enhance regeneration and hopefully improve the outcomes of these challenging injuries.

CLINICS CARE POINTS

- Timely management of peripheral nerve injury is important, as irreversible end-organ atrophy and fibrosis may occur within 12 to 18 months of denervation
- Although primary repair of peripheral nerve injury remains the standard of care, satisfactory functional outcomes are seldom achieved, and primary repair is often not possible due to excessive tension from significant nerve gaps
- Autografts are the gold standard for larger nerve defects, but challenges include increased operative time from harvest as well as donor site morbidity
- Allografts and conduits avoid donor site morbidity, but evidence for their use is limited to injuries of small nerves with short gaps
- In cases where primary repair or grafting may not be reliable such as brachial plexus injuries and other proximal lesions with a long distance from the target motor end plate, nerve transfers can be considered. However, challenges include sacrifice of the donor nerve as well as limited salvage options following transfer
- There are currently no pharmacologic agents clinically available to augment axonal regeneration, but there are many molecular and cellular targets for which potential therapeutics may play a role in peripheral nerve injury in the future

REFERENCES

1. Lanier ST, Hill JR, Dy CJ, et al. Evolving Techniques in Peripheral Nerve Regeneration. J Hand Surg Am 2021;46:695–701.
2. Vastamäki M, Kallio PK, Solonen KA. The results of secondary microsurgical repair of ulnar nerve injury. J Hand Surg Br 1993;18:323–6.
3. Dy CJ, Lingampalli N, Peacock K, et al. Direct Cost of Surgically Treated Adult Traumatic Brachial Plexus Injuries. J Hand Surg Glob Online 2020;2:77–9.
4. Hong TS, Tian A, Sachar R, et al. Indirect Cost of Traumatic Brachial Plexus Injuries in the United States. J Bone Joint Surg Am 2019;101:e80.

5. Kretschmer T, Ihle S, Antoniadis G, et al. Patient satisfaction and disability after brachial plexus surgery. Neurosurgery 2009;65:A189–96.

6. Noble J, Munro CA, Prasad VS, et al. Analysis of upper and lower extremity peripheral nerve injuries in a population of patients with multiple injuries. J Trauma 1998;45:116–22.

7. Seddon HJ. A Classification of Nerve Injuries. Br Med J 1942;2:237–9.

8. Moore AM, Wagner IJ, Fox IK. Principles of nerve repair in complex wounds of the upper extremity. Semin Plast Surg 2015;29(1):40–7.

9. Flores AJ, Lavernia CJ, Owens PW. Anatomy and physiology of peripheral nerve injury and repair. Am J Orthop (Belle Mead NJ) 2000;29:167–73.

10. Lee SK, Wolfe SW. Peripheral nerve injury and repair. J Am Acad Orthop Surg 2000;8:243–52.

11. Boecker AH, Lukhaup L, Aman M, et al. Evaluation of MR-neurography in diagnosis and treatment in peripheral nerve surgery of the upper extremity: A matched cohort study. Microsurgery 2022;42(2):160–9.

12. Mackinnon SE. New directions in peripheral nerve surgery. Ann Plast Surg 1989;22:257–73.

13. Campbell WW. Evaluation and management of peripheral nerve injury. Clin Neurophysiol 2008;119:1951–65.

14. Riddoch G, Medical Research Council (Great Britain). University of Edinburgh. *Aids to the Investigation of Peripheral Nerve Injuries*. Revised. Second edition. London: Her Majesty's Stationery Office; 1943.

15. Mackinnon S, Dellon A. Surgery of the peripheral nerve. New York: Thieme Publishing Group; 1988.

16. Arnold DMJ, Wilkens SC, Coert JH, et al. Diagnostic Criteria for Symptomatic Neuroma. Ann Plast Surg 2019;82:420–7.

17. Thesleff S. Trophic functions of the neuron. II. Denervation and regulation of muscle. Physiological effects of denervation of muscle. Ann N Y Acad Sci 1974;228:89–104.

18. Robinson LR. Traumatic injury to peripheral nerves. Muscle Nerve 2000;23:863–73.

19. Stewart JD. Electrodiagnostic techniques in the evaluation of nerve compressions and injuries in the upper limb. Hand Clin 1986;2:677–87.

20. Koenig RW, Pedro MT, Heinen CP, et al. High-resolution ultrasonography in evaluating peripheral nerve entrapment and trauma. Neurosurg Focus 2009;26:E13.

21. Bendszus M, Stoll G. Technology insight: visualizing peripheral nerve injury using MRI. Nat Clin Pract Neurol 2005;1:45–53.

22. Chhabra A, Ahlawat S, Belzberg A, et al. Peripheral nerve injury grading simplified on MR neurography: As referenced to Seddon and Sunderland classifications. Indian J Radiol Imaging 2014;24:217–24.

23. Grinsell D, Keating CP. Peripheral nerve reconstruction after injury: a review of clinical and experimental therapies. BioMed Res Int 2014;2014:698256.

24. Kurze T. Microtechniques in neurological surgery. Clin Neurosurg 1964;11:128–37.

25. Smith JW. Microsurgery of peripheral nerves. Plast Reconstr Surg 1964;33:317–29.

26. Martin AR, Gittings DJ, Levin LS, et al. Acute Radial Nerve Repair with Humeral Shaft Shortening and Fixation Following a Closed Humeral Shaft Fracture: A Case Report. JBJS Case Connect 2018;8:e109.

27. Griffin JW, Hogan MV, Chhabra AB, et al. Peripheral nerve repair and reconstruction. J Bone Joint Surg Am 2013;95:2144–51.

28. Beris A, Gkiatas I, Gelalis I, et al. Current concepts in peripheral nerve surgery. Eur J Orthop Surg Traumatol 2019;29:263–9.

29. Hirasawa Y. Peripheral nerve suture. J Orthop Sci 1996;1:214–29.

30. Lundborg G, Rosén B, Dahlin L, et al. Tubular versus conventional repair of median and ulnar nerves in the human forearm: early results from a prospective, randomized, clinical study. J Hand Surg Am 1997;22:99–106.

31. Laubscher M, Held M, Maree M, et al. Radial nerve lacerations–the outcome of end-to-end repairs in penetrating trauma. Hand Surg 2015;20:67–72.

32. Gürbüz Y, Kayalar M, Bal E, et al. Long-term functional results after radial nerve repair. Acta Orthop Traumatol Turc 2011;45:387–92.

33. Post R, de Boer KS, Malessy MJ. Outcome following nerve repair of high isolated clean sharp injuries of the ulnar nerve. PLoS One 2012;7:e47928.

34. Lundborg G. A 25-year perspective of peripheral nerve surgery: evolving neuroscientific concepts and clinical significance. J Hand Surg Am 2000;25:391–414.

35. Tarasidis G, Watanabe O, Mackinnon SE, et al. End-to-side neurorrhaphy: a long-term study of neural regeneration in a rat model. Otolaryngol Head Neck Surg 1998;119:337–41.

36. Lundborg G, Zhao Q, Kanje M, et al. Can sensory and motor collateral sprouting be induced from intact peripheral nerve by end-to-side anastomosis? J Hand Surg Br 1994;19:277–82.

37. Yu Q, Lin ZK, Ding J, et al. Functional motor nerve regeneration without motor-sensory specificity following end-to-side neurorrhaphy: an experimental study. J Hand Surg Am 2011;36:2010–6.

38. Isaacs JE, McDaniel CO, Owen JR, et al. Comparative analysis of biomechanical performance of available "nerve glues". J Hand Surg Am 2008;33:893–9.

39. Ornelas L, Padilla L, Di Silvio M, et al. Fibrin glue: an alternative technique for nerve coaptation–Part II. Nerve regeneration and histomorphometric assessment. J Reconstr Microsurg 2006;22:123–8.

40. Whitlock EL, Kasukurthi R, Yan Y, et al. Fibrin glue mitigates the learning curve of microneurosurgical repair. Microsurgery 2010;30:218–22.

41. Sallam A, Eldeeb M, Kamel N. Autologous Fibrin Glue Versus Microsuture in the Surgical Reconstruction of Peripheral Nerves: A Randomized Clinical Trial. J Hand Surg Am 2022;47(1):89.e1-11.

42. Danielsen N, Varon S. Characterization of neurotrophic activity in the silicone-chamber model for nerve regeneration. J Reconstr Microsurg 1995;11:231–5.

43. Isaacs J, Safa B, Evans PJ, et al. Technical Assessment of Connector-Assisted Nerve Repair. J Hand Surg Am 2016;41:760–6.

44. Ducic I, Safa B, DeVinney E. Refinements of nerve repair with connector-assisted coaptation. Microsurgery 2017;37:256–63.

45. Rebowe R, Rogers A, Yang X, et al. Nerve Repair with Nerve Conduits: Problems, Solutions, and Future Directions. J Hand Microsurg 2018;10:61–5.

46. Colen KL, Choi M, Chiu DT. Nerve grafts and conduits. Plast Reconstr Surg 2009;124:e386–94.

47. Millesi H, Meissl G, Berger A. The interfascicular nerve-grafting of the median and ulnar nerves. J Bone Joint Surg Am 1972;54:727–50.

48. Frykman GK, Cally D. Interfascicular nerve grafting. Orthop Clin North Am 1988;19:71–80.

49. Taylor GI, Ham FJ. The free vascularized nerve graft. A further experimental and clinical application of microvascular techniques. Plast Reconstr Surg 1976;57:413–26.

50. Terzis JK, Kostopoulos VK. Vascularized nerve grafts and vascularized fascia for upper extremity nerve reconstruction. Hand (N Y) 2010;5:19–30.

51. Slutsky DJ. A practical approach to nerve grafting in the upper extremity. Atlas Hand Clin 2005;10:e92.

52. Bamba R, Loewenstein SN, Adkinson JM. Donor site morbidity after sural nerve grafting: A systematic review. J Plast Reconstr Aesthet Surg 2021;74:3055–60.

53. Ehretsman RL, Novak CB, Mackinnon SE. Subjective recovery of nerve graft donor site. Ann Plast Surg 1999;43:606–12.

54. Mauch JT, Bae A, Shubinets V, et al. A Systematic Review of Sensory Outcomes of Digital Nerve Gap Reconstruction With Autograft, Allograft, and Conduit. Ann Plast Surg 2019;82:S247–55.

55. Ansselin AD, Pollard JD. Immunopathological factors in peripheral nerve allograft rejection: quantification of lymphocyte invasion and major histocompatibility complex expression. J Neurol Sci 1990;96:75–88.

56. Lassner F, Schaller E, Steinhoff G, et al. Cellular mechanisms of rejection and regeneration in peripheral nerve allografts. Transplantation 1989;48:386–92.

57. Mackinnon SE, Doolabh VB, Novak CB, et al. Clinical outcome following nerve allograft transplantation. Plast Reconstr Surg 2001;107:1419–29.

58. Brenner MJ, Lowe JB, Fox IK, et al. Effects of Schwann cells and donor antigen on long-nerve allograft regeneration. Microsurgery 2005;25:61–70.

59. Ray WZ, Kale SS, Kasukurthi R, et al. Effect of cold nerve allograft preservation on antigen presentation and rejection. J Neurosurg 2011;114:256–62.

60. Hudson TW, Zawko S, Deister C, et al. Optimized acellular nerve graft is immunologically tolerated and supports regeneration. Tissue Eng 2004;10:1641–51.

61. Karabekmez FE, Duymaz A, Moran SL. Early clinical outcomes with the use of decellularized nerve allograft for repair of sensory defects within the hand. Hand (N Y) 2009;4:245–9.

62. Giusti G, Willems WF, Kremer T, et al. Return of motor function after segmental nerve loss in a rat model: comparison of autogenous nerve graft, collagen conduit, and processed allograft (AxoGen). J Bone Joint Surg Am 2012;94:410–7.

63. Whitlock EL, Tuffaha SH, Luciano JP, et al. Processed allografts and type I collagen conduits for repair of peripheral nerve gaps. Muscle Nerve 2009;39:787–99.

64. Safa B, Shores JT, Ingari JV, et al. Recovery of Motor Function after Mixed and Motor Nerve Repair with Processed Nerve Allograft. Plast Reconstr Surg Glob Open 2019;7:e2163.

65. Dunn JC, Tadlock J, Klahs KJ, et al. Nerve Reconstruction Using Processed Nerve Allograft in the U.S. Military. Mil Med 2021;186:e543–8.

66. Rbia N, Shin AY. The Role of Nerve Graft Substitutes in Motor and Mixed Motor/Sensory Peripheral Nerve Injuries. J Hand Surg Am 2017;42:367–77.

67. Isaacs J. Treatment of acute peripheral nerve injuries: current concepts. J Hand Surg Am 2010;35:491–7 [quiz: 498].

68. Chiu DT, Strauch B. A prospective clinical evaluation of autogenous vein grafts used as a nerve conduit for distal sensory nerve defects of 3 cm or less. Plast Reconstr Surg 1990;86:928–34.

69. Deal DN, Griffin JW, Hogan MV. Nerve conduits for nerve repair or reconstruction. J Am Acad Orthop Surg 2012;20:63–8.

70. Shin RH, Friedrich PF, Crum BA, et al. Treatment of a segmental nerve defect in the rat with use of bioabsorbable synthetic nerve conduits: a comparison of commercially available conduits. J Bone Joint Surg Am 2009;91:2194–204.

71. Bushnell BD, McWilliams AD, Whitener GB, et al. Early clinical experience with collagen nerve tubes in digital nerve repair. J Hand Surg Am 2008;33:1081–7.

72. Lohmeyer JA, Siemers F, Machens HG, et al. The clinical use of artificial nerve conduits for digital nerve repair: a prospective cohort study and literature review. J Reconstr Microsurg 2009;25:55–61.

73. Klein S, Vykoukal J, Felthaus O, et al. Collagen Type I Conduits for the Regeneration of Nerve Defects. Materials 2016;9.

74. Meek MF, Coert JH. US Food and Drug Administration/Conformit Europe- approved absorbable nerve conduits for clinical repair of peripheral and cranial nerves. Ann Plast Surg 2008;60:466–72.

75. Weber RA, Breidenbach WC, Brown RE, et al. A randomized prospective study of polyglycolic acid conduits for digital nerve reconstruction in humans. Plast Reconstr Surg 2000;106:1036–45 [discussion: 1046–8].

76. Battiston B, Geuna S, Ferrero M, et al. Nerve repair by means of tubulization: literature review and personal clinical experience comparing biological and synthetic conduits for sensory nerve repair. Microsurgery 2005;25:258–67.

77. Rinker B, Liau JY. A prospective randomized study comparing woven polyglycolic acid and autogenous vein conduits for reconstruction of digital nerve gaps. J Hand Surg Am 2011;36:775–81.

78. Bertleff MJ, Meek MF, Nicolai JP. A prospective clinical evaluation of biodegradable neurolac nerve guides for sensory nerve repair in the hand. J Hand Surg Am 2005;30:513–8.

79. Ray WZ, Mackinnon SE. Management of nerve gaps: autografts, allografts, nerve transfers, and end-to-side neurorrhaphy. Exp Neurol 2010;223: 77–85.

80. Samardzic M, Grujicic D, Rasulic L, et al. Transfer of the medial pectoral nerve: myth or reality? Neurosurgery 2002;50:1277–82.

81. Panagopoulos GN, Megaloikonomos PD, Mavrogenis AF. The Present and Future for Peripheral Nerve Regeneration. Orthopedics 2017;40: e141–56.

82. Tung TH, Mackinnon SE. Nerve transfers: indications, techniques, and outcomes. J Hand Surg Am 2010;35:332–41.

83. Kobayashi J, Mackinnon SE, Watanabe O, et al. The effect of duration of muscle denervation on functional recovery in the rat model. Muscle Nerve 1997;20:858–66.

84. von Guionneau N, Sarhane KA, Brandacher G, et al. Mechanisms and outcomes of the supercharged end-to-side nerve transfer: a review of preclinical and clinical studies. J Neurosurg 2020;134:1590–8.

85. Dengler J, Dolen U, Patterson JMM, et al. Supercharge End-to-Side Anterior Interosseous-to-Ulnar Motor Nerve Transfer Restores Intrinsic Function in Cubital Tunnel Syndrome. Plast Reconstr Surg 2020;146:808–18.

86. Barbour J, Yee A, Kahn LC, et al. Supercharged end-to-side anterior interosseous to ulnar motor nerve transfer for intrinsic musculature reinnervation. J Hand Surg Am 2012;37:2150–9.

87. Power HA, Kahn LC, Patterson MM, et al. Refining Indications for the Supercharge End-to-Side Anterior Interosseous to Ulnar Motor Nerve Transfer in Cubital Tunnel Syndrome. Plast Reconstr Surg 2020;145:106e–16e.

88. Kang JR, Zamorano DP, Gupta R. Limb salvage with major nerve injury: current management and future directions. J Am Acad Orthop Surg 2011;19(Suppl 1):S28–34.

89. Yan Y, Sun HH, Hunter DA, et al. Efficacy of short-term FK506 administration on accelerating nerve regeneration. Neurorehabil Neural Repair 2012;26: 570–80.

90. Konofaos P, Terzis JK. FK506 and nerve regeneration: past, present, and future. J Reconstr Microsurg 2013;29:141–8.

91. Tajdaran K, Shoichet MS, Gordon T, et al. A novel polymeric drug delivery system for localized and sustained release of tacrolimus (FK506). Biotechnol Bioeng 2015;112:1948–53.

92. Mekaj AY, Morina AA, Bytyqi CI, et al. Application of topical pharmacological agents at the site of peripheral nerve injury and methods used for evaluating the success of the regenerative process. J Orthop Surg Res 2014;9:94.

93. Odaci E, Kaplan S. Chapter 16: Melatonin and nerve regeneration. Int Rev Neurobiol 2009;87:317–35.

94. Atik B, Erkutlu I, Tercan M, et al. The effects of exogenous melatonin on peripheral nerve regeneration and collagen formation in rats. J Surg Res 2011; 166:330–6.

95. Mohammad JA, Warnke PH, Pan YC, et al. Increased axonal regeneration through a biodegradable amnionic tube nerve conduit: effect of local delivery and incorporation of nerve growth factor/hyaluronic acid media. Ann Plast Surg 2000;44: 59–64.

96. Fairbairn NG, Meppelink AM, Ng-Glazier J, et al. Augmenting peripheral nerve regeneration using stem cells: A review of current opinion. World J Stem Cells 2015;7:11–26.

97. Gautam M, Noakes PG, Moscoso L, et al. Defective neuromuscular synaptogenesis in agrin-deficient mutant mice. Cell 1996;85:525–35.

98. Werle MJ. Cell-to-cell signaling at the neuromuscular junction: the dynamic role of the extracellular matrix. Ann N Y Acad Sci 2008;1132:13–8.

99. Zuo KJ, Gordon T, Chan KM, et al. Electrical stimulation to enhance peripheral nerve regeneration: Update in molecular investigations and clinical translation. Exp Neurol 2020;332:113397.

Approach to Tendinopathies of the Upper Limb: What Works

Ronald D. Brown, MD[a], Stephen A. Kennedy, MD[b],*

KEYWORDS

- Tendinopathy • Tenosynovitis • Tendon • Instability • Anconeus • Flap

KEY POINTS

- Pain after tendinopathy surgery can come from multiple sources and requires consideration of bio-psychosocial influences and pitfalls of accurate diagnosis.
- Trigger finger can persist proximal or distal to the A1 pulley and can be treated by further releasing the sheath or reducing the contents of the sheath by excising a slip of superficialis.
- De Quervain tenosynovitis can remain symptomatic due to an unreleased subsheath or first extensor compartment instability requiring stabilization.
- Tendon stability can be achieved with multiple techniques, and salvage options include tenodesis or tenotomy.
- Persistent lateral epicondylitis can be effectively treated with repeat debridement, denervation, and/or anconeus flap reconstruction.

INTRODUCTION

Tendinopathy is a broad term that encompasses tenosynovitis, tendinitis, epicondylitis, split tears, and enthesopathy. Although the term includes any tendon disease resulting from inflammation, metabolic disease, endocrine disease, or other causes, it is most commonly related to noninflammatory thickening and/or disorganization of tendon. Common tendinopathies treated by the hand surgeon include trigger digits (stenosing tenosynovitis), de Quervain tenosynovitis, extensor carpi ulnaris (ECU) tendinopathy at the wrist, and epicondylitis of the elbow. Fortunately, the hand surgeon is often successful in treating these tendinopathies using nonoperative techniques and minor surgical procedures. Some patients, however, will return with reduced motion, persistent or recurrent mechanical symptoms, instability, pain, or other complications related to their treatment. These can be challenging scenarios and require special consideration.

EVALUATION

In approaching the patient with persistent symptoms, it is important to consider the bio-psychosocial paradigm of patient evaluation.[1-6] Healing timelines can differ between patients and psychosocial factors influence treatment response.[7-11] The strongest predictors of outcome for several hand surgeries are related to psychosocial factors.[4,8,10,11] Patients can benefit from consideration of psychosocial influences and are more open to these discussions than we often realize.[12] They may benefit from both multidisciplinary management and revision surgery, so they need not be exclusionary of one another.

[a] Department of Plastic and Reconstructive Surgery, The Ohio State University Hand and Upper Extremity Center, The Ohio State University, 915 Olentangy River Road, Suite 3200, Columbus, OH 43212, USA; [b] Department of Orthopaedics and Sports Medicine, University of Washington, Harborview Medical Center, 325 Ninth Avenue, MS 359798, Seattle, WA 98104, USA
* Corresponding author.
E-mail address: sajk@uw.edu

Hand Clin 39 (2023) 417–425
https://doi.org/10.1016/j.hcl.2023.02.010
0749-0712/23/© 2023 Elsevier Inc. All rights reserved.

Recalcitrant cases of tendinopathy also deserve consideration of misdiagnosis. Misdiagnosis is more common than drug errors in medicine.[2] Most Americans will receive a misdiagnosis or late diagnosis in their lifetime.[1,6] Conditions like tendinopathy are prevalent in hand clinics so the diagnosis can be misapplied to conditions with similar presentation. Recalcitrant "trigger finger" might actually be snapping lateral bands or chronic sesamoiditis[3] (**Box 1**). For patients with ongoing symptoms, it is important to avoid cognitive tunneling. Mnemonics that involve body systems or tissues can prompt us to consider a differential diagnosis and our own biases.

When missed or misdiagnosed conditions have been excluded, recalcitrant cases are often due to joint stiffness from adhesions or contractures, persistent tenosynovitis, or tendon or joint instability.

Tendon Adhesions and Contractures

The most common complications after surgical management of tendinopathy are related to stiffness and/or limited range of motion.[13] Tendon adhesions may be present as a component of trigger finger even before treatment and can be a significant cause of loss of motion (**Fig. 1**).[14] Despite improvement in triggering symptoms, range of motion limitations may persist or worsen as a result of capsular contracture and/or tendon adhesions. Such complications can also manifest as persistent pain, and they may coexist with persistent triggering.[13]

Tendon adhesions can be categorized as loose or dense and can adhere tendon to tendon sheath or tendon to tendon.[15] Adhesions most commonly occur at the surgical site, but evaluation of the whole digit can help better identify where such adhesions are located. When present, the patient may experience a pulling sensation at the site. Clues may also be gleaned from passive motion of individual joints and the effect on adjacent joint motion. If joint contracture is unaffected by position of other joints of the finger, hand, or wrist, the contracture is likely localized closely adjacent to that specific joint and possibly capsuloligamentous. Palpation combined with motion may also reveal nodules, persistent triggering, or masses.

In tendinopathies occurring at larger joints, such as those at the wrist and elbow, tendon adhesions and contractures following surgery are rare and are usually the result of prolonged immobilization or disuse.

Persistent Tenosynovitis

Despite best efforts to relieve tendon sheath tendon entrapment and resolve triggering, tenosynovitis can persist or recur at the same location or elsewhere in the same digit. The A1 pulley is recognized as a critical structure for trigger finger release, but recent evidence indicates the importance of proximal fibrous tissue referred to as the "A0 pulley."[16] Studies of patients undergoing

---

Box 1
Differential diagnoses to consider for common tendinopathies

Trigger finger
- Snapping lateral bands
- Chronic sesamoiditis
- Inflammatory tenosynovitis
- Infectious tenosynovitis

De Quervain tenosynovitis
- Basal thumb arthritis
- Radioscaphoid instability or arthritis
- Scaphoid fracture or nonunion

Epicondylitis
- Collateral ligament pathology
- Arthritis or loose bodies
- Inflammatory enthesopathy
- Cubital tunnel syndrome or other entrapment
- Snapping triceps
- Olecranon bursitis

ECU tendinopathy
- TFCC tear
- Distal Radioulnar Joint (DRUJ) instability
- Ulnocarpal impaction
- Lunotriquetral ligament tear or instability
- Ulnotriquetral split tear

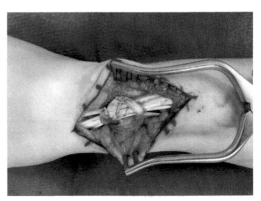

Fig. 1. Brachioradialis flap for APL and EPB stabilization. (*Courtesy of* Sonu Jain, MD, Columbus, OH.)

trigger finger release using Wide Awake, Local Anesthetic, No Tourniquet (WALANT) technique have shown the A0 pulley to influence motion similarly to the A1 pulley.[16] Thus, one advantage of performing tenosynovitis surgery using the WALANT technique is that patient cooperation can demonstrate confirmation of satisfactory motion before closing the incision.

In persistent triggering, it is also important to evaluate for less common sites of trigger digit for entrapment. Tendon nodules can occur distal to the A2 or A3 pulleys near the proximal interphalangeal joint and may cause similar bothersome symptoms. Sometimes these findings can go unnoticed when there is a larger nodule proximally in the more typical A1 pulley location. Alternatively, other conditions, such as snapping lateral bands, chronic sesamoiditis, or arthritis, can imitate some trigger digit symptoms.

Persistent tenosynovitis related to de Quervain tenosynovitis deserves special attention. The first dorsal compartment has variable anatomy and may have a septum or subsheath separating the extensor pollicis brevis (EPB) from the abductor pollicis longus (APL).[17,18] It is possible to have persistent tenosynovitis of one of these sheaths. Finkelstein's test and Eichhoff's test are the classically described maneuvers for evaluating these tendons but primarily evaluate APL[19].[19] If the tendon sheath of APL is released without releasing the EPB, Finkelstein and Eichhoff's tests may improve while pain persists.[19] To test the EPB specifically, resisted thumb extension at the metacarpophalangeal joint can be performed. If this results in pain localized to the area of the first dorsal compartment, it suggests persistent EPB tenosynovitis.

Tendon Instability

ECU instability can occur following a traumatic injury or may follow a more chronic course. It can be associated with ulnar-sided wrist pain, palpable subluxation, instability, and/or snapping on examination. Other tendons can also undergo instability after surgical procedures, including the first dorsal compartment tendons after de Quervain release.[20–23] It is also possible for flexor tendons to bowstring or deviate ulnarly after trigger finger release.[13]

An evaluation of tendon instability involves focused history and physical examination. With ECU and first dorsal compartment instability, patients may describe subluxation or snapping.[21–26] More often, they will describe pain and instability and/or a sense of not being able to trust their wrist. During ulnar deviation of the wrist, the ECU tendon experiences ulnar translational forces, and if stabilizing structures are deficient, subluxation can occur. Supination and/or flexion can similarly cause subluxation.[24–26] A specific examination maneuver for ECU tenosynovitis is the "ECU synergy test."[27] The patient is asked to place their elbow on a table and perform resisted abduction of the middle finger and the thumb. In a positive test, the patient will describe pain in the area of the dorsal aspect of the ulnar head at the ECU tendon sheath[27] related to the activation of ECU and Flexor Carpi Ulnaris (FCU). This is achieved without direct contact to the area, and so a positive finding is more specific for the diagnosis than local palpation and may distinguish it from Triangular Fibrocartilage Complex (TFCC) pathology.[27]

In the case of finger flexor tendon instability or bowstringing, pain may be present over the flexor sheath, particularly at a site of instability. Patients may often have a concomitant flexion contracture.[20–22]

Neuropathic Pain and Other Causes of Pain (Infection, Inflammatory, Neoplastic, Metabolic, and Vascular)

It is also important to be considerate of other potential sources of persistent pain. Surgery for tendinopathy can be complicated by neuropathic pain at the surgical site. This can be associated with partial or complete injury to nerves, but it can also be attributed to nerve retraction or blunt dissection. The radial sensory nerve is prone to postoperative neuritis at least partially due to its superficial location under the skin. Complex regional pain syndrome may develop, with or without nerve injury or entrapment. Focused examination for hyperesthesia, dermatomal numbness, Tinel sign, trophic changes, and fixed contractures should all be part of the evaluation.

THERAPEUTIC OPTIONS
Nonoperative Treatments

Hand therapy involving motion, strengthening, and edema management can significantly improve motion, strength, pain, and coping skills.[7,8,10–12,28] Tendon adhesions and contractures can benefit greatly from supervised motion, strengthening, and static progressive stretching regimens. Acute tendon instability may be treated with a trial period of rest and immobilization, with generic or custom splints that address the site of instability. In many settings, the hand therapist facilitates not only the management of the physical findings such as edema and contracture, but also the mental aspects such as cognitions and behaviors.

In some cases, the mental aspects of the injury are more difficult than the physical aspects, and this is an important time to consider referral to a psychologist.[7,11,28] Psychological factors can be measured using validated tools.[7-11] Depression, anxiety, pain catastrophizing, posttraumatic stress disorder, and other factors are often underrecognized in surgical clinics and can be treated using conventional multidisciplinary teams to improve mental and physical health.[7,8,10,11,28,29]

Tenolysis and Contracture Release

In cases of persistent contracture due to tendon adhesions and/or capsular contracture, tenolysis may be indicated.[30,31] Not all patients will be candidates for such procedures. Tenolysis is a demanding procedure, not only in terms of technical skill required, but also in terms of the necessary postoperative therapy and postoperative therapy standpoint.[30,31] If the patient is unable or unwilling to participate in an extensive hand therapy program, surgery can result in no benefit or even a worse outcome. Patients with diffuse scarring and contracture, such as is seen in complex regional pain syndrome, are also less likely to have successful improvement in their symptoms. If surgery is undertaken for tenolysis, WALANT techniques or local anesthesia with short-acting sedation can allow the patient to demonstrate adequacy of motion at the completion of the procedure.

Tendon Stabilization Procedures

Tendon instability after tendinopathy surgery is a rare complication after trigger finger release or de Quervain tenosynovitis.[20-22,32,33] Only about 2% of patients experience first dorsal compartment tendon instability after surgical release for de Quervain tenosynovitis. Tendon instability after trigger finger release is more likely related to tendon bowstringing from excessive release of the A2 pulley. Recurrent instability after ECU stabilization is a more common problem.[24-26] However, not all tendon instability will be symptomatic, and some can be treated successfully with a course of immobilization. Acute pulley rupture or instability in the fingers can be treated with pulley orthoses. There are, however, cases that will require repeat or salvage stabilization. In order of frequency, this includes ECU instability, first dorsal compartment instability, and digit flexor tendon bowstringing.

Stabilization of a persistently unstable ECU tendon has been described using multiple techniques.[24-26,34] This can include the so-called anatomic reconstructions with or without deepening of the ECU tendon groove or loop reconstructions using slips of extensor retinaculum or tendon grafts (**Fig. 2**). It can also include tenodesis procedures, securing tendon to bone in the groove, and/or tenotomy of the ECU distal to the ulna.[34]

In the case of first dorsal compartment instability, a more dorsal incision in the tendon sheath has been proposed to help guard against volar subluxation. Retinaculum repair, sheath reconstruction, or alternative decompression techniques have also been suggested.[21,22,35] Data suggest, however, that such a dorsal ulnar incision may serve to increase risk of dorsal subluxation, so a midline incision has been recommended.[20,21,23,35]

When instability occurs, the main form of stabilization involves reconstruction of the tendon sheath using extensor retinaculum or tendon autograft. Brachioradialis tendon inserts immediately adjacent to the first dorsal compartment and can be released proximally and turned over the tendons and sutured dorsally to recreate the tendon sheath (see **Fig. 1**).[22]

Flexor tendon bowstringing following surgical management of trigger digit is a rare complication. In the case of tendon bowstringing of the fingers, pulley reconstruction can be performed using local or regional tendon grafts. Most commonly this involves a tendon graft looped around the proximal phalanx (see **Fig. 2**), but it can also be sutured to bone at the bony attachment sites of the tendon pulleys. Pulley orthoses can support the reconstruction in the immediate postoperative period.

Tenotomy and Debridement

In persistent cases of epicondylitis, tenotomy and debridement, with or without reattachment, can provide symptom relief.[36-42] Case series report

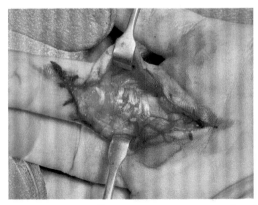

Fig. 2. Finger A2 pulley reconstruction using palmaris longus graft. (*Courtesy of* Sonu Jain, MD, Columbus, OH.)

varying degrees of success with the surgery, with estimates varying from about 70% to over 90%. Epicondylectomy is also described.[40] Denervation of the region can also be effective in up to 80% of cases.[40,42] In cases where such procedures are unsuccessful, and therapy and activity modification has been exhausted, an anconeus flap reconstruction can be considered.[38,39,41] In cases of persistent symptoms, it is important to evaluate for other possible sources of pain. When revision surgery is undertaken, consideration is given to possible collateral ligament injury or insufficiency and the adequacy of debridement.

Neurolysis, Grafts, and Flaps

Surgical exposure in reoperation is made more difficult by postsurgical scarring and altered anatomy. Care should be taken to avoid incidental injury to nerves and vessels, and the surgeon needs to be alert to findings such as neuroma, neuroma in continuity, nerve entrapment, and nerve scarring that may require neurolysis. In recalcitrant cases of pain, especially neuropathic pain, there may also be utility of other soft tissue procedures to address postsurgical scarring and neuroma, such as local, regional, or free tissue transfers. Flap reconstruction has specifically been recommended in relation to persistent lateral epicondylitis pain after tenotomy and debridement. The anconeus flap has demonstrated significant improvement in case series.[38,39,41]

SURGICAL TECHNIQUES

The following examples are the authors' preferred techniques for revision surgeries following failed upper extremity tendinopathy management.

Tenolysis for Adhesions or Contractures Following Trigger Digit Release

When tenolysis is undertaken, the extent and nature of the adhesions will influence the result.[29] Patients with highly localized adhesions and good preparation for postoperative therapy are best suited for surgery. Risks are communicated and hand therapy is scheduled days after surgery.[30,31] Tenolysis can be performed under regional or general anesthetic, but our preference is wide awake using WALANT. Local anesthetic with epinephrine adequately controls pain for the procedure and can safely reduce bleeding in the surgical field, minimizing the need for a noxious tourniquet. When awake, a patient can be instructed to open and close the fist, confirming the adequacy of the releases.

The prior incision is reopened and extended as needed in a Bruner or midlateral incision. Meticulous dissection and bipolar electrocautery is performed to avoid neuroascular injury or postoperative bleeding. Tenolysis instruments, such as Meals tenolysis knives, are passed between tendon and pulley within the flexor tendon sheath to release adhesions (**Fig. 3**). In simple cases, an Allis clamp can be placed around the tendon and rotated in order to pull the tendon out of scar tissue. Great care should be taken to avoid avulsing the tendon from its musculotendinous junction proximally. The A2 pulley may be vented partially, or fully in some severe cases. If bowstringing results, acute pulley reconstruction using local or regional tendon graft is performed to ensure adequate stability of the tendons after surgery.

Once the adhesions have been released, the patient is instructed to demonstrate full motion in the operating room. If limited range of motion persists, further tenolysis or capsular release may be required. Following tenolysis and/or capsular release, a soft bandage is applied and formal hand therapy is initiated within 3 to 5 days of surgery. Therapy should focus on the range of motion and strengthening. Ancillary modalities such as scar massage and relative motion splinting may be implemented to prevent additional adhesion or contracture formation.

Excision of a Slip of Flexor Digitorum Superficialis for Persistent Triggering Following Trigger Digit Release

Persistent triggering after trigger release is also preferably performed using WALANT. Previous

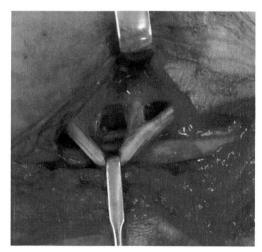

Fig. 3. Flexor tendon adhesions. Adhesions may be short and dense or longer and more loose.

incisional scars are used and extended as needed. The persistent triggering of a digit can be related to several anatomic structures. Frequently, the fibrous bands proximal to the A1 pulley, or the "A0 pulley," result in persistent triggering. Full release of these proximal fibrous bands and the A1 pulley is important to confirm.[16] If there is chronic inflammatory tenosynovium, tissue, it can be excised and sent for culture and sensitivity as well as histopathology. When triggering persists, triggering may be occurring distally at the cruciform and A3 pulleys.

For persistent triggering, our preferred technique is to excise a slip of flexor digitorum superficialis (FDS).[43] The advantage of this technique is that it reduces the area of soft tissue dissection to limit subsequent scarring, it does not result in any new or additional bowstringing, and it does not result in a loss of finger flexion strength. Traction is applied to FDS, and the Proximal Interphalangeal (PIP) joint is maximally flexed. The FDS is split at the Camper's chiasm, and a tenotomy is performed at the most distal extent of one FDS slip and excised proximally. The patient is then asked to flex and extend the digit.

The ulnar slip of FDS is more frequently excised than the radial slip due to the tendency for fingers to develop ulnar drift (ie, in inflammatory arthropathy). It is postulated that a retained ulnar slip might contribute to such an imbalance. This has not been demonstrated in clinical studies, and the effective function of FDS as a finger flexor may supersede this concern, particularly in noninflammatory cases, so both FDS slips should be evaluated before excision. Radial slip excision may be preferred in some circumstances. Following resolution of the triggering, a soft dressing can be applied and early active motion initiated.

In persistent de Quervain tenosynovitis, revision surgery can also be performed under local anesthetic. Careful dissection is extended proximally or distally as needed. Injury to the radial sensory nerve is avoided, and neurolysis may be necessary to mobilize a scarred nerve. The first dorsal compartment may give the appearance of an unopened tendon sheath due to healing. The compartment is opened, and tendons are identified and freed. Great care is taken to identify subsheaths.[17,22,44] If there is no tendon instability, a soft dressing can be applied and early motion can be initiated. This avoids tendon and nerve scarring, with little risk of tendon instability.

Extensor Retinaculum Reconstruction for Extensor Carpi Ulnaris Instability

The ECU will tend to undergo subluxation from its normal position in ulnar deviation, flexion, and supination of the wrist.[24,25] Exposure is achieved through an ulnar or dorsal ulnar incision. Dorsal cutaneous branches of the ulnar nerve are identified and protected. Neurolysis of these branches from the extensor retinaculum may be performed. After tendon sheath incision, the ECU tendon may be evaluated to perform synovectomy, debridement, and/or repair of split tears in the tendon. If there is a tear of the triangular fibrocartilage complex, this may also require debridement and osseous repair.

Multiple techniques have been described for revision stabilization of the ECU.[24] A small amount of deepening of the groove is likely low risk, but may increase risk of hematoma, weakened bone, and fracture. Our preferred technique involves anatomic repair of the ECU subsheath using suture anchors at the ulnar border of the ECU groove. An effective alternative technique includes a radial-based extensor retinaculum sling procedure. Extensor retinaculum can be elevated off the fourth compartment and wrapped around the ECU as a sling and then sutured back on itself (**Fig. 4**).[24] This can provide significant stability to the tendon.[24–26,34]

In cases of multiple reoperations for ECU instability, it may be necessary to consider tenotomy of the tendon, with or without tenodesis to the ulna. In these scenarios, connective tissue disorders, or other circumstances, this procedure can be simple and effective.[34] Wrist extension will require the maintenance of at least one intact wrist extensor tendon, and avoidance of a radial deviation wrist deformity will require an intact flexor carpi ulnaris.

First Dorsal Compartment Reconstruction for Instability After De Quervain Release

In cases of instability of the first dorsal compartment, an effective reconstruction option involves

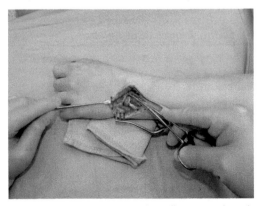

Fig. 4. An extensor retinaculum flap passed under and over the ECU tendon for stabilization. (*From* Byrd JN, Sasor SE, Chung KC. Extensor Carpi Ulnaris Subluxation. Hand Clin. 2021 Nov;37(4):487-491. Elsevier; with permission.)

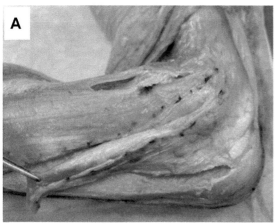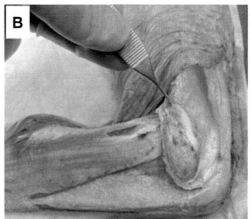

Fig. 5. An anconeus flap for persistent lateral epicondylitis. (*A*) The flap is dissected between anconeus and ECU. (*B*) The flap is turned over the defect at the origin of extensor carpi radialis brevis.

the use of brachioradialis tendon as a donor.[21–23] The insertion of brachioradialis is volar at the level of the first dorsal compartment. The tendon can be transposed dorsal to the tendon and secured to the extensor retinaculum of the second compartment. This creates an effective barrier to volar translation. The same tendon can be used to stabilize the second and fourth compartments when needed for bowstringing. The harvest of brachioradialis tendon has little negative consequence in regard to patient-reported outcomes. Alternatively, a sling of retinaculum can be used, similar to ECU stabilization. Other authors have advocated for excision of the radial ridge to avoid the painful snapping.[44]

Anconeus Flap for Persistent Lateral Epicondylitis

In cases of persistent lateral epicondylitis symptoms despite surgery, reconstruction with flap coverage can provide satisfactory results. The anconeus muscle has proximal and distal vascular pedicle perfusion.[38,39,41] It can be released from its distal pedicle and transposed to cover the lateral epicondyle region (**Fig. 5**A). This has been shown to provide satisfactory relief in recalcitrant cases for the majority of patients and is the authors' preferred technique in these scenarios.[38] Alternatively, denervation has been described as an effective technique.[40,42]

Anconeus flap for persistent lateral epicondylitis is best performed under tourniquet control through a 5- to 6-cm lateral incision from the lateral epicondyle toward the distal insertion of the anconeus on the ulna. Subcutaneous dissection is then performed to expose the muscle origin and insertion. The distal insertion is sharply elevated and this sharp dissection is continued proximally until the anconeus can be rotated over the common

extensor origin and inset in a tension-free manner (**Fig. 5**B). The elbow is taken through a full flexion/extension arc to ensure no excess tension before tourniquet release and evaluation of hemostasis. We do not routinely see the vascular pedicle in our flap elevation. Patients are then immobilized in a long-arm splint for 5 to 7 days, after which elbow range of motion (ROM) is initiated. Strengthening is initiated at 8 weeks postoperatively.

SUMMARY

The care of patients with persistent or worsened symptoms following previous surgical intervention is challenging in many respects. There are disease factors, patient factors, and surgical factors that may all contribute. It is important to avoid cognitive tunneling and to ensure that all diagnostic options and nonoperative treatments have been considered.

Revision surgery for tendinopathy is uncommon. Reported surgical techniques are usually described in relation to small surgical case series, often with heterogeneity between patients, and are prone to bias. It is important in such cases to adhere to the best principles of anatomy, physiology, and careful surgical technique. It is also most important to communicate such limitations to the patient.

CLINICS CARE POINTS

- Pain and disability in the acute period after upper extremity surgery is most strongly predicted by psychosocial influences.
- Focused examination and consideration of alternative diagnoses minimize bias and misdiagnosis.

- Wide Awake, Local Anesthetic, No Tourniquet techniques allow for safe and effective release combined with active motion
- Revision surgery for epicondylitis can be successful using denervation and/or anconeus flap coverage.

DISCLOSURE

Dr S.A. Kennedy and Dr R.D. Brown have no financial relationships with companies or entities.

REFERENCES

1. Berner ES, Graber ML. Overconfidence as a Cause of Diagnostic Error in Medicine. Am J Medicine 2008;121(5):S2–23.
2. Boodman, S.G. "Misdiagnosis is more common than drug errors or wrong-site surgery" The Washington Post. May 7, 2013. Available at: https://www.washingtonpost.com/national/health-science/misdiagnosis-is-more-common-than-drug-errors-or-wrong-site-surgery/2013/05/03/5d71a374-9af4-11e2-a941-a19bce7af755_story.html. Accessed March 4, 2023.
3. Graber ML, Wachter RM, Cassel CK. Bringing Diagnosis Into the Quality and Safety Equations. JAMA 2012;308(12):1211–2.
4. Ring D. Pearls: Effective Communication Strategies for the Biopsychosocial Paradigm of Musculoskeletal Medicine. Clin Orthop Relat Res 2020;478(12):2720–1.
5. Singh H, Giardina TD, Meyer AND, et al. Types and Origins of Diagnostic Errors in Primary Care Settings. JAMA Intern Med 2013;173(6):418–25.
6. Sun L. Most Americans will get a wrong or late diagnosis at least once in their lives. Wash Post 2015.
7. De SD, Vranceanu AM, Ring DC. Contribution of Kinesophobia and Catastrophic Thinking to Upper-Extremity-Specific Disability. J Bone Jt Surg 2013;95(1):76–81.
8. Miner H, Rijk L, Thomas J, et al. Mental-Health Phenotypes and Patient-Reported Outcomes in Upper-Extremity Illness. J Bone Joint Surg 2021;103(15):1411–6.
9. Moussavi S, Chatterji S, Verdes E, et al. Depression, chronic diseases, and decrements in health: results from the World Health Surveys. Lancet 2007;370(9590):851–8.
10. Ring D, Kadzielski J, Fabian L, et al. Self-Reported Upper Extremity Health Status Correlates with Depression. J Bone Jt Surg 2006;88(9):1983–8.
11. Vranceanu AM, Jupiter JB, Mudgal CS, et al. Predictors of Pain Intensity and Disability After Minor Hand Surgery. J Hand Surg 2010;35(6):956–60.
12. Mallette P, Ring D. Attitudes of Hand Surgeons, Hand Surgery Patients, and the General Public Regarding Psychologic Influences on Illness. J Hand Surg 2006;31(8):1362.e1–6.
13. Everding NG, Bishop GB, Belyea CM, et al. Risk factors for complications of open trigger finger release. Hand 2015;10(2):297–300.
14. Chuang XL, McGrouther DA. Adhesions as a component of the trigger finger: a dynamic sonographic study. J Hand Surg European 2020;46(8):852–6.
15. Tang JB. Clinical Outcomes Associated with Flexor Tendon Repair. Hand Clin 2005;21(2):199–210.
16. Wu RT, Walker ME, Peck CJ, et al. Differential Pulley Release in Trigger Finger: A Prospective, Randomized Clinical Trial. Hand 2021. https://doi.org/10.1177/1558944721994231. 155894472199423.
17. Abi-Rafeh J, Jaberi MM, Kazan R, et al. Utility of Ultrasonography and Significance of Surgical Anatomy in the Management of de Quervain Disease: A Systematic Review and Meta-Analysis. Plast Reconstr Surg 2022;149(2):420–34.
18. Andring N, Kennedy SA, Iannuzzi NP. Anomalous Forearm Muscles and Their Clinical Relevance. J Hand Surg 2018;43(5):455–63.
19. Wu F, Rajpura A, Sandher D. Finkelstein's Test Is Superior to Eichhoff's Test in the Investigation of de Quervain's Disease. J Hand Microsurg 2018;10(2):116–8.
20. Horn BJ, Zondervan R, Shafer-Crane G, et al. Prevention of Tendon Subluxation in Dequervain's Tenosynovitis Release Using Retinacular Repair. Spartan Medical Res J 2016;1(1):4705.
21. Kim JH, Yang SW, Ham HJ, et al. Tendon Subluxation After Surgical Release of the First Dorsal Compartment in De Quervain Disease. Ann Plas Surg 2019;82(6):628–35.
22. McMahon M, Craig SM, Posner MA. Tendon subluxation after de Quervain's release: Treatment by brachioradialis tendon flap. J Hand Surg 1991;16(1):30–2.
23. Renson D, Mermuys K, Vanmierlo B, et al. Pulley Reconstruction for Symptomatic Instability of the Tendons of the First Extensor Compartment Following de Quervain's Release. J Wrist Surg 2017;7(1):31–7.
24. Byrd JN, Sasor SE, Chung KC. Extensor Carpi Ulnaris Subluxation. Hand Clin 2021;37(4):487–91.
25. Ghatan AC, Puri SG, Morse KW, et al. Relative Contribution of the Subsheath to Extensor Carpi Ulnaris Tendon Stability: Implications for Surgical Reconstruction and Rehabilitation. J Hand Surg 2016;41(2):225–32.
26. Ruchelsman DE, Vitale MA. Extensor Carpi Ulnaris Subsheath Reconstruction. J Hand Surg 2016;41(11):e433–9.
27. Ruland RT, Hogan CJ. The ECU Synergy Test: An Aid to Diagnose ECU Tendonitis. J Hand Surg 2008;33(10):1777–82.

28. Starr AJ, Smith WR, Frawley WH, et al. Symptoms of Posttraumatic Stress Disorder After Orthopaedic Trauma. J Bone Jt Surgery-american Volume 2004; 86(6):1115–21.

29. Straszewski AJ, Lee CS, Dickherber JL, et al. Temporal Relationship of Corticosteroid Injection and Open Release for Trigger Finger and Correlation With Postoperative Deep Infections. J Hand Surg 2021. https://doi.org/10.1016/j.jhsa.2021.08.017.

30. Kher S, Graham DJ, Symes M, et al. Outcomes of Isolated Digital Flexor Tenolysis: A Systematic Review. J Hand Surg Asian-pacific 2021;26(4):580–7.

31. Azari KK, Meals RA. Flexor Tenolysis. Hand Clin 2005;21(2):211–7.

32. Pompeu Y, Almeida BA, Kunze K, et al. Current Concepts in the Management of Advanced Trigger Finger: A Critical Analysis Review. Jbjs Rev 2021; 9(9). https://doi.org/10.2106/jbjs.rvw.21.00006.

33. Gil JA, Hresko AM, Weiss APC. Current Concepts in the Management of Trigger Finger in Adults. J Am Acad Orthop Sur 2020;15:e642–50.

34. Smith WR, Lutsky KF, Gallant G, et al. Extensor Carpi Ulnaris Tenodesis to the Distal Ulna for the Treatment of Recalcitrant Instability and Tendinopathy. American Association for Hand Surgery 2019. Available at: https://meeting.handsurgery.org/abstracts/2019/HSEP93.cgi. Accessed May 12, 2022.

35. Bakhach J, Sentucq-Rigal J, Mouton P, et al. La plastie d'expansion en Oméga « Ω » : une nouvelle technique de traitement chirurgical de la ténosynovite de De Quervain. Ann De Chir Plastique Esthétique 2006;51(1):67–73.

36. Calfee RP, Patel A, DaSilva MF, et al. Management of Lateral Epicondylitis: Current Concepts. J Am Acad Orthop Sur 2008;16(1):19–29.

37. Lindenhovius A, Henket M, Gilligan BP, et al. Injection of Dexamethasone Versus Placebo for Lateral Elbow Pain: A Prospective, Double-Blind, Randomized Clinical Trial. J Hand Surg 2008; 33(6):909–19.

38. Ruch DS, Orr SB, Richard MJ, et al. A comparison of débridement with and without anconeus muscle flap for treatment of refractory lateral epicondylitis. J Shoulder Elb Surg 2015;24(2):236–41.

39. Luchetti R, Atzei A, Brunelli F, et al. Anconeus Muscle Transposition for Chronic Lateral Epicondylitis, Recurrences, and Complications. Techniques Hand Up Extremity Surg 2005;9(2):105–12.

40. Berry N, Neumeister MW, Russell RC, et al. Epicondylectomy versus Denervation for Lateral Humeral Epicondylitis. Hand 2011;6(2):174–8.

41. Degreef I, Raebroeckx AV, Smet LD. Anconeus muscle transposition for failed surgical treatment of tennis elbow: preliminary results. Acta Orthop Belg 2005;71(2):154–6.

42. Rose NE, Forman SK, Dellon AL. Denervation of the Lateral Humeral Epicondyle for Treatment of Chronic Lateral Epicondylitis. J Hand Surg 2013;38(2): 344–9.

43. Bickham R, Carr L, Butterfield J, et al. Current Management of Trigger Digit in Rheumatoid Arthritis Patients: A Survey of ASSH Members. Hand 2020. https://doi.org/10.1177/1558944720975137. 155894472097513.

44. Collins ED. Radial Ridge Excision for Symptomatic Volar Tendon Subluxation Following de Quervain's Release. Techniques Hand Up Extremity Surg 2014;18(3):143–5.

Flexor Tendon Repair
Avoidance and Management of Complications

Sally Jo, MD, Christopher J. Dy, MD, MPH*

KEYWORDS

- Flexor tendon repair • Complications • Repair site rupture • Flexor tendon adhesions

KEY POINTS

- Repair site rupture and adhesion formation are the most common complications after a flexor tendon repair.
- The principal strategy for preventing complications is ensuring a stout repair without repair site gapping at time zero, which will enable the accrual of repair site strength and intrinsic healing through the early initiation of postoperative motion.
- Intraoperative strategies for confirming tendon gliding and strength at the time of repair, such as Wide Awake Local Anesthesia No Tourniquet hand surgery, are becoming increasingly prevalent.

INTRODUCTION

Flexor tendon injuries occur at a rate of less than 1% of all hand injuries per year.[1] These injuries most commonly occur in the young, working population, creating a significant impact on the productivity of both the individual and society at large. Although flexor tendon repair is one of the most frequently published topics in orthopedic literature, the rates of complications and reoperation have remained stable.[1,2] Increasing efforts are therefore warranted in understanding how to avoid and properly manage these complications.

GENERAL PRINCIPLES OF REPAIR

The primary repair of lacerated flexor tendons in the hand and forearm is a relatively modern practice. In the 1910s, surgeons coined the term "no man's land" after recognizing the difficulty in gaining range of motion after primary repair of flexor tendons. Advancements since that time have shown that a strong repair that can withstand early rehabilitation is the key to successful outcomes.

The flexor tendon is divided into anatomic zones according to a classification system by Kleinert.[3]

The anatomy of zone 2 is unique in that both the flexor digitorum superficialis (FDS) and flexor digitorum profundus (FDP) tendons must glide past each other in a tight fibro-osseous tunnel. This anatomy makes repairs in zone 2 prone to complications such as adhesion formation and repair site rupture. Tendon repairs in this zone tend to have the most variable outcomes, although complications can occur in other zones as well.

The Strickland criteria are one of the more commonly used tools to assess outcomes after flexor tendon repair.[4] With these criteria, outcome is measured based on the degree of active proximal interphalangeal (PIP) and distal interphalangeal (DIP) joint flexion. Combined motion arc of greater than 150° or 85% of normal is rated as excellent, motion between 125° and 149° or 70% to 84% of normal is rated as good, motion between 90° and 124° or 50% to 69% of normal is rated as fair, and motion less than 90° or less than 50% of normal is rated as poor. Multiple digits injuries, age, smoking history, delay to surgery, and concomitant FDS and nerve injuries are more likely to lead to poor outcomes.[5-9] Furthermore, there is still variability in surgical technique,

Department of Orthopaedic Surgery, Washington University in St. Louis, St Louis, MO, USA
* Corresponding author. Washington University in St. Louis, 660 South Euclid Avenue, Campus Box 8233, St. Louis, MO 63110.
E-mail address: dyc@wustl.edu

Hand Clin 39 (2023) 427–434
https://doi.org/10.1016/j.hcl.2023.03.003
0749-0712/23/© 2023 Elsevier Inc. All rights reserved.

suture choice, and post-op rehabilitation that could be contributing to the variability in patient outcomes.[10]

DISCUSSION
Complications After Flexor Tendon Repair

In a state-wide database study, the rate of reoperation after primary repair has been reported to be around 6% due to various complications or unsatisfactory outcomes.[2] Risk factors that are associated with greater overall rate of reoperation include older age and workers' compensation status. Although with the potential disadvantage of underreporting complications not captured by administrative coding, the above study remains without any publication bias toward underreporting and is likely a good estimate of general complication rates. In this article, the authors discuss the most common complications associated with flexor tendon repair as well as ways to prevent and manage these complications.

Repair Site Rupture

Repair site rupture, occurring at a rate of 4%, is one of the most common and dreaded complications of flexor tendon repair. Patients typically present with a sudden loss of digital motion or grip strength. The diagnosis of a repair site rupture is usually a clinical one, although ultrasound can aid in the diagnosis.

Repair site rupture typically occurs between 0 and 9 weeks after surgery.[11,12] This supports the clinical practice of continuous splint wear for 5 to 6 weeks, followed by activity restrictions to light grasping activities for the subsequent 6 weeks. Possible causes of repair site rupture include patient noncompliance with splint wear or activity restrictions, repair technique (eg, not using at least four strands in the core suture configuration), and not using an epitendinous suture.[13] Age and sex of patients, smoking, or delay in primary repair have not been linked with rupture rates.[11] Delayed repair site rupture beyond the 9 weeks can occur if there is gapping greater than 3 mm at the time of the initial repair.[14] Although early mobilization can be achieved even if gapping is present due to the strength of the suture itself, the tendon will not accrue strength and is predisposed to rupture.

Prevention of Repair Site Rupture

The main strategy for preventing repair site rupture is ensuring a strong repair without gapping at the time of the index surgery. Optimizing the time-zero biomechanical strength and minimizing any repair gapping will enable the accrual of tensile strength at the repair site during rehabilitation. A gap formation of greater than 3 mm at time zero has been associated with insufficient strength to withstand early mobilization.[14]

Numerous technical variables and their impact on repair site strength have been studied. These variables include core suture strand number, caliber, purchase, suture configuration, epitendinous suture purchase, and locking versus grasping loop configurations. Techniques that ensure adequate strength at the repair site include using a minimum of four strands of core suture with a running epitendinous suture. This repair construct has been shown to have increased loads to failure. Core suture placement of 7 to 10 mm from the tendon edge is also important for sufficient tissue purchase.

Wide Awake Local Anesthesia No Tourniquet (WALANT) hand surgery has been increasingly used in efforts to prevent repair site ruptures. In WALANT surgery, a local anesthetic mixture of lidocaine and epinephrine is injected proximal to the operative area. Tumescence is achieved, which means that there is a sufficiently large volume of injected material that the tissues become slightly firm.[15] By avoiding tourniquet use and sedation, the repair construct can be tested, whereas the patient is comfortable and awake. Intraoperative Total Active Movement Examination can be performed, in which the patient is asked to fully extend and flex the operative digit before skin closure.[16] This examination helps detect gapping at the repair site. Gapping can occur when the sutures are tied with inadequate tension, causing bunching of the suture at the repair site with flexion of the digit. If detected, this gapping should be repaired before leaving the operating room.

Treatment of Repair Site Rupture

Management of repair site rupture primarily depends on the amount of tendon end displacement and the chronicity of the rupture. If there is less than 1 cm of displacement of the tendon ends, a revision of the repair construct with scar excision can be performed. If there is more than 1 cm of displacement, however, tendon reconstruction with grafting should be considered, as excessive advancement of the proximal tendon end can lead to the quadriga effect. Grafting is also considered if the rupture occurs in a delayed manner, greater than 6 to 8 weeks from the index surgery.

ADHESION FORMATION

Adhesion formation, occurring at a rate of 4%, is another common complication following flexor tendon repair. Adhesions can form between the FDP and FDS tendons or between the tendon and the pulley system. Patients with adhesion formation commonly present with decreased finger motion. On clinical examination, a passive range of motion will be greater than active motion. Decreased passive range of motion indicates tightness of the dorsal capsule, volar plate, or collateral ligaments, rather than an isolated flexor tendon pathology. Such contractures should be addressed before consideration of flexor tenolysis.[17] Patients with adhesions may also complain of decreased grip strength and finesse of digit movement.[18]

Prevention of Adhesion Formation

Immaculate soft tissue handling during the index surgery is the first step to preventing adhesion formation. Inadvertent damage can be done to the pulley or the tendon while trying to retrieve retracted tendon ends. Flexion of the digit at the metacarpophalangeal (MCP) joint for zone 2 injuries or the PIP joint for zone 1 injuries can often help deliver the proximal end of the tendon into the operating field. One should avoid blind attempts to grasp the tendon. Often, a separate incision can be made proximally where there is a soft tissue bulk indicating a retracted tendon end. A pediatric catheter can be passed proximally, and the tendon end can be sutured onto the catheter then passed distally. Surgeon expertise has been linked with lower rates of adhesions requiring flexor tenolysis, suggesting that deft handling of soft tissues is an important factor in preventing adhesions.[19]

Bulkiness at the repair site is another important consideration. Concomitant repair of both the FDS and FDP tendons has been shown to be associated with increased rates of adhesions and subsequent flexor tenolysis.[20] The increased pressure in a tight fibro-osseous tunnel impairs tendon healing and increases the risk for tendon rupture and adhesion formation. FDS slip excision in cases of concomitant FDS and FDP injury has been advocated.[21]

Postoperative rehabilitation is one of the most important factors in preventing adhesions, but it is also one of the most variable practices. In the 1940s, arguments were made for total immobilization of the digit after flexor tendon repair, and this remained standard practice for 20 to 30 years.[22] Although the flexor tendon would heal, there would be an excessive amount of extrinsic healing and adhesion to the surrounding tissue that limited motion. Controlled passive motion was first introduced with rubber band traction immobilization in 1960, and then popularized with the publication of the Louisville protocol in 1977.[23,24] These protocols introduced the concepts of early passive flexion and early active extension of the digits. Bench research showed that early mobilization helps promote the ingrowth of epitenon cells that synthesize collagen at the repair site (intrinsic healing of the tendon). This contrasts with immobilized tendons, which heal by the ingrowth of adhesions and delayed proliferation of endotenon cells (extrinsic healing of the tendon).[25] On microscopic examination, repaired tendons subjected to early motion show reorientation of the collagen fibers in a longitudinal direction that closely replicates that of normal tendons.[25]

The next phase of rehabilitation research focused on synergistic wrist motion to augment the total tendon excursion.[26,27] The Indiana protocol incorporated synergistic wrist motion and place and hold exercises.[28] Place and hold exercises involve a 5-second hold, whereas the digit was passively flexed and the wrist extended. The next phase of flexor tendon rehabilitation research has involved early active motion, in which active flexion exercises are done for the affected digit.[29,30] Subsequent studies have found that early active motion does not lead to superior outcomes compared with place and hold exercises.[31] Furthermore, there is a theoretic risk of catastrophic failure with aggressive active motion.

Postoperative rehabilitation after flexor tendon repair typically begins within 4 to 7 days after the index surgery. Motion before 4 days is discouraged as postsurgical edema may cause undue stress on the repair site. Rehabilitation initiated more than 7 days from surgery increases the risk for adhesion formation.[32] Postsurgical rehabilitation is modified according to the patient's concurrent injuries, repair site integrity, and projected compliance of the patient. More excursion and force do not necessarily mean less adhesion; as little as 1.7 mm of excursion and force application of less than 10 N may be sufficient to prevent adhesions.[33]

At our institution, rehabilitation typically consists of passive range of motion with place-and-hold exercises in a dorsal blocking splint for the first 3 weeks. This is followed by a gradual increase of active motion, then removal of the splint by 6 weeks post-op. No difference in functional outcomes has been found between patients who practice active mobilization and those who primarily exercise passive movement with place-and-hold at terminal flexion.[31,34]

Management of Adhesion Formation

Flexor tenolysis can be considered if there is a lack of improvement in active range of motion relative to passive range of motion 3 to 6 months after repair. Waiting at least 3 months is recommended to prevent tendon devascularization and weakening of the repair site.[35] Patient selection for flexor tenolysis is critical. For example, noncompliance with postoperative rehabilitation after the initial surgery may be a relative contraindication for flexor tenolysis, which requires patient's willingness to once again undergo a regimented rehabilitation program.

The surgical approach for flexor tenolysis usually uses the same incision as the index surgery. Adhesion is often encountered between the FDS and FDP tendons, and this is carefully teased apart. Sacrificing the FDS tendon may be necessary for FDP gliding, and this excision of tendon has not been shown to impact total active motion.[36] Adhesions may also form between the tendon and the pulley. A beaver blade can be used to carefully tease apart the two structures circumferentially. The pulley can also be dilated with a pediatric catheter. There are dedicated surgical instruments such as tenolysis knives and pulley dilator that can be used in these scenarios.

Inducing anesthesia and hemostasis with WALANT is useful during flexor tenolysis, as the surgeon can ask the patient to actively move the digit in the operating room. This has a twofold effect. It helps ensure that there are no remaining adhesions blocking range of motion. It can also demonstrate the arc of motion to the patient, and thereby motivate the patient to maintain the degree of motion achieved during surgery.

Rehabilitation after flexor tenolysis typically depends on intraoperative findings. If the tendon repair site is sufficiently healed, active and passive motion is resumed within days. If the repair is not fully healed, a more gradual protocol of passive flexion and place-and-hold exercises at terminal flexion can be used.

TRIGGERING

Triggering of the repaired tendon is commonly attributed to repair site bulkiness and inadequate venting of pulleys. Patients present with a clicking or locking sensation while moving the affected digit, in a manner similar to triggering in native flexor tendons.

It is worth noting that triggering is a complication that is especially associated with partial lacerations. The beveled edge of a partially cut tendon can catch on the proximal border of the A2 pulley, causing a triggering sensation.[37] Delayed presentations have also been described, which occur due to a nodule of scar tissue forming at the site of the partial tendon injury.[38]

Prevention of Triggering

In cases of partial tendon injuries, surgical treatment focuses on smoothing out the tendon edges to prevent catching, rather than on maximizing tensile strength at the repair site. In fact, the repair of partial flexor tendons has been shown to yield poorer tensile strength and higher likelihood of rupture than unrepaired tendons.[39–43] Attempts to prevent triggering include trimming the tendon edge, excising the pulley that is causing impingement, and repairing the injured flexor sheath to prevent further catching.[44,45] Most surgeons agree that partial tendon lacerations involving greater than 50% of the tendon should be treated operatively.[46]

In cases of full diameter tendon injuries, traditional principles of a stout repair construct combined with early rehabilitation still stand as the primary way to prevent bulbous scar formation. Excess bulk of the repair site should be avoided particularly in zone 2, where both the FDS and FDP tendons must glide through a tight fibroosseous tunnel. For injuries proximal to the Camper's chiasm, repair of both FDS and FDP could lead to excess bulkiness. In these circumstances, isolated repair of FDP and slip excision of FDS has been advocated.[47] Digital extension–flexion test advocated by Tang can be performed in the operating room to ensure that there is no triggering at time zero.[48] WALANT also enables the assessment of active motion in the OR and early detection of any bulkiness to the repair that could lead to triggering.

Treatment of Triggering

Corticosteroid injections can be considered once the repair site is sufficiently healed. The revision of the repair site with scar debulking is alternatives. Partial excision of a pulley may also be needed.

Quadriga Syndrome

Quadriga syndrome is a phenomenon in which there is a decreased flexion of the uninjured digits. In short, the range of motion of the neighboring digits becomes limited by the shortest tendon length. This occurs when the injured tendon is over-advanced or if adhesions limit the range of motion of the injured digit. The anatomic basis of this phenomenon is the shared muscle belly of FDP tendons to the middle, ring, and small fingers as well as the dense fibrous interconnections between the FDP tendons.[49] Patients with quadriga often present with weakness of grip strength.

Prevention of Quadriga Syndrome

Avoiding over-advancement of the tendon is the primary strategy for preventing quadriga. A 1 cm of tendon advancement may be the maximum amount that is tolerated.[50] This limit may be greater in the index finger due to the independent muscle belly of FDP to the index. Early postoperative rehabilitation is also critical for preventing the formation of adhesions that could cause quadriga.

Primary tendon grafting rather than primary repair should be considered if there is greater than 1 cm of gapping between the tendon ends at the index surgery. Tendon grafting is also considered when the patient presents in a delayed manner, more than 3 weeks after injury. In tenotomized tendons, sarcomere degeneration and fibrosis cause tendon retraction, which can leave a gap between the proximal and distal stumps.[51] Rather than attempting a tensioned repair, tendon grafting should be performed in these instances. Commonly used grafts include the palmaris longus and plantaris tendons. The graft is typically secured to the proximal stump of the injured FDP tendon. If this is unavailable, the graft can be sutured in an end-to-side fashion to adjacent FDS or FDP tendons.

Staged tendon grafting is indicated in cases of significant soft tissue defects, joint contracture, or pulley incompetence. The first stage of staged grafting involves reconstructing the pulley with a silicone rod, which triggers an inflammatory response that creates a pseudo-sheath around the rod. Any soft tissue defects should be addressed in this stage as well. The second stage involves removal of the rod and placement of the graft.

Treatment of Quadriga Syndrome

If the weakness caused by quadriga is clinically apparent, surgical treatment can be considered. Any adhesions tethering the tendon can be released. The FDP tendon can also be released proximally near the origin of the lumbrical muscles to increase its excursion.[52]

Joint Stiffness

Patients with joint stiffness in the DIP or PIP joint present with limitations in both active and passive ranges of motion. Causes of joint stiffness can be variable. These include a concomitant volar plate injury, neurovascular injury or fracture, skin contracture, prolonged immobilization, tendon adhesions, inadequate rehabilitation, and pulley incompetence. If caused by extrinsic factors, increased PIP joint extension with MCP joint flexion can be seen.

Prevention of Joint Stiffness

Preventable causes of joint stiffness include prolonged immobilization. Fabrication of an intrinsic plus splint with MCP joint flexion and extension at the IP joints is important. Stiffness due to other concomitant soft tissue injuries can be difficult to prevent.

Treatment of Joint Stiffness

Conservative treatment starts with extension splinting. If the patient has persistent stiffness despite conservative measures, extrinsic causes of joint stiffness are addressed next. Skin contractures and tendon adhesions can be managed with contracture release and flexor tenolysis. PIP joint release can be performed if the patient has residual stiffness, which may include a release of the checkrein ligaments, collateral ligaments, and volar plate in ascending order.

BOWSTRINGING

Tendon bowstringing occurs when there is a concomitant injury to the pulley system, or if there is excessive venting of the pulleys during surgery. This leads to decreased efficiency of tendon excursion and increased force requirements for joint rotation.[53] Patients with tendon bowstringing present with decreased grip strength.

Prevention of Bowstringing

During the approach for primary repair, release of the fibro-osseous sheath through cruciate pulleys is recommended, although judicious release of the A2 and A4 pulleys has also been advocated in the literature.[54–56] Balance must be weighed between the risk for excessive pulley excision causing bowstringing versus the need to vent the pulleys adequately to prevent adhesion formation and triggering.

Treatment of Bowstringing

Pulley reconstruction can be considered with cases of persistent bowstringing that leads to weakness. Reconstruction with the extensor retinaculum has been shown to provide the least resistance to tendon gliding.[57] Pulley reconstruction with tissues extrinsic to the injured digit such as palmaris longus graft has been shown to be associated with increased excursion resistance.

SWAN NECK DEFORMITY

Swan neck deformity can result from an unrecognized FDS and volar plate injury. Patients present with hyperextension at the PIP joint and flexion at the DIP joint. Patients are rarely symptomatic from this, however, as flexion through the FDP tendon often provides sufficient grip strength.

Prevention of Swan Neck Deformity

Prevention mainly consists of careful preoperative examination to ascertain levels of injury and intra-operative examination for volar plate or FDS injury. If injury to these structures is identified, they should be repaired.

Treatment of Swan Neck Deformity

Tenodesis of a slip of the FDS tendon can be considered for correction of swan neck deformity.

LUMBRICAL PLUS DEFORMITY

Lumbrical plus deformity occurs when the FDP tendon is too long and thereby nonfunctional, leading to the lumbricals being recruited during active flexion and causing extension in the IP joints via the lateral bands. Lumbrical plus is caused by a pathology opposite that of quadriga syndrome, where the FDP tendon is excessively shortened.

Treatment can include tendon grafting and lumbrical release.

SUMMARY

Despite numerous advances in flexor tendon surgery over the past 50 years, outcomes of flexor tendon repair remain variable, especially in zone 2. Adhesion formation and repair site rupture are the most common complications. Modern advances such as WALANT have enabled the early detection of problems before leaving the OR. Above all, adhering to basic principles for a strong repair remains paramount.

DISCLOSURES

No financial disclosures relevant to this publication.

REFERENCES

1. Hill C, Riaz M, Mozzam A, et al. A regional audit of hand and wrist injuries. A study of 4873 injuries. J Hand Surg Br 1998;23(2):196–200.
2. Dy CJ, Daluiski A, Do HT, et al. The epidemiology of reoperation after flexor tendon repair. J Hand Surg Am 2012;37(5):919–24.
3. Kleinert HE, Spokevicius S, Papas NH. History of flexor tendon repair. J Hand Surg Am 1995;20(3 Pt 2):S46–52.
4. Strickland JW, Glogovac SV. Digital function following flexor tendon repair in Zone II: A comparison of immobilization and controlled passive motion techniques. J Hand Surg Am 1980; 5(6):537–43.
5. Trumble TE, Vedder NB, Seiler JG 3rd, et al. Zone-II flexor tendon repair: a randomized prospective trial of active place-and-hold therapy compared with passive motion therapy. J Bone Joint Surg Am 2010;92(6):1381–9.
6. Elhassan B, Moran SL, Bravo C, et al. Factors that influence the outcome of zone I and zone II flexor tendon repairs in children. J Hand Surg Am 2006; 31(10):1661–6.
7. Kasashima T, Kato H, Minami A. Factors influencing prognosis after direct repair of the flexor pollicis longus tendon: multivariate regression model analysis. Hand Surg 2002;7(2):171–6.
8. McFarlane RM, Lamon R, Jarvis G. Flexor tendon injuries within the finger. A study of the results of tendon suture and tendon graft. J Trauma 1968; 8(6):987–1003.
9. Silfverskiold KL, May EJ, Oden A. Factors affecting results after flexor tendon repair in zone II: a multivariate prospective analysis. J Hand Surg Am 1993;18(4):654–62.
10. Gibson PD, Sobol GL, Ahmed IH. Zone II Flexor Tendon Repairs in the United States: Trends in Current Management. J Hand Surg Am 2017;42(2): e99–108.
11. Harris SB, Harris D, Foster AJ, et al. The aetiology of acute rupture of flexor tendon repairs in zones 1 and 2 of the fingers during early mobilization. J Hand Surg Br 1999;24(3):275–80.
12. Elliot D, Moiemen NS, Flemming AF, et al. The rupture rate of acute flexor tendon repairs mobilized by the controlled active motion regimen. J Hand Surg Br 1994;19(5):607–12.
13. Dy CJ, Hernandez-Soria A, Ma Y, et al. Complications after flexor tendon repair: a systematic review and meta-analysis. J Hand Surg Am 2012;37(3): 543–551 e1.
14. Gelberman RH, Boyer MI, Brodt MD, et al. The effect of gap formation at the repair site on the strength and excursion of intrasynovial flexor tendons. An experimental study on the early stages of tendon-healing in dogs. J Bone Joint Surg Am 1999;81(7): 975–82.
15. Lalonde DH. Wide-awake flexor tendon repair. Plast Reconstr Surg 2009;123(2):623–5.
16. Higgins A, Lalonde DH, Bell M, et al. Avoiding flexor tendon repair rupture with intraoperative total active movement examination. Plast Reconstr Surg 2010; 126(3):941–5.
17. Strickland JW. Flexor tendon surgery. Part 2: Free tendon grafts and tenolysis. J Hand Surg Br 1989; 14(4):368–82.
18. Moriya K, Yoshizu T, Tsubokawa N, et al. Incidence of tenolysis and features of adhesions in the digital

flexor tendons after multi-strand repair and early active motion. J Hand Surg Eur Vol 2019;44(4): 354–60.

19. Tang JB. Outcomes and evaluation of flexor tendon repair. Hand Clin 2013;29(2):251–9.

20. Civan O, Gursoy MK, Cavit A, et al. Tenolysis rate after zone 2 flexor tendon repairs. Jt Dis Relat Surg 2020;31(2):281–5.

21. Tang JB. Flexor tendon repair in zone 2C. J Hand Surg Br 1994;19(1):72–5.

22. Mason ML, Allen HS. The Rate of Healing of Tendons: An Experimental Study of Tensile Strength. Ann Surg 1941;113(3):424–59.

23. Young RE, Harmon JM. Repair of tendon injuries of the hand. Ann Surg 1960;151:562–6.

24. Lister GD, Kleinert HE, Kutz JE, et al. Primary flexor tendon repair followed by immediate controlled mobilization. J Hand Surg Am 1977;2(6):441–51.

25. Gelberman RH, Vande Berg JS, Lundborg GN, et al. Flexor tendon healing and restoration of the gliding surface. An ultrastructural study in dogs. J Bone Joint Surg Am 1983;65(1):70–80.

26. Cooney W, Lin G, An K-N. Improved tendon excursion following flexor tendon repair. J Hand Ther 1989;2(2):102–6.

27. Zhao C, Amadio PC, Momose T, et al. Effect of synergistic wrist motion on adhesion formation after repair of partial flexor digitorum profundus tendon lacerations in a canine model in vivo. J Bone Joint Surg Am 2002;84(1):78–84.

28. Strickland JW, Schmidt CC. Repair of flexor digitorum profundus lacerations: the Indiana method. Operat Tech Orthop 1998;8(2):73–80.

29. Coats RW 2nd, Echevarria-Ore JC, Mass DP. Acute flexor tendon repairs in zone II. Hand Clin 2005; 21(2):173–9.

30. Clancy SP, Mass DP. Current flexor and extensor tendon motion regimens: a summary. Hand Clin 2013;29(2):295–309.

31. Neiduski RL, Powell RK. Flexor tendon rehabilitation in the 21st century: A systematic review. J Hand Ther 2019;32(2):165–74.

32. Wu YF, Tang JB. Tendon healing, edema, and resistance to flexor tendon gliding: clinical implications. Hand Clin 2013;29(2):167–78.

33. Boyer MI, Gelberman RH, Burns ME, et al. Intrasynovial flexor tendon repair. An experimental study comparing low and high levels of in vivo force during rehabilitation in canines. J Bone Joint Surg Am 2001; 83(6):891–9.

34. Chevalley S, Tenfalt M, Ahlen M, et al. Passive Mobilization With Place and Hold Versus Active Motion Therapy After Flexor Tendon Repair: A Randomized Trial. J Hand Surg Am 2022;47(4):348–57.

35. Wray RC Jr, Moucharafieh B, Weeks PM. Experimental study of the optimal time for tenolysis. Plast Reconstr Surg 1978;61(2):184–9.

36. Breton A, Jager T, Dap F, et al. Effectiveness of flexor tenolysis in zone II: A retrospective series of 40 patients at 3 months postoperatively. Chir Main 2015; 34(3):126–33.

37. Frewin PR, Scheker LR. Triggering secondary to an untreated partially-cut flexor tendon. J Hand Surg Br 1989;14(4):419–21.

38. Schlenker JD, Lister GD, Kleinert HE. Three complications of untreated partial laceration of flexor tendon–entrapment, rupture, and triggering. J Hand Surg Am 1981;6(4):392–8.

39. Reynolds B, Wray RC Jr, Weeks PM. Should an incompletely severed tendon be sutured? Plast Reconstr Surg 1976;57(1):36–8.

40. Cooney WP, Weidman K, Malo D, et al. Management of acute flexor tendon injury in the hand. Instr Course Lect 1985;34:373–81.

41. Boardman ND 3rd, Morifusa S, Saw SS, et al. Effects of tenorraphy on the gliding function and tensile properties of partially lacerated canine digital flexor tendons. J Hand Surg Am 1999;24(2):302–9.

42. Bishop AT, Cooney WP 3rd, Wood MB. Treatment of partial flexor tendon lacerations: the effect of tenorrhaphy and early protected mobilization. J Trauma 1986;26(4):301–12.

43. Ollinger H, Wray RC Jr, Weeks PM. Effects of suture on tensile strength gain of partially and completely severed tendons. Surg Forum 1975;26:63–4.

44. al-Qattan MM. Conservative management of zone II partial flexor tendon lacerations greater than half the width of the tendon. J Hand Surg Am 2000;25(6): 1118–21.

45. Erhard L, Zobitz ME, Zhao C, et al. Treatment of partial lacerations in flexor tendons by trimming. A biomechanical in vitro study. J Bone Joint Surg Am 2002;84(6):1006–12.

46. McCarthy DM, Boardman ND 3rd, Tramaglini DM, et al. Clinical management of partially lacerated digital flexor tendons: a survey [corrected] of hand surgeons. J Hand Surg Am 1995;20(2):273–5.

47. Tang JB, Xie RG, Cao Y, et al. A2 pulley incision or one slip of the superficialis improves flexor tendon repairs. Clin Orthop Relat Res 2007;456:121–7.

48. Tang JB. New Developments Are Improving Flexor Tendon Repair. Plast Reconstr Surg 2018;141(6): 1427–37.

49. Leijnse JN, Walbeehm ET, Sonneveld GJ, et al. Connections between the tendons of the musculus flexor digitorum profundus involving the synovial sheaths in the carpal tunnel. Acta Anat 1997;160(2):112–22.

50. Malerich MM, Baird RA, McMaster W, et al. Permissible limits of flexor digitorum profundus tendon advancement–an anatomic study. J Hand Surg Am 1987;12(1):30–3.

51. Jamali AA, Afshar P, Abrams RA, et al. Skeletal muscle response to tenotomy. Muscle Nerve 2000;23(6): 851–62.

52. Neu BR, Murray JF, MacKenzie JK. Profundus tendon blockage: quadriga in finger amputations. J Hand Surg Am 1985;10(6 Pt 1):878–83.

53. Peterson WW, Manske PR, Bollinger BA, et al. Effect of pulley excision on flexor tendon biomechanics. J Orthop Res 1986;4(1):96–101.

54. Tang JB. How to vent the pulley properly without tendon bowstringing in zone 2 repair. Chir Main 2015;34:395–6.

55. Tang JB. Release of the A4 pulley to facilitate zone II flexor tendon repair. J Hand Surg Am 2014;39(11):2300–7.

56. Tang JB. Recent evolutions in flexor tendon repairs and rehabilitation. J Hand Surg Eur 2018;43(5):469–73.

57. Nishida J, Amadio PC, Bettinger PC, et al. Flexor tendon-pulley interaction after pulley reconstruction: a biomechanical study in a human model in vitro. J Hand Surg Am 1998;23(4):665–72.

Extensor Tendon Repair
Avoidance and Management of Complications

R Adams Cowley II, MD[a], Curtis M. Henn, MD[a],*

KEYWORDS

- Extensor • Tendon • Repair • Complications

KEY POINTS

- The most common complication following extensor tendon repair is loss of range of motion.
- Loss of range of motion occurs despite early range of motion protocols.
- Outcomes following extensor tendon repair are significantly affected by the location of the injury and the presence or absence of associated injuries.
- Managing complications following extensor tendon repair primarily involves nonsurgical treatment of the stiff finger and rarely leads to surgical intervention in the form of extensor tenolysis with or without capsulotomy.

INTRODUCTION

The extensor mechanism is composed of a delicate network of interrelated structures that function together to facilitate normal hand function. The normal function of the extensor tendons is vital for normal hand function. Extension of the wrist facilitates increased grip strength, extension of the digits allows the hand to grasp larger objects, normal excursion of the extensor tendons allows grasping smaller objects, and so forth. It follows, then, that dysfunction of the extensor mechanism can be as devastating, if not more devastating, to hand function as dysfunction of the flexor mechanism.

Injuries to the extensor tendon range from closed injuries and simple sharp lacerations to complex crush injuries that may include extensive soft tissue, bony, and neurovascular compromise. Not surprisingly, the presence of associated injuries significantly affects surgical treatment, postoperative rehabilitation protocols, complications, and outcomes. The location of the injury also significantly affects treatment options and outcomes. The

extensor tendon over the hand, wrist, and distal forearm is amenable to core sutures, similar to flexor tendon repairs, whereas the extensor tendon distal to the metacarpophalangeal (MCP) joint is often surprisingly thin. Extensor tendon injuries in the digits are often complicated by traumatic arthrotomies into the distal interphalangeal (DIP), proximal interphalangeal (PIP), or MCP joints.

Management of extensor tendon injuries requires a robust understanding of the intrinsic and extrinsic extensor mechanism anatomy and their complex interactions. This is even more true when managing extensor tendon repair complications, when scar tissue from the original injury or from previous surgery affects the surgeon's ability to easily identify individual structures.

This article will first highlight anatomic pearls that are vital in treating extensor tendon injuries; review extensor tendon repair outcomes and complications by zone of injury and provide pearls to avoid those complications; then ultimately discuss the management of complications following extensor tendon repair.

a Department of Orthopedic Surgery, MedStar Georgetown University Hospital, Georgetown University School of Medicine, Washington, DC, USA
* Corresponding author. Medstar Georgetown University Hospital, 1st floor, Main Building, 3800 Reservoir Road NW, Washington, DC 20007.
E-mail address: Curits.M.Henn@gunet.georgetown.edu

Hand Clin 39 (2023) 435–446
https://doi.org/10.1016/j.hcl.2023.03.004
0749-0712/23/© 2023 Elsevier Inc. All rights reserved.

ANATOMY

The extensor tendon system has been divided into 9 distinct zones to simplify discussion of injuries and treatment options (**Fig. 1**).

The Forearm (Zones VIII and IX)

Injuries to the extensor mechanism in the forearm may include injuries to the tendon, musculotendinous junction, the muscles themselves, and/or the nerves supplying the extrinsic extensors.

The Wrist and Hand (Zones VI and VII)

The extensor tendons at this level pass through the synovial-lined 6 dorsal compartments under the extensor retinaculum, which facilitates gliding of the extensor tendons and improves their mechanical efficiency (**Fig. 2**).[1] The tendons run longitudinally, except the extensor pollicis longus (EPL) tendon, which makes an abrupt turn toward the thumb around Lister tubercle at the level of the radiocarpal joint. The extensor indicis proprius (EIP) and extensor digiti minimi (EDM) lie ulnar to their respective extensor digitorum communis (EDC) tendons and are capable of independent index and small finger extension. Over the dorsum of the hand, intertendinous connections between the EDC tendons, called juncturae tendinae, allow active MCP extension of the injured digit despite a complete EDC laceration proximally. Variation in number of EIP and EDM slips, variation in number and location of juncturae, and absence of EDC to the small finger, which occurs in more than half of patients, contribute to the challenge of surgical planning and repair of lacerated extensor tendons in the hand, particularly when multiple tendons have been injured.

The Fingers (Zones I–V)

The extrinsic extensor tendons travel dorsal to the MCP joint where radial and ulnar sagittal bands centralize the tendons and provide a yoke to extend the MCP (**Fig. 3**). There is no direct EDC connection to the proximal phalanx, yet the EDC is the primary extensor of the MCP joint through its extensor hood. Across the dorsum of the proximal phalanx, the extrinsic tendon trifurcates, sending fibers centrally to the central slip, which also receives contributing fibers from the intrinsic mechanism and serves to extend the PIP joint. The remaining extrinsic fibers radially and ulnarly join with the remaining intrinsic fibers to form the lateral bands and ultimately the terminal extensor, which inserts on the dorsal base of the distal phalanx and extends the DIP joint.

The intrinsic tendons, which are composed of contributions from the lumbrical and interosseous muscles, travel volar to the MCP center of rotation and consequently are the prime flexors of the MCP joints. After the intrinsic tendons join the lateral bands, they pass dorsal to the center of rotation of the PIP and DIP joints and are consequently the prime extensors of the interphalangeal joints.

EXTENSOR TENDON REPAIR OUTCOMES AND COMPLICATIONS

The surgeon must understand the expected outcomes and likelihood of possible complications, not only to provide adequate informed consent but also to take steps to avoid these complications. Even after impeccable extensor tendon repair under the most optimal conditions, injury characteristics, patient factors, and other unknown factors may lead to complications and less than ideal outcomes.

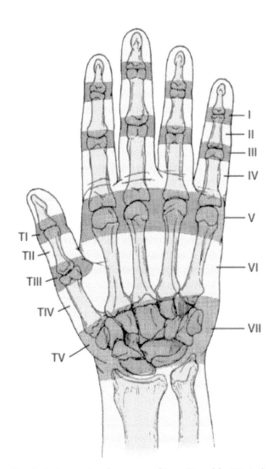

Fig. 1. Extensor tendon zones. (*From* Trumble TE et al, editors: Core knowledge in orthopaedics: hand, elbow, and shoulder, Philadelphia, 2006, Mosby; with permission.)

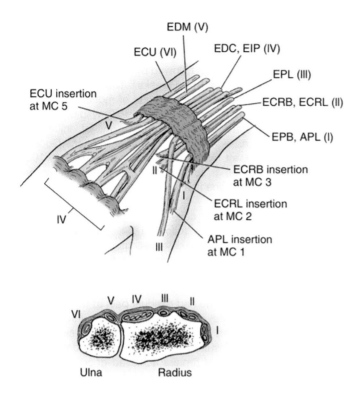

Fig. 2. The 6 dorsal compartments of the extensor tendons. (Reavy P, Rafijah G. Anatomy and Examination of the Hand, Wrist, Forearm, and Elbow. In: Principles of Hand Surgery and Therapy, Third Edition, Elsevier, 2016.)

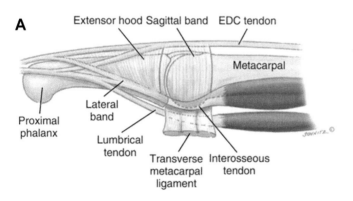

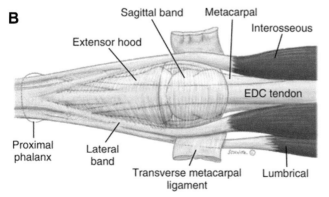

Fig. 3. The lateral (*A*) and dorsal (*B*) view of the extensor mechanism at the MCP joint. (*From* Kenneth R. Means, Jr., Rebecca J. Saunders, Thomas J. Graham, Nancy M. Cannon, Imran Yousaf. Pathophysiology and Surgical Management of the Stiff Hand; Postoperative Management of Metacarpophalangeal Joint and Proximal Interphalangeal Joint Capsulectomies. In: Rehabilitation of the Hand and Upper Extremity, Seventh Edition, 2021 Elsevier, Inc.)

General Considerations

Complications following extensor tendon repair include loss of active, and often passive, range of motion of the affected digits and potentially the neighboring digits. Patients may lose flexion, extension, or both. Depending on the degree of loss of motion and which joints are affected, these complications may or may not be functionally significant.

Loss of flexion may occur because of any combination of the following: extensor tendon adhesions, excessively shortening the extensor tendon, joint contracture, or secondary flexor tendon adhesions. Loss of extension may be attributable to any combination of the following: gapping at the repair site, extensor tendon adhesions, joint contracture, extensor tendon rerupture, and secondary flexor tendon adhesions. Loss of flexion has been shown to be a more common problem following extensor tendon repair than the loss of extension. Newport and colleagues showed a greater percentage of extensor tendon repairs exhibited loss of flexion compared with the percentage of digits that lost extension. They also noted the amount of lost flexion was greater than the amount of lost extension, highlighting the importance of focusing on restoring flexion following extensor tendon repair.[2]

Avoiding these complications requires optimizing repair strength, initiating early range of motion, and avoiding excessive shortening of the repair. Fortunately, extensor tendon lacerations often do not significantly retract proximally, except for the EPL over the dorsum of the hand, which commonly retracts proximal to the wrist. If the tendon has retracted and the repair is not performed acutely, then the surgeon should consider interposition grafting or tendon transfer, such as is often the case for an EPL rupture.

Optimal repair strength and early range of motion are more readily possible in zones V to VIII, given the caliber of the extensor tendon, which allows core suture repair. In the digits, the extensor tendon is flat and often cannot accept core sutures. As a result, distal repairs are often protected with prolonged static splinting or extension pinning, whereas more proximal repairs can be treated either with early controlled active range of motion or with a relative motion orthosis or dynamic extension splint (**Fig. 4**).

The results following extensor tendon repair are superior in zones V to VIII compared with zones I to IV,[2] regardless of whether the postoperative protocol uses static splinting[2,3] or dynamic splinting.[4]

Several studies have evaluated outcomes following extensor tendon repair across all zones, and there are few reported complications other than decreased range of motion.[2–5] Carl and colleagues evaluated the outcomes of 203 extensor tendon repairs followed by static splinting postoperatively for 4 to 6 weeks.[3] The authors reported outcomes based on range of motion and did not comment on complications. They did, however, correlate increased complexity of injury with decreased ultimate range of motion. Good to excellent results were obtained in 87% to 100% of cases in zones I, II, IV, and V, whereas only 43% in zone III and 54% in zone VI were good or excellent.

Purcell and colleagues reported similarly positive outcomes following 44 repairs, with 95% achieving good or excellent range of motions.[5] Only 2 of these cases had associated injuries, and most repairs were in zones V to VIII. Reported complications included one repair required a tenolysis, one had residual pain at the repair site, and one developed a postoperative infection.

Newport and colleagues reported significantly inferior results in 101 extensor tendon repairs. Only 50% of repairs achieved good or excellent range of motion in zones I to IV, and 63% to 83% achieved good or excellent range of motion in zones V to VIII.[2] However, 60% of the cases in this series included an associated injury (fracture, dislocation, joint capsule, or flexor tendon damage), whereas only 2 patients in the Purcell series had associated injuries. Reported complications included 4 repair failures but the failures were not defined or otherwise discussed further. One repair also required a tenolysis, and there were 2 superficial wound infections.

Hung and colleagues reported results after using a dynamic splinting protocol following 48 repairs.[4] They found similar results with final total active motion of 220 (range 95–207) across all repairs. They reported one revision for a persistent buttonhole deformity at the PIP. Two repairs required tenolysis and capsulotomy, and both injuries were segmental tendon defects over the MCP in the same hand.

Considered together, the available evidence confirms that the most common complication following extensor tendon repairs is stiffness. However, the ability to counteract stiffness with early range of motion and other techniques highly depends on the location of the injury. Therefore, it is also useful to discuss the outcomes and complications organized by location of the injury.

Zones I and II

Most extensor tendon injuries at this level are closed injuries that are treated nonsurgically. In a

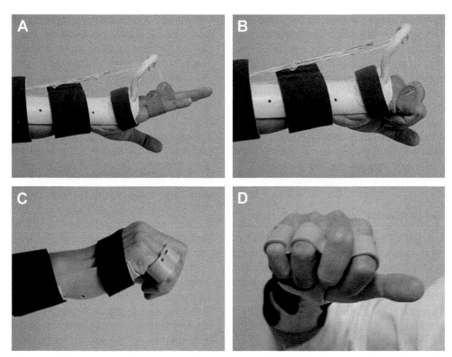

Fig. 4. (*A, B*) Dynamic extension splint. (*C, D*) Relative motion orthosis. (*From* David Netscher, Nikhil Agrawal, Nicholas A. Fiore II. Hand Surgery. In: Sabiston Textbook of Surgery: The Biological Basis of Modern Surgical Practice, Twenty First Edition, 2022, Elsevier Inc.)

systematic review, Lin and Samora found that the complication rate following closed treatment of mallet injuries was 12.8%, most commonly cold intolerance and skin complications related to the splint.[6] Several randomized trials have compared various splints and reported on outcomes and complications. One of the trials found a significantly decreased risk of complications and treatment failure with thermoplastic splints compared with Stax splints or dorsal aluminum splints (**Fig. 5**).[7]

A second randomized trial compared volar aluminum, dorsal aluminum, and custom thermoplastic splints and found no significant difference in complications but they noticed a trend in decreased extensor lag with the thermoplastic splints.[8] A third randomized trial compared Stax splinting to custom-padded aluminum cap splints and found no difference in correcting the deformity, but there were significantly more skin complications in the Stax splint group.[9] Considered together, the available data suggest avoiding Stax splints and using a custom thermoplastic splint to minimize complications.

Open injuries in zone I and II and injuries with associated volar subluxation of the DIP typically are treated surgically. Options include standard repair of the extensor tendon with a running suture, repair of the extensor tendon and skin together

with figure-of-8 sutures, or debridement and closure of the skin alone followed by extension pinning. Regardless of the repair technique, extension pinning is typically necessary to protect the repair of the paper-thin tendon at this level.[10]

Lin and Samora reported a 14.5% complication rate in surgically treated patients, most commonly nail deformities and infection.[6] Infections may

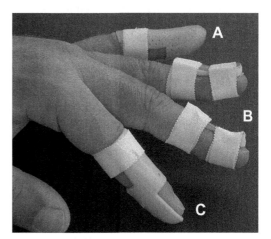

Fig. 5. Mallet orthoses. (A) Custom thermoplastic. (B) AlumaFoam. (C) Stax. (*From* Burke, S. L., Higgins, J., McClinton, M. A., et al. [2006]. Hand and upper extremity rehabilitation: A practical guide [3rd ed.]. St. Louis, MO: Churchill Livingstone; with permission.)

range from minor pin site infections to septic DIP joints. Avoiding open reduction of fractures may decrease the risk of nail deformity, without sacrificing clinical or radiographic outcomes. Various techniques have been described for percutaneous reduction and fixation and exhibit satisfactory outcomes with low complication rates.[11,12]

Historically, larger mallet fractures of greater than one-third of the joint mandated open reduction and internal fixation. However, satisfactory outcomes of these injuries treated nonsurgically have been shown even with larger fragments.[13,14]

Zone III and IV (Central Sip Injury)

Extensor tendon injuries in zone III may also be closed or open injuries. There is a paucity of literature supporting treatment and reporting complications following closed treatment of closed injuries. Most texts recommend 4 to 6 weeks of extension splinting of the PIP. Allowing active and passive flexion of the DIP may limit DIP stiffness following treatment.

In contrast, open injuries or avulsion fractures that are displaced or rotated are typically treated surgically with exploration, drainage of the interphalangeal joint, followed by repair of the tendon. At this level, core sutures may be possible but often reinserting the central slip is necessary with a pull-out suture through bone tunnels or with a small suture anchor. The PIP joint can then be transfixed with a K-wire in full extension (**Fig. 6**).

With only approximately 5 to 7 mm of excursion with flexion and extension, the central slip is quite sensitive to changes in length.[15] Gapping at the repair site leads to extensor lag and can lead to a progressive boutonniere deformity following palmar migration of the lateral bands.

To prevent this complication, repairs can be protected with prolonged extension pinning or splinting for 4 to 6 weeks.[16] However, tendon to bone adhesions in zone IV begin to increase tension at zone III repairs when flexion is initiated after 4 weeks,[17] which can then lead to attenuation of the repair and subsequent extensor lag (**Fig. 7**). Furthermore, the loss of 2 mm of tendon excursion at Zone 3 may result in 50% loss in range of motion,[18] highlighting the negative effects of any extensor adhesions following prolonged immobilization.

Several studies have reported outcomes following central slip repair with a variety of techniques and postoperative protocols.[15,16,19–23] The most common complications are lack of full flexion, extensor lag, or development of a boutonniere deformity.

Two studies compared static splinting protocols with early motion protocols.[16,23] Walsh and colleagues retrospectively compared outcomes and complications between central slip repairs that underwent an early motion protocol (n = 12) versus those that underwent static splinting (n = 19). Although the study was underpowered, they showed no differences in total active motion, total passive motion, or the incidence of extensor lag.[16]

Evans similarly compared an early active motion protocol (n = 38) with 3 to 6 weeks of static extension splinting (n = 26) following central slip repair.[23] The early motion protocol group exhibited significantly superior outcomes, including greater PIP range of motion at 6 weeks and at discharge, greater total active motion at discharge, and greater DIP range of motion at discharge. The early motion did not lead to increased extensor lag or boutonniere deformity. Early motion protocol patients were also discharged from therapy significantly sooner than the static group.

Considered together, it seems the most reliable method surgeons may use to avoid the complications of loss of flexion or residual extensor lag would be to adopt an early motion protocol following extensor tendon repair in zone III.

Zone V (Sagittal Band)

Injuries in zone V most commonly include closed sagittal band injuries. Acute closed injuries are treated nonsurgically with relative motion splinting. If treatment is instituted within 3 weeks, one can expect a greater than 95% success rate.[24–26] Delayed treatment may result in recurrent or persistent EDC subluxation.

Chronic EDC subluxation is treated with either direct repair or reconstruction of the sagittal band. One can expect restoration of full range of motion and few, if any, complications. Minor complications that have been reported include asymptomatic recurrent subluxation in a patient with ligamentous laxity and loss of 10° of flexion in another.[24] Failure of repair with recurrent subluxation has also been reported, requiring 2 subsequent reconstructions in one patient.[27] This failure, though, noted significant suture reaction and may be related to patient factors rather than surgical technique or postoperative protocol. To our knowledge, no other complications or failures are reported in the literature.

Zones V (Extensor Digitorum Communis)—VIII

Open injuries in Zone V include lacerations or penetrating injuries to the EDC, the sagittal band, or both. These injuries often include a traumatic arthrotomy and can occur via a clenched fist mechanism. Provided that the wound is clean, treatment

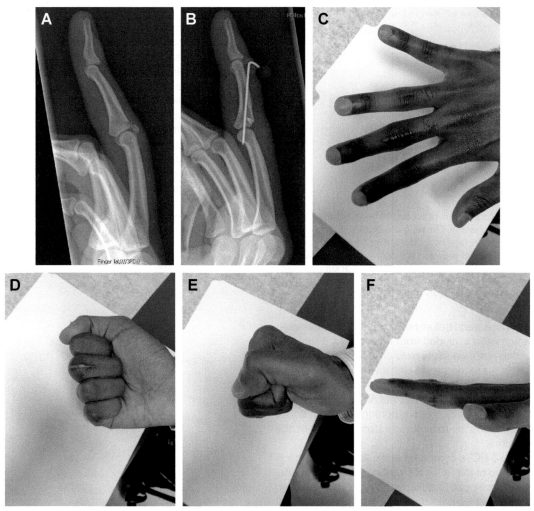

Fig. 6. Case example of central slip avulsion fracture. (*A*) Lateral radiograph demonstrating displaced central slip avulsion fracture and developing boutonniere deformity. (*B*) Postoperative lateral radiograph demonstrating excision of the avulsed fragment, repair of the central slip with a suture anchor, and protection of the repair with a K wire. (*C–F*) Clinical photographs at 3 months postoperatively demonstrating excellent range of motion.

entails debridement and repair of the extensor tendon, followed by either static extension splinting or an early active motion protocol with or without a relative motion orthosis.

Two small case series have evaluated repairs in zones IV and V: one with a running interlocking horizontal mattress suture technique[28] (**Fig. 8**) and the other with a core suture repair.[29] Both series allowed controlled early active motion. The studies included a total of 28 repairs. Twenty repairs regained full extension and flexion, 3 exhibited less than 5° of flexion loss, 2 exhibited less than 10° of both extension lag and flexion loss, and 1 lost 25° of flexion. There were no other complications reported. Both repair techniques and early motion can reliably restore nearly full range of motion with few complications.

Several larger series reported extensor tendon repair outcomes across zones IV to VIII, including 3 randomized controlled trials (RCTs)[30–32] and 2 case series.[33,34] Overall, these studies include 337 repairs in zones IV to VII, and a total of 14 complications were reported. Three repairs required a tenolysis, 1 in a dynamic splinting group and 2 in a static group. Two repairs developed wound infections treated with oral antibiotics, and 6 had persistent swelling. Three repairs ruptured, 1 in the dynamic splinting group and 2 in a static splinting group.

The ruptures were reported in the Khandwala series, which was a randomized trial of 100 extensor tendon repairs that were treated postoperatively with either palmar blocking splint versus a dynamic outrigger splint. The authors reported an additional 5 ruptures that occurred between discharge from

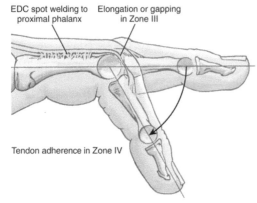

EDC spot welding to   Elongation or gapping
proximal phalanx   in Zone III

Tendon adherence in Zone IV

Fig. 7. The problem of tendon to bone adhesions at the proximal phalanx. The repaired central slip may gap or attenuate in late mobilization programs because its more proximal segment is adherent. (*From* Evans RB, Thompson DE. An analysis of factors that support early active short arc motion of the repaired central slip. J Hand Ther. 1992;5:190; with permission.)

the hospital and before presentation to the therapist, which were excluded from analysis. All 8 ruptures underwent immediate revision surgery, 7 with rere-pair of the tendon and 1 with an EIP transfer. Range of motion results of these patients was good in 5 and fair in 3. The authors acknowledge that their group is the only group reporting results of active mobilization of extensor tendons to experience ruptures.

The 3 RCTs compared static to dynamic splint-ing. Two of the RCTs showed no difference in total active motion at final follow-up and recommended static splinting over dynamic splinting because of ease of use and cost.[30,31] Interestingly, the Mowl-avi study did show improved total active motion at 4, 6, and 8 weeks but no difference at 6 months. The Khandwala study showed no difference at 8 weeks, despite having significantly more patients in the study (n = 100 vs n = 34). Kitis and col-leagues reported significantly improved total active motion in the dynamic splinting group compared with static splinting group at 1, 3, and 6 months. They concluded dynamic splinting improved func-tional outcomes compared with static splinting.[32]

Considered together, the available evidence in-dicates that dynamic splinting may improve func-tional outcomes, particularly early in the postoperative period, and dynamic splinting does not seem to increase the chance of extensor lag or extensor tendon rupture in zones IV to VII.

MANAGING COMPLICATIONS
Loss of Motion

The tenets of managing complications following extensor tendon repair follow the principles of

managing the stiff finger from any cause, which has been meticulously described previously.[35]

Loss of motion following extensor tendon repair due to stiffness and scarring should be initially, and often definitively, treated nonoperatively. All available tools should be unutilized to optimize motion, including formal hand therapy, static and dynamic splinting, and at least 6 months have passed since the tendon repair.

A small subset of extensor tendon repairs ulti-mately undergoes an extensor tenolysis due to persistent and functionally limiting stiffness. Although no consensus exists regarding the indica-tions for this procedure, Schneider identified 6 criteria to identify ideal candidates for extensor tenolysis: (1) failed nonsurgical management

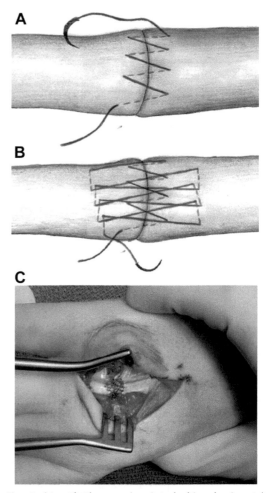

Fig. 8. (*A* , *B*) The running interlocking horizontal mattress suture technique. (*C*) Repair of an extensor tendon using this technique. (Spencer Skinner, Jona-than Isaacs, Extensor Tendon Injuries in the Athlete, Clinics in Sports Medicine, 39 (2), 2020, 259-277. https://doi.org/10.1016/j.csm.2019.12.005.)

greater than 6 months, (2) anatomic fracture alignment, (3) full passive range of motion, (4) pliable, well-healed skin, (5) uninvolved joint surfaces, and (6) cooperative patient with access to therapy.[36]

In practice patients rarely, if ever, satisfy all 6 criteria. Extensor tendon repairs that develop adhesions and subsequent contractures often lose both active and passive flexion. Joint contracture may be the result of direct trauma to the joint, prolonged postoperative immobilization, or extensor tendon adhesions. Surgical treatment should proceed in a stepwise manner, starting with an extensor tenolysis. If passive flexion is not restored, then capsulotomy and possibly incremental collateral ligament release may be necessary (**Fig. 9**).[37]

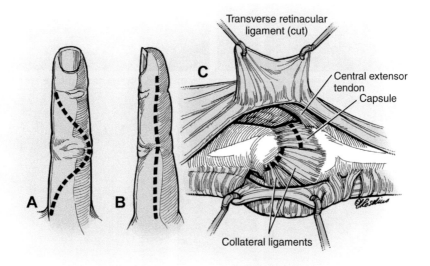

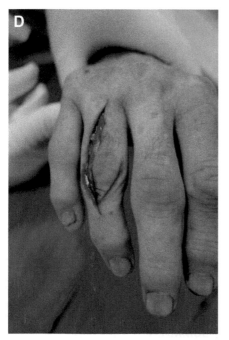
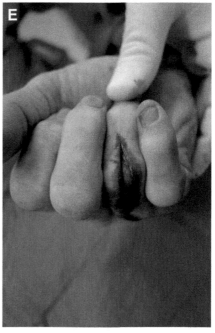

Fig. 9. (*A–C*) Extension contracture release of the PIP joint can be performed through a dorsal curvilinear or midlateral approach. Once the skin is elevated and mobilized, the transverse retinacular ligament is divided to expose the joint. Extensor tenolysis is performed, and a dorsal capsulotomy is made. The collateral ligaments are then released at their origin on the proximal phalanx. (*D*) A 58-year-old man with ring finger PIP extension contracture. (*E*) Passive flexion following extensor tenolysis and PIP dorsal capsulotomy. (*A–C*, Copyright © Elizabeth Martin.)

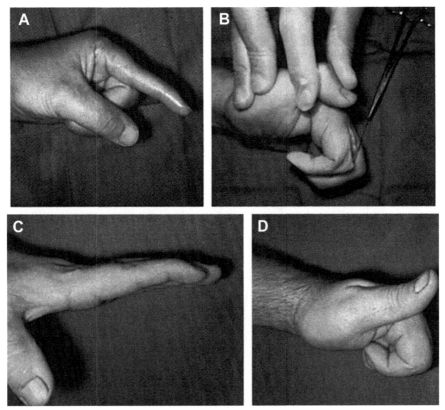

Fig. 10. A 42-year-old man severed his extensor mechanism over the PIP joint of his left index finger. Extension contracture persisted despite an active exercise program. (*A*) Fixed extension posture of the finger preoperatively (*B*) On an operating table, after tenolysis of tendon adhesions and release of dorsal capsule of the PIP joint. (*C, D*) Range of motion was restored with therapy at 3 months following tenolysis. (*From* Culp R, Feldscher S, Rodriguez S. Flexor and Extensor Tenolysis: Surgeon's and Therapist's Management. In: Rehabilitation of the Hand and Upper Extremity, Sixth Edition, 2011, Elsevier.)

Before proceeding with an extensor tenolysis, it is imperative the surgeon, the patient, and the therapist have realistic expectations. Patients rarely, if ever, achieve full flexion, and often sacrifice some extension to improve flexion (**Fig. 10**).[38] One can expect some improvement in motion at final follow-up but improvement ranges from 20° to 50°, and occasionally, there is little or no improvement in motion.[35,37]

Rerupture and Extensor Lag

An extensor lag may be the result of a completely ruptured repair or gapping of the repair. Gapping may be accompanied by, and in fact result from extensor tendon adhesions. Therefore, it can be difficult to determine preoperatively whether the extensor tendon repair has ruptured, is attenuated, or is completely adherent. Any active function of the tendon rules out rupture. In this instance, the treatment would be what is described above for the stiff finger. If there has been a sudden loss of function,

the diagnosis of rerupture is straightforward. Although this is a rare occurrence, most would favor reexploration and rerepair of the ruptured tendon. If sufficient tendon is not available, then tendon transfer or grafting may be necessary.

Tendon Imbalance (Boutonniere or Swan Neck)

Extensor tendon injury and repair can lead to an imbalance of extrinsic and intrinsic tendons in the digit, leading to either a swan neck or a boutonniere deformity. Management of these deformities when they occur following extensor tendon repair is the same as that of managing these chronic deformities from any cause.[39]

SUMMARY

Avoiding complications following extensor tendon repair requires balancing protection of the repair with facilitation of early range of motion to prevent loss of motion. If the repair is not sufficiently protected, attenuation or rupture of the repair may result, which is rarely reported in the literature. Even with early controlled active motion, one can expect some repairs will lose flexion, extension, or both. This loss of range of motion, though, rarely leads to tenolysis or revision surgery.

CLINICS CARE POINTS

- Utilize cores sutures when possible to optimize repair strength and facilitate early range of motion.
- When repair strength allows, early range of motion may limit the most common complication of stiffness following extensor tendon repair.
- Static splinting, when necessary, may also lead to satisfactory outcomes following extensor tendon repair.

DISCLOSURE

The authors have no conflicts of interest to report.

REFERENCES

1. Leversedge F, Goldfarb C, Boyer M. Primus manus. 1 edition. Philadelphia, PA: Wolters Kluwer Health/Lippincott Williams & Wilkins; 2010. p. 36–42.
2. Newport ML, Blair WF, Steyers CM Jr. Long-term results of extensor tendon repair. J Hand Surg Am 1990;15(6):961–6.
3. Carl HD, Forst R, Schaller P. Results of primary extensor tendon repair in relation to the zone of injury and pre-operative outcome estimation. Arch Orthop Trauma Surg 2007;127(2):115–9.
4. Hung LK, Chan A, Chang J, et al. Early controlled active mobilization with dynamic splintage for treatment of extensor tendon injuries. J Hand Surg Am 1990;15(2):251–7.
5. Purcell T, Eadie PA, Murugan S, et al. Static splinting of extensor tendon repairs. J Hand Surg Br 2000; 25(2):180–2.
6. Lin JS, Samora JB. Surgical and nonsurgical management of mallet finger: A systematic review. J Hand Surg Am 2018;43(2):146–63.e2.
7. O'Brien LJ, Bailey MJ. Single blind, prospective, randomized controlled trial comparing dorsal aluminum and custom thermoplastic splints to stack splint for acute mallet finger. Arch Phys Med Rehabil 2011;92(2):191–8.
8. Pike J, Mulpuri K, Metzger M, et al. Blinded, prospective, randomized clinical trial comparing volar, dorsal, and custom thermoplastic splinting in

treatment of acute mallet finger. J Hand Surg Am 2010;35(4):580–8.
9. Maitra A, Dorani B. The conservative treatment of mallet finger with a simple splint: A case report. Arch Emerg Med 1993;10(3):244–8.
10. Netscher DT, Henn CM. Textbook of hand & upper extremity surgery, second edition. Chapter 27: extensor injuries: acute and chronic. Chicago, IL: American Society for Surgery of the Hand; 2019. p. 611–39.
11. Lee YH, Kim JY, Chung MS, et al. Two extension block kirschner wire technique for mallet finger fractures. J Bone Joint Surg Br 2009;91(11):1478–81.
12. Tetik C, Gudemez E. Modification of the extension block kirschner wire technique for mallet fractures. Clin Orthop Relat Res 2002;404:284–90.
13. Wehbé MA, Schneider LH. Mallet fractures. J Bone Joint Surg Am 1984;66(5):658–69.
14. Stern PJ, Kastrup JJ. Complications and prognosis of treatment of mallet finger. J Hand Surg Am 1988;13(3):329–34.
15. Saldana MJ, Choban S, Westerbeck P, et al. Results of acute zone III extensor tendon injuries treated with dynamic extension splinting. J Hand Surg Am 1991;16(6):1145–50.
16. Walsh MT, Rinehimer W, Muntzer E, et al. Early controlled motion with dynamic splinting versus static splinting for zones III and IV extensor tendon lacerations: A preliminary report. J Hand Ther 1994;7(4):232–6.
17. Evans RB, Thompson DE. An analysis of factors that support early active short arc motion of the repaired central slip. J Hand Ther 1992;5(4):187–201.
18. Lovett WL, McCalla MA. Management and rehabilitation of extensor tendon injuries. Orthop Clin North Am 1983;14(4):811–26.
19. Maddy LS, Meyerdierks EM. Dynamic extension assist splinting of acute central slip lacerations. J Hand Ther 1997;10(3):206–12.
20. Pratt AL, Burr N, Grobbelaar AO. A prospective review of open central slip laceration repair and rehabilitation. J Hand Surg Br 2002;27(6):530–4.
21. O'Dwyer FG, Quinton DN. Early mobilisation of acute middle slip injuries. J Hand Surg Br 1990;15(4):404–6.
22. Zhang X, Yang L, Shao X, et al. Treatment of bony boutonniere deformity with a loop wire. J Hand Surg Am 2011;36(6):1080–5.
23. Evans RB. Early active short arc motion for the repaired central slip. J Hand Surg Am 1994;19(6):991–7.
24. Rayan GM, Murray D. Classification and treatment of closed sagittal band injuries. J Hand Surg Am 1994;19(4):590–4.
25. Peelman J, Markiewitz A, Kiefhaber T, et al. Splintage in the treatment of sagittal band incompetence and extensor tendon subluxation. J Hand Surg Eur 2015;40(3):287–90.

26. Catalano LW 3rd, Gupta S, Ragland R 3rd, et al. Closed treatment of nonrheumatoid extensor tendon dislocations at the metacarpophalangeal joint. J Hand Surg Am 2006;31(2):242–5.

27. Kettelkamp DB, Flatt AE, Moulds R. Traumatic dislocation of the long-finger extensor tendon. A clinical, anatomical, and biomechanical study. J Bone Joint Surg Am 1971;53(2):229–40.

28. Altobelli GG, Conneely S, Haufler C, et al. Outcomes of digital zone IV and V and thumb zone TI to TIV extensor tendon repairs using a running interlocking horizontal mattress technique. J Hand Surg Am 2013;38(6):1079–83.

29. Neuhaus V, Wong G, Russo KE, et al. Dynamic splinting with early motion following zone IV/V and TI to TIII extensor tendon repairs. J Hand Surg Am 2012;37(5):933–7.

30. Mowlavi A, Burns M, Brown RE. Dynamic versus static splinting of simple zone V and zone VI extensor tendon repairs: A prospective, randomized, controlled study. Plast Reconstr Surg 2005;115(2):482–7.

31. Khandwala AR, Webb J, Harris SB, et al. A comparison of dynamic extension splinting and controlled active mobilization of complete divisions of extensor tendons in zones 5 and 6. J Hand Surg Br 2000;25(2):140–6.

32. Kitis A, Ozcan RH, Bagdatli D, et al. Comparison of static and dynamic splinting regimens for extensor tendon repairs in zones V to VII. J Plast Surg Hand Surg 2012;46(3–4):267–71.

33. Howell JW, Merritt WH, Robinson SJ. Immediate controlled active motion following zone 4-7 extensor tendon repair. J Hand Ther 2005;18(2):182–90.

34. Svens B, Ames E, Burford K, et al. Relative active motion programs following extensor tendon repair: A pilot study using a prospective cohort and evaluating outcomes following orthotic interventions. J Hand Ther 2015;28(1):11–8 [quiz: 19].

35. Yang G, McGlinn EP, Chung KC. Management of the stiff finger: Evidence and outcomes. Clin Plast Surg 2014;41(3):501–12.

36. Schneider LH. Tenolysis and capsulectomy after hand fractures. Clin Orthop Relat Res 1996;327:72–8.

37. Guelmi K, Sokolow C, Mitz V, et al. Dorsal tenolysis and arthrolysis of the proximal interphalangeal joint. 19 cases. Ann Chir Main Memb Super 1992;11(4):307–12 [discussion: 312-3].

38. Inoue G. Lateral band release for post-traumatic extension contracture of the proximal interphalangeal joint. Arch Orthop Trauma Surg 1991;110(6):298–300.

39. Elzinga K, Chung KC. Managing swan neck and boutonniere deformities. Clin Plast Surg 2019;46(3):329–37.

Tendon Transfers
Techniques to Minimize Complications

Kanu Goyal, MD[a],*, Kyle J. Chepla, MD[b]

KEYWORDS

- Tendon • Transfer • Complications • Revision • Management

KEY POINTS

- Tendon transfers are a commonly performed surgical technique to restore upper extremity function after nerve injury or traumatic loss of muscle-tendon units.
- Complications after tendon transfer commonly arise from inadequate patient education, poor timing of surgery, inappropriate donor muscle selection, incorrect tensioning, inadequate strength of the repair, and prolonged postoperative immobilization.
- Complications after tendon transfer can be minimized through thoughtful preoperative surgical planning and patient education, appropriate execution of the transfer with proper tensioning, and advanced postoperative rehabilitation protocols.

 Video content accompanies this article at http://www.hand.theclinics.com.

INTRODUCTION

Refined indications, improved donor nerve selection and increasing reports of good outcomes have increased the popularity of nerve transfers to restore upper extremity function. However, tendon transfers still remain the "gold standard" to restore upper extremity function after peripheral nerve injury and central neurologic deficits including stroke, cerebral palsy, and spinal cord injury. Tendon transfers are also the most used reconstructive option for traumatic or oncologic loss of muscle tendon units and attritional ruptures as a result of rheumatoid arthritis or after distal radius fracture. Tendon transfers can be used to replace a single motion for grasp, pinch, release, and eliminate deforming force that can result in imbalance or restore balance for improved functional use.[1] They have been used for decades, and as a result, outcomes have been widely studied and are both predictable and reproducible if several key surgical tenets are observed. These include (1) supple joints with full passive range of motion; (2) soft-tissue equilibrium; (3) choosing an expendable synergistic donor of adequate strength and excursion; (4) creating a straight line of pull between the donor and recipient; and (5) assigning a single function per transfer.

Each of these criteria needs to be assessed preoperatively and if necessary, corrected as part of the preoperative planning process. Patients with joint contracture are commonly referred to occupational therapy for an exercise program and orthotic fabrication. Surgical release can be considered in the setting of more severe contractures and usually precedes tendon transfers in a staged fashion. To allow for appropriate tendon gliding, soft-tissue equilibrium can be restored with therapy and tends to improve with time through scar maturation; however, regional or flap reconstruction may be required. Alternatively, tendon transfers that avoid an unhealthy wound bed can be considered. In some cases, inadequate donor excursion may be present, but can

[a] Division of Hand Surgery, Department of Orthopaedic Surgery, The Ohio State University Wexner Medical Center, 915 Olentangy River Road, Suite 3200, Columbus, OH 43212, USA; [b] Division of Plastic Surgery – MetroHealth Hospital, 2500 MetroHealth Drive, Columbus, OH 44109, USA
* Corresponding author.
E-mail address: kanu.goyal@osumc.edu

Hand Clin 39 (2023) 447–453
https://doi.org/10.1016/j.hcl.2023.03.005

be increased by releasing part of the muscle origin (eg, flexor carpi ulnaris or brachioradialis [BR]). If, however, a mismatch in excursion still exists it can be compensated for using a tenodesis effect. As an example, in the common scenario of a wrist flexor (33 mm excursion) being used to restore finger extension (50 mm excursion), full digital extension can be achieved as the wrist flexes and passively tensions the donor tendon.

In addition to these "classic" concepts, recent advances have created further opportunities to increase the predictability of outcomes after tendon transfer. A review of all possible tendon transfers is beyond the scope of this article, and instead the authors have chosen to focus on how an expanded standardized approach starting with preoperative evaluation, patient education, surgical planning, intraoperative techniques, and postoperative therapy can build on these historic principles and improve outcomes. These additional concepts and approaches can help treating surgeons further minimize potentially preventable complications that are common after tendon transfer and minimize the need for revision surgery.

PREOPERATIVE MANAGEMENT

Similar to many of the principles of tendon transfer reviewed in the introduction, improving outcomes after tendon transfers starts before surgery. Many patients who may benefit from tendon transfers have several upper extremity pathologies. However, the surgeon should discuss with the patient their current function and uses of the extremity, motivation for surgery, and their specific functional goals. Through this, the surgeon will be better able to not only restore the desired function but also avoid diminishing the patient's current function. As an example, a patient who relies on active forearm pronation for wheelchair propulsion may not do well with transfer of their pronator teres. There should also be a focus on patient education. This includes discussions not only of risks and expected outcomes but also postoperative restrictions, splint requirements, and therapy. Finally, the surgeon should be careful to identify patients who are not psychologically ready for surgery or who lack a support network for appropriate postoperative care.

Early, preoperative referral to occupational therapy is a helpful adjunct in this process as meeting with the therapist creates another opportunity for further discussion of postoperative restrictions and requirements. Postoperative splints can also be fabricated at this time, or if concomitant arthrodesis is planned, splints to model expected limitations can be created for the patient to trial. Treating therapists are instructed to relay any concerns that may arise during this evaluation, and patients who are thought to be unwilling or unable to comply with postoperative requirements are observed until psychologically ready. During this observation period, serial visits with the surgeon and/or therapist may still be necessary to identify and prevent deteriorating neurologic or functional losses. Additional indicated treatments, such as chemodenervation (onabotulinumtoxinA) to prevent or correct muscle contracture formation, are also common during this time.

Timing of surgery is another important preoperative variable to consider and the decision to proceed with surgery often depends on the etiology of the injury. Indications for early tendon transfer include situations where recovery is not expected to occur naturally such as in the loss of an entire muscle unit or where recovery may be significantly delayed such as with a high nerve transection. In the latter scenario, early tendon transfers may limit the need for orthoses and allow for restoration of function early in the post-injury period while awaiting nerve recovery. It may also help stimulate reeducation and improve coordination of the residual muscle tendon units. Studies have demonstrated that the combined results of early tendon transfer and nerve repair are superior to either procedure alone.[2] The muscle chosen to act as an internal splint should be synergistic which allows for spinal reflex arcs and other autonomic feedback to further enhance reeducation.

For those patients who sustain neuropraxic type injury, where the nerve remains in continuity, 85% will recover in 1 to 4 months with a fracture/dislocation mechanism, and 70% will recover in 3 to 9 months after a gunshot mechanism.[3] Thus, for nerves that are known to be in continuity, the authors typically recommend a period of observation with serial clinical evaluation every 3 months and electrodiagnostic studies to support physical examination findings as needed. If, on examination or electrodiagnostic testing, there is concern that nerve recovery has stalled at a known compression point, such as at the leading edge of the supinator or carpal tunnel for radial and median nerve injury, respectively, the authors recommend exploration with decompression/neurolysis and intraoperative nerve stimulation. Because of the high rate of spontaneous recovery, the authors do not routinely recommend "baby-sitter" tendon transfer for these patients and rather choose to prevent deformity through splinting, home exercises, and therapy.

When it is decided between the provider and patient to proceed with tendon transfer surgery, careful planning needs to take place. Creating a table of potential donor muscles and recipient tendons/desired function can aid in this process. Although any functioning muscle can serve as a potential donor, the "ideal" donor should have similar power (cross-sectional area) and excursion to the recipient, acts across a single joint with a straight line of pull, and is expendable. The strength of all potential donor muscles should be evaluated and graded using the British Medical Research Council grading system (**Box 1**). Donors that sustained complete or partial denervation, even those that have recovered, should be used with caution as changes in muscle fiber length and fibrosis can impact excursion and power.

Another factor to consider when selecting a donor includes the anticipated path of the transfer. Care should be taken to avoid placing transfers directly over bone, and when fascial planes or the interosseous membrane need to be crossed a large opening should be created to minimize scarring and subsequent loss of excursion. Minimizing the angle of approach between the donor and recipient tendons is also critical and can be accomplished by dividing the recipient tendons to better align them with the donor. Studies have demonstrated that a 40° change of direction will result in a clinically significant loss of force, as only a component of the donor force vector will be transferred to the recipient. As an example, in a radial nerve injury, it is common to transfer flexor carpi radialis (FCR) to extensor digitorum communis (EDC) for restoration of finger extension. The division of the recipient EDC tendons at the musculotendinous junction before transfer allows for a more direct line of repair to the FCR tendon, especially for the most ulnar EDC to the small finger, thereby optimizing the force transfer and simplifying the tensioning process. Force is also

potentially lost when a pulley needs to be created to reroute the donor to the recipient (as it can lead to friction) and should only be used if no better donors exist.

INTRAOPERATIVE MANAGEMENT

Sterling Bunnell famously referred to tendon transfers as "muscle balance operations." Four main biomechanical force concepts are at play in patients undergoing tendon transfers: muscle-tendon unit excursion, muscle-tendon unit force-generation, moment arm, and tendon transfer tension. The most critical of these is the determination of the correct tension for the transfer. The appropriate tension after tendon transfer depends on mean fiber length, cross-sectional area, and total muscle volume[4,5] and has been studied using cadaveric dissections[6] and intraoperatively during tendon transfer.[7]

To achieve optimal force generation which is a combination of active and passive force as seen with Blix's curve (**Fig. 1**), the donor muscle should be set as closely as possible to its native resting state where maximal overlap of the actin–myosin occurs. This muscle length should be set at the mid-range of desired joint motion so that on muscle activation and shortening the joint will move in one direction but will still be able to move in the opposite direction with passive muscle stretch. Historically, setting appropriate muscle length was done through a combination of techniques including tenodesis, accepted positioning of the joints, and movement achieved through direct traction on the donor. Some surgeons will place sutures in the muscle belly at prescribed lengths before harvest so that on inset, it is set at the same muscle length. However, despite all these techniques, incorrect tensioning can still occur and is one of the most common reasons for revision surgery after tendon transfer. Transfers that are too "loose" may fail to generate adequate excursion or force for the transfer to be useful. Setting them too "tight" may restrict motion at adjacent joints and impair function.

Although advances such as laser diffraction allowed for intraoperative measurement of sarcomere length change these were cumbersome and never gained popularity.[8] However, recent advances have improved our ability to assess tension intraoperatively and have been shown to improve early outcomes and reduce the need for revision surgery. Surgery using wide-awake local anesthesia with or without tourniquet control (WALA and WALANT, respectively) rather than general anesthesia was first popularized for office-based procedures such as mass excision, trigger finger,

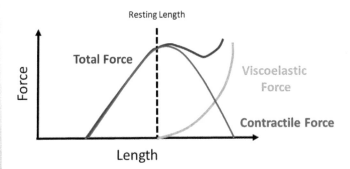

Fig. 1. Blix Curve: the total force generated by a muscle depends on the muscle fiber length and is the sum of the passive (viscoelastic) and the active (contractile) forces.

and carpal tunnel release. Comparative studies of patients undergoing surgery under local only to those receiving general anesthesia have demonstrated equivalent outcomes, low complication rates, and high patient satisfaction.[9,10] As a result, surgery under local anesthesia is now being offered for an increasing number of procedures including thumb basal joint arthroplasty, fixation of phalangeal and distal radius fractures and even for tendon transfers.

The advantages of an awake patient who has retained motor control of the donor muscle/tendon are enormous as it enables immediate and accurate feedback on the set tension and repair strength. Although not all patients are candidates for tendon transfer under local anesthesia only, it is very useful for simple and single transfers that do not require extensive soft tissue dissection. A good example is the extensor indicis proprius (EIP) to extensor pollicis longus (EPL) transfer for attritional EPL rupture after closed management of a distal radius fracture. Intraoperative activation of the transfer by the patient allows for direct confirmation that tension is appropriate, and the repair has sufficient strength to withstand an early active motion protocol (Video 1). A recent study compared outcomes after EIP to EPL tendon transfer using either a wide-awake approach or conventional transfer under general anesthesia.[11] Although no differences were seen between grip and pinch strength, those done using a wide-awake approach had significantly better interphalangeal joint flexion and total arc of motion at 6 weeks and 2, 4, and 6 months postoperatively. Significantly better metacarpophalangeal joint flexion and total arc of motion was improved at all-time points (up to 1 year postoperatively). Transfers that require more extensive muscle mobilization and dissection may require more local anesthesia and therefore lead to partial motor block—this would mitigate the benefits of the patient remaining awake for surgery as they would

not be able to completely activate the donor muscle. So though wide-awake tendon transfers are in many ways the best way of assessing proper tension, it is not possible in every circumstance.

Another method to assess intraoperative tension is by stimulating the donor muscle intraoperatively and creating a tetanic contraction using a commercially available hand-held nerve stimulator (Checkpoint Surgical, Cleveland, OH). Intraoperative stimulation of tendon transfers was evaluated by Omer and Vogel,[1] which allows for direct assessment of transfer tension when patients are under general anesthesia. Although outcomes after tendon transfer using intraoperative stimulation have not been assessed for upper extremity tendon transfer, improvements have been seen in patients undergoing facial reanimation using a one-stage temporalis myoplasty.[12] Intraoperative stimulation resulted in intraoperative changes to the position of the insertion point of the muscle transfer into the nasolabial fold, upper lip, and oral commissure in 55% of patients undergoing primary surgery and all patients undergoing revision surgery.

This technique can be used in any patient undergoing tendon transfer. However certain variables must be considered: (1) No paralysis can be used during surgery; (2) Prolonged tourniquet use, and the resulting muscle ischemia, may affect stimulation; (3) Stimulation may not be possible or difficult depending on the size/location of the muscle; and (4) The patient may not be able to volitionally reproduce the muscle activation as seen intraoperatively with direct stimulation.

When using this technique, an estimate of the appropriate tension is first made using tenodesis and joint positioning before the transfer is temporized with a surgical clamp or one to two sutures. The muscle is then stimulated directly using 20 mA and by gradually increasing the pulse width up to 150 ms. Stimulation of the muscle is best done at the junction of the proximal and middle one-thirds which corresponds to the entry point of the motor nerve. If this area was not exposed as part of the surgical dissection a separate incision can be made proximally and a small fascial window can be created. More complete stimulation of the muscle can be achieved if both the grounding lead and stimulating lead are placed into the donor muscle. Intraoperative stimulation, similar to active motion during WALANT, allows for the surgeon to visualize expected range of motion generated and can be used to confirm that the transfer repair has sufficient strength to withstand an early motion protocol (Video 2). Intraoperative stimulation is also very useful for transfers that are not performed as commonly and for which no accepted positioning of the joints or tenodesis movements are described to ensure appropriate tension (Video 3). Finally, intraoperative stimulation may also help the surgeon to identify muscles that may lack sufficient strength or excursion to serve as an adequate donor and supplements visual inspection where it is sometimes difficult to discern denervated, pale, fibrotic muscle with disuse atrophy.

Even appropriately tensioned transfers can fail if they are not secured properly or if they become scarred. Several methods of tendon transfer repair have been described, though the most commonly performed are the Pulvertaft (3 or 4 weave) and side-to-side. The investigators prefer the side-to-side repair, as it has been demonstrated to be stronger and appears to have a less bulky appearance enabling smoother glide.[13] Regardless of the repair technique chosen, care should be taken to avoid creating a stress riser within the tendon repair site, such as by using too many stitches or by using necrosing stitches, as this can lead to rupture. The suture used should always be braided and nonabsorbable; however, the caliber will depend on the tendon's size. A stronger repair will enable earlier range of motion, which will help decrease postoperative adhesions and improved tendon excursion. In addition, as mentioned earlier, the transfer repair should be performed in an area that is less likely to lead to adhesions. This includes avoiding repairs over bone and through fascial planes. If the repair has to be passed through a fascial plane, a large window should be created. Finally, it is ideal if the skin repair is not directly over the tendon repair as this too can lead to unwanted early adhesions.

POSTOPERATIVE MANAGEMENT

Early postoperative mobilization is one of the key tenets to optimizing results. Early protected motion prevents scarring of the transfer to the surrounding wound bed and allows for earlier retraining of the tendon transfers (Video 4). A systematic review of early mobilization of tendon transfers found that an early mobilization protocol was associated with reduced total cost, total rehabilitation time, and that it was safe without increased rates of tendon rupture or pull out.[14] Range of motion, grip strength, pinch strength, total active digit motion, deformity correction, and integration of tendon transfers were significantly superior with early mobilization when compared with immobilization at 4 weeks. However, despite this very short-term difference, outcomes evaluated 2 to 12 month postoperatively were similar. Another multicenter study of pinch force strength after BR to flexor pollicis longus (FPL) tendon transfer in patients with tetraplegia demonstrated that early cast removal was associated with increased pinch force and that pinch force was associated with improved performance and patient satisfaction.[15]

COMPLICATION MANAGEMENT

Despite the best efforts by the surgeon and patient, complications can still occur after tendon transfer. Nonspecific complications such as postoperative bleeding, wound healing complications, and infection are rare but should be discussed preoperatively. More specific to tendon transfer surgeries and more commonly, the surgeon may be faced with rupture of the transfer, inappropriate tensioning of the transfer, or loss of motion secondary to scarring. Some postoperative complications are easier to diagnose such as rupture of the transfer. In these cases, patients will likely notice a sudden loss of active motion and on physical examination tenodesis will no longer be present. In these cases, early re-repair with or without interpositional graft is an option; however, if the donor muscle/tendon unit no longer has appropriate excursion (due to retraction/scarring) then consideration for another donor or tenodesis alone should be given.

Inadequate tensioning of tendon transfers can be more difficult to diagnose early. The inability to activate the expected range of motion after tendon transfer may be related to poor cognitive control, tendon adhesions, or inadequate tensioning. In these cases, time and therapy are usually recommended first so that the patient has the opportunity to learn the transfer more and so that tendon adhesions can be minimized before committing the patient to a second operation to address any issues related to tensioning. If reoperation for inadequate tensioning is performed, the soft tissue dissection needed during the index operation usually is not necessary. Therefore, these operations are much more amenable to wide awake and local anesthesia only surgery enabling enhanced and accurate feedback on appropriate tensioning.

SUMMARY

Tendon transfers are a well-established surgical option to restore functional loss. Historically, outcomes have been very good, and if done correctly, reproducible. We have described our expanded pre, intra and postoperative approach to further minimize the common complications of stiffness, incorrect tensioning, and rupture of the transfer through an expanded focus on patient evaluation, donor selection, augmented assessment of transfer tension and strength, and an early mobilization protocol.

CLINICS CARE POINTS

Outcomes after tendon transfer can be improved:

- With thoughtful history and examination of each patient and tailoring surgery to their particular desired function
- If performed when timing is right, the patient is psychologically ready, and the soft tissues and joints are supple
- With careful surgical planning including identification of donor muscles/tendons that suit the desired function
- With the patient wide awake as this enables immediate and accurate feedback on appropriate tensioning and strength of repair
- With intraoperative muscle stimulation to assess appropriate tensioning and strength of repair
- With careful attention to the tendon transfer route, repair technique, and location of the repair relative to other tissues to help avoid scarring
- With an early postoperative mobilization protocol

DISCLOSURE

No funding was provided for this work. K.J. Chepla is a consultant for Checkpoint Surgical and Polynovo. K. Goyal has received research funding from Skeletal Dynamics and Acumed.

SUPPLEMENTARY DATA

Supplementary data related to this article can be found online at https://doi.org/10.1016/j.hcl.2023.03.005.

REFERENCES

1. Omer GE Jr, Vogel JA. Determination of physiological length of a reconstructed muscle-tendon unit through muscle stimulation. J Bone Joint Surg Am 1965;47:304–12.
2. Burkhalter WE. Median nerve palsy. In: Green DP, editor. Operative hand surgery. 3rd edition. New York: Churchill-Livingstone; 1993. p. 1419–48.
3. Omer GE Jr. Injuries to nerves of the upper extremity. J Bone Joint Surg Am 1974;56(8):1615–24.
4. Brand PW. The motor: muscles. In: Brand PW, editor. Clinical mechanics of the hand. St. Louis: CV Mosby; 1985. p. 11–29.
5. Brand PW. Biomechanics of tendon transfers. Hand Clin 1988;4(2):137–54.
6. Brand PW, Beach RB, Thompson DE. Relative tension and potential excursion of muscles in the forearm and hand. J Hand Surg Am 1981;6(3):209–19.
7. Freehafer AA, Peckham PH, Keith MW. Determination of muscle-tendon unit properties during tendon transfer. J Hand Surg Am 1979;4(4):331–9.
8. Fleeter TB, Adams JP, Brenner B, Podolsky RJ. A laser diffraction method for measuring muscle sarcomere length in vivo for application to tendon transfers. J Hand Surg Am 1985;10(4):542–6.
9. Moscato L, Helmi A, Kouyoumdjian P, Lalonde D, Mares O. The impact of WALANT anesthesia and office-based settings on patient satisfaction after carpal tunnel release: a patient reported outcome study. Orthop Traumatol Surg Res 2021;103134. https://doi.org/10.1016/j.otsr.2021.103134.
10. Pina M, Cusano A, LeVasseur MR, Olivieri-Ortiz R, Ferreira J, Parrino A. Wide Awake Local Anesthesia No Tourniquet Technique in Hand Surgery: The Patient Experience. Hand (N Y) 2021. https://doi.org/10.1177/15589447211058838. 15589447211058838.
11. Hong J, Kang HJ, Whang JI, et al. Comparison of the Wide-Awake Approach and Conventional Approach in Extensor Indicis Proprius-to-Extensor Pollicis Longus Tendon Transfer for Chronic Extensor Pollicis Longus Rupture. Plast Reconstr Surg 2020;145(3):723–33.
12. Har-Shai Y, Gil T, Metanes I, Labbé D. Intraoperative muscle electrical stimulation for accurate positioning of the temporalis muscle tendon during dynamic, one-stage lengthening temporalis myoplasty for

facial and lip reanimation. Plast Reconstr Surg 2010; 126(1):118–25.

13. Brown SH, Hentzen ER, Kwan A, et al. Mechanical strength of the side-to-side versus Pulvertaft weave tendon repair. J Hand Surg Am 2010; 35(4):540–5.

14. Sultana SS, MacDermid JC, Grewal R, Rath S. The effectiveness of early mobilization after tendon transfers in the hand: a systematic review. J Hand Ther 2013;26(1):1–21.

15. Johanson ME, Jaramillo JP, Dairaghi CA, Murray WM, Hentz VR. Multicenter Survey of the Effects of Rehabilitation Practices on Pinch Force Strength After Tendon Transfer to Restore Pinch in Tetraplegia. Arch Phys Med Rehabil 2016;97(6 Suppl):S105–16.

Advanced Dupuytren Contracture
Approach to Management

Jill Putnam, MD

KEYWORDS

• Dupuytren disease • Contracture • Recurrence • Complications

KEY POINTS

- Recurrence of Dupuytren contracture is more common in younger patients and associated with an increased risk of complications.
- The most common complications in surgical management of Dupuytren disease include recurrence, nerve injury, wound problems, and deformity related to extensor tendon imbalance.
- Associated proximal interphalangeal joint contractures may be managed with arthrolysis, extension splinting, distraction with external fixators, or arthrodesis.
- A variety of surgical techniques may help to relieve contractures and prevent recurrences.

INTRODUCTION

Dupuytren disease challenges hand surgeons with fascinating and often hazardous pathologic condition. The purpose of this article is to review techniques for the management of difficult Dupuytren cases, especially cases that involve recurrence or significant contracture.

PATHOANATOMY

Dupuytren disease is an inherited condition that causes aberrant collagen processing and progressive tissue contracture.[1–3] The condition is autosomal dominant with variable penetrance.[2–4] Fibroblasts and myofibroblasts play key roles in the development of Dupuytren disease, and various genes have been found to contribute to the pathophysiology.[4] The thickened tissue either may cause nodular disease or may lead to contractures in the palm. Nodules have been shown to progress to cords in approximately 50% of patients, and this conversion is associated with fibroblast contracture and conversion to a relatively acellular collagen matrix over time.[1,5]

PRESENTATION AND EVALUATION

Men are more likely to be affected and prevalence may be as high as 22% in northern European populations such as the Netherlands.[6,7] Other factors associated with Dupuytren disease may include heavy smoking or drinking, and patients with type 1 or 2 diabetes.[8]

Patients may present with painless palmar nodules or pitting, or a developing flexion contracture.[1] The greatest risk factor for the progression of disease is younger age (typically <50 years).[5] "Dupuytren diathesis" has been used to describe patients who present with more serious disease and are more likely to exhibit recurrence; this diathesis is defined by age less than 50 years at onset, male sex, bilateral involvement, family history, Garrod pads, and Northern European descent.[9] Patients with Dupuytren diathesis may have a recurrence risk as high as 71% and should be counseled accordingly.[9] Logically, patients with a greater initial deformity have a higher risk of contracture recurrence, and a greater risk of complications, as do patients with more

The Hand and Upper Extremity Center, The Ohio State University, 915 Olentangy River Road, Suite 3200, Columbus, OH 43212, USA
E-mail address: Jill.Putnam.22@gmail.com

Hand Clin 39 (2023) 455–463
https://doi.org/10.1016/j.hcl.2023.03.006
0749-0712/23/© 2023 Elsevier Inc. All rights reserved.

involvement in the proximal interphalangeal joint (PIPJ) than in the metacarpophalangeal joint (MCPJ).[10]

The initial evaluation of a patient with Dupuytren disease should prompt discussion of family history and the presence of other nodules, such as plantar nodules, to determine risk of disease progression and recurrence.[11]

COMMON OPTIONS FOR MANAGEMENT

Observation is generally suggested for nodular disease, which is typically painless. If the nodules are sensitive or painful, a steroid injection may help to soften and flatten nodules.[12] A single study of 37 patients demonstrated 50% improvement in nodules 5 years after injection of triamcinolone acetonide.[13]

Contracture can also be managed conservatively, although therapy, braces, and stretching have not been shown to significantly change disease progression. Many patients are asked to consider the "table top" test and return when they have difficulty getting a flat palm on the table.[14]

Needle aponeurotomy (NA) is a relatively simple technique involving the use of a small needle to rupture a cord, without the removal of diseased tissue. The procedure can be readily done in the clinic setting with limited equipment. Elderly patients with prominent palmar cords are the ideal candidates for this procedure because rupture of these cords puts tendons and nerves at minimal risk (**Fig. 1**).[15] Relative contraindications for NA include flattened, nodular disease and severe PIPJ contracture.[16] Patients should be cautioned that skin tears are common (5%–38%), and typically heal well primarily with good local wound care.[16] The following steps are recommended.

- About 1 to 2 cc of lidocaine with or without epinephrine is injected very superficially about the planned regions for cord rupture.
- About 2 to 3 locations are typically selected, based on where the cord is most prominent. Locations approaching the PIPJ may put the digital nerves at higher risk.
- The skin is prepared with alcohol or other cleaning solution.
- An 18 to 22G needle is introduced subdermally, and dermal tissue is swept off of the prominent cord with the needle.
- A "sawing" motion is used to rupture the cord, with very gentle extension pressure on the contracted digit. Overly aggressive extension pressure could bring the neurovascular bundles and tendons closer to the procedure. Once the tense cord is palpated with the needle, deep to superficial "sawing" is often most effective.
- The procedure should be kept superficial, generally within 1 to 3 mm of the skin, to protect tendon, nerve, and artery.
- The needle is removed, and the digit is maximally extended, and the cord maximally ruptured. A bandage or light dressing is placed.
- Manual manipulation of the PIPJ may be performed for volar capsular contractures.
- The patient is taught local wound care and may benefit from the use of a nighttime splint.

Recurrence rates of 12% to 85% have been described at 5 years for NA, although the definition of recurrence is heterogenous.[17–19] Other complications including nerve and tendon injuries have been reported to occur less than 0.5% and less than 0.05%, respectively.[20] The author thinks that NA can be an excellent first step in the management of complex contractures. Primary NA, followed by fasciectomy in a staged fashion 2 to 10 weeks later, may allow for therapy and splinting of difficult interphalangeal joint contractures.

Collagenase injections are another less-invasive option for Dupuytren contracture. Although collagenase is best described for prominent palmar cords causing MCPJ contractures, they can be effective for the PIPJ as well with careful technique.[21,22] Complications include edema, localized rash, blistering, and skin tears.[21–23] Contraindications for collagenase injections include nodular disease and known sensitivity to collagenase. These injections involve a minimum of 2 visits: the first visit involves the injection of the collagenase enzyme in typically 2 to 3 locations along a cord and the second visit 1 to 4 days later involves manual rupture of the cord. Local wound care and soft dressings are applied as needed, and a nighttime splint is typically recommended to limit recurrence. Patients should be aware of the potential for significant cost of the injections.[18,22] Recurrence rates are reported at 33% to 83% at 2 to 5-year follow-up.[22,24,25]

Subtotal or limited palmar fasciectomy is the most common surgical procedure indicated for Dupuytren disease. This involves excision of the majority of a cord causing significant contracture. The approach is performed with either a Bruner style incision or a longitudinal incision followed by Z-plasty; neither has been shown to be superior in terms of recurrence or complications.[26] The cord is removed with careful attention to the neurovascular bundles.

The open-palm technique, or modification thereof, has also been described. This involves

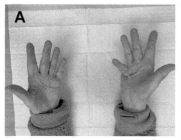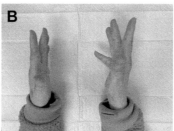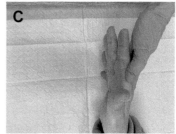

Fig. 1. This elderly female with an isolated MCPJ contracture is an ideal candidate for NA. (*A, B*) Pre-NA maximum digital extension. (*C*) Postprocedure extension.

making transverse incisions in the palm and fingers, releasing contractures, and allowing the wound to heal secondarily (**Fig. 2**). This can potentially decrease the risk for hematoma, contracture, or flap necrosis. There is the risk of delayed wound healing. This technique can also be used in cases where the goal is not to perform a complete palmar fasciectomy and minimal dissection is desired.[27]

MANAGEMENT OF RECURRENT DISEASE

Management of recurrent Dupuytren contracture is fraught with troublesome scar management, a higher risk of neurovascular injury, and diminishing returns for patient satisfaction. The surgeon should have a variety of tools in his or her armamentarium to increase the odds of success in these cases.

Recurrence can be due to a variety of factors. Early recurrence, especially of PIPJ contractures, may be due to an attenuated central slip or tight lateral bands; the latter is more likely to improve with therapy and splinting. Later recurrence can be due to a new or recurrent cord, hypertrophic scarring, or noncompliance with splinting or therapy. Recognition of the cause guides management.[28]

The use of a skin graft coupled with fasciectomy has long been used as an option to theoretically decrease the risk of primary or secondary recurrence, or to aid in wound closure for severe contracture. In 2009, a randomized study of fasciectomy with or without skin grafting did not demonstrate any significant difference in recurrence between groups.[29] Dermatofasciectomy describes the excision of skin involved in Dupuytren contracture along with the underlying cord. Theoretically, introducing skin that is uninvolved in the Dupuytren pathologic condition might reduce the risk of recurrence by inhibiting myofibroblast contraction.[30] If the need for a skin graft is identified, the following is recommended.

- Full-thickness skin grafts are typically obtained from the antecubital fossa, the ulnar forearm, or the hypothenar eminence.

- The donor site is prepared, measured according to the deficit needing coverage, and a full thickness skin graft is harvested. The donor site is closed primarily.
- The recipient site is prepared by ensuring that meticulous hemostasis has been achieved to prevent hematoma that would threaten the graft. Deflation of tourniquet before graft inset is recommended to ensure a dry recipient bed.
- The graft is sutured in place with minimal tension, and a bolster dressing is applied.

Management of recurrent disease after NA or collagenase injection is becoming more common. In a survey of surgeons managing these recurrent cases after nonsurgical management, most surgeons did not think that there was significant distortion of anatomy.[31] In the authors' experience with these cases, the surgeon will encounter not only a longitudinal cord but also longitudinal *segments* of a thickened cord, representing where segments of ruptured, unexcised pathologic tissue caused contracture recurrence. These cases are accordingly managed with fasciectomy and routine caution around the neurovascular bundles.

MANAGEMENT OF PROXIMAL INTERPHALANGEAL JOINT CONTRACTURES

Contracture of the PIPJ initially occurs because of the Dupuytren's cord and tends to recur because of contracture of the volar plate and collateral ligaments, and later attenuation of the central slip. The patient should be aware of the higher rate of recurrence when significant contracture of the PIPJ is involved.[10,28] Recurrence of PIPJ contractures has also been associated with therapy noncompliance postoperatively.[32]

Release of the volar plate and collateral ligaments will allow for immediate correction at the time of surgery but recurrence is high because of edema and subsequent scar tissue and, frequently, the inability of the attenuated central slip to maintain extension after correction. Further,

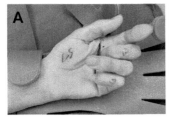 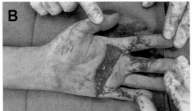 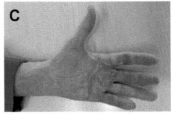

Fig. 2. Using the open-palm technique. (*A*) This elderly male has severe contracture of his left small, ring, and middle finger PIPJ and MPJ. (*B*) Intraoperative release of contractures with open wound in palm. (*C*) Healing of palm wound 6 weeks after surgery with local wound care, range of motion, and night splinting. (*Courtesy Sonu Jain, MD, Columbus, OH.*)

exposing and releasing the PIPJ involves dissection of the flexor sheath and pulley system; even with careful manipulation, this approach may cause adhesions. Splints may help to prevent recurrence after arthrolysis; however, maintenance of extension should not occur at the expense of flexion loss, which ultimately limits grip strength. Rarely, an excessive excision of the volar plate and/or collateral release may cause overcorrection in the form of a swan neck deformity, which is poorly tolerated by the patient.

Progressive extension of the PIPJ may help to maintain correction.[33,34] A variety of dynamic external fixators, or extension torque devices, can be fashioned by the surgeon, or are available from a variety of companies.[33,35] These fixators are typically used in a staged fashion but can also achieve some correction in a single stage if the patient is inclined to avoid further open surgery.[35]

- First, pins are placed intraoperatively into the middle phalanx, with or without open volar approach to the PIPJ for volar plate release (**Fig. 3**).[34]
- As an adjunct in the first stage, some surgeons prefer to perform NA at the time of external fixator application. This provides further immediate correction and allows for better MCPJ motion while awaiting the second stage.
- Postoperatively, increasingly thick rubber bands are used to progressively extend the digit during a 4-to-8-week time frame, or until satisfactory extension is achieved.
- In the second stage, the patient returns to the operating room for formal fasciectomy and implant removal.

Early results described for this technique are encouraging. One study of checkrein ligament release and distraction with an external fixator reported a mean 57° PIPJ contracture improvement in contractures greater than 60°, at a mean follow-up of 18 months.[34]

Similarly, NA before formal fasciectomy for severe PIPJ contractures may allow for more effective splinting and therapy before formal fasciectomy (**Fig. 4**). In the authors' experience, NA 4 to 8 weeks before formal fasciectomy for severe PIPJ contractures allows the patient to engage in therapy for formal PIPJ stretching and splinting. This acts similarly in a staged fashion to extension stretching with an external fixator. Once the patient's wounds are well healed and motion improved, fasciectomy is performed. The authors rarely find the need for a skin graft when this technique is used because it affords soft tissues time to stretch, and small wounds time to granulate.[35]

Uncommonly, arthrodesis is used as a salvage procedure to treat recalcitrant PIPJ contracture. Aggressive preparation of the joint to cancellous bone is always performed followed by fixation with pins, cerclage wires, screws, or a plate, depending on the bone quality and size. The small finger is more likely than other digits to exhibit recurrent contracture and to be indicated for arthrodesis.[28,36] Rarely, amputation may be considered for severe disease recurrence in a digit that is dystrophic and contracted.[37]

COMPLICATIONS: WOUNDS AND HEMATOMA

Wound healing complications are reported in up to 22% of fasciectomy cases and most commonly involve hematoma or skin necrosis from thin flaps or unsuccessful grafts.[38]

All patients undergoing NA, collagenase injections, or surgery should be aware that correction of a contracture requires increasing the surface area or stretching of volar skin. Patients with more severe primary disease or recurrence should be counseled regarding the possible need for skin grafts, should insufficient tissue be present at the time of wound closure. In general, small wounds (less than 3–4 mm) granulate well and do not require grafting. Dermatofasciectomy to prevent

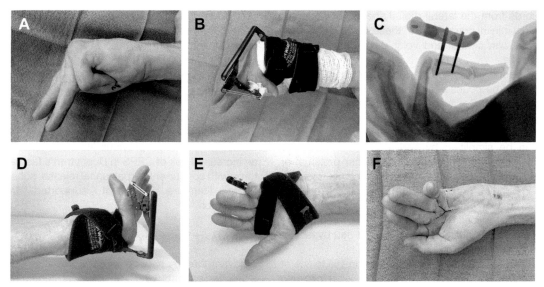

Fig. 3. Management of a severe PIPJ contracture using a dynamic external fixator. (*A*) Preoperative contracture. (*B*) Postoperative appearance of the digit after placement of the external fixator (Stage 1). (*C*) Intraoperative radiograph demonstrating appropriate pin placement in the middle phalanx. (*D, E*) Maximum PIPJ extension before Stage 2. (*F*) Digit that is now prepared for Stage 2. (*Courtesy* James Chang, MD, Stanford, CA.)

the recurrence in primary disease has not been shown to decrease the recurrence.[29]

Hematoma is reported to occur in 2% of fasciectomy cases.[38] This is typically managed with close observation and local wound care. Hematoma prevention is key. Tourniquet release should be routinely performed before wound closure; if desired, the tourniquet can be reinflated for wound closure after hemostasis is achieved.

Many patients undergoing surgery for Dupuytren contracture are anticoagulated. Although no break in anticoagulation is recommended for NA or collagenase injection, the authors recommend holding rivaroxaban or apixaban for 24 to 48 hours before fasciectomy, and 24 hours postoperatively, to decrease the risk of hematoma.[39] Warfarin is frequently bridged with heparin in the perioperative period.

COMPLICATIONS: NERVE AND ARTERY INJURY

Nerve injury has been reported in up to 20% of recurrent Dupuytren fasciectomy.[38] Temporary dysesthesia or neurapraxia has been noted in 4% to 18% of fasciectomy cases.[29,40] Nerve injury has been reported in 3% to 4% of fasciectomy cases.[29,38] Injuries to digital neurovascular bundles have been reported to be 10 times higher in revision fasciectomy cases compared with primary cases.[38] Displacement of the neurovascular bundle is more common in spiral cords, lateral

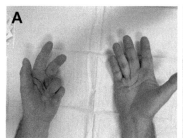
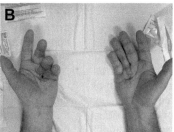
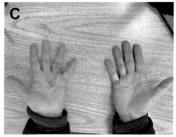

Fig. 4. This middle-aged man has a severe left small finger PIPJ contracture and mild Boutonniere deformity, with maximum digital flexion depicted. (*A*) The right hand has more minor disease. (*B*) Postaponeurotomy, with dramatically improved digital extension and improvement in the Boutonniere deformity. The patient engaged in therapy before formal left small finger fasciectomy. (*C*) Post-fasciectomy result, 4 months status post aponeurotomy, and 2 months status post fasciectomy.

cords from the lateral digital sheath, or abductor digiti minimi cords.[41] All of these cords are associated with central and volar displacement of the bundle.

Preoperatively, patients with recurrent disease should be counseled about the increased risk of numbness. Because of the thickened scar tissue and adherent diseased fascia, identification of the neurovascular bundles may be difficult. This can be simplified by finding "normal" anatomy that is free of prior dissection, either proximal or distal to the zone of recurrence. Once neurovascular bundles are clearly identified, these are followed longitudinally through the entire plane of the dissection. Recurrent disease should not be excised without first localizing the neurovascular bundles.

Arterial injury has been reported in 1% to 3% of fasciectomy cases.[29,38] Digital extension following contracture release may cause significant vasospasm. The digit typically recovers from this vasospasm. Injection of plain lidocaine or warm saline may help to resolve vasospasm. If vasospasm does not correct in the intraoperative or immediate postoperative period following tourniquet deflation, then the typical extension splint should be relaxed to allow some digital flexion.

BOUTONNIERE DEFORMITY IN DUPUYTREN DISEASE

Boutonniere deformity in Dupuytren disease can be related to attenuation of the central slip with increasing contracture, or from contracture of the transverse retinacular ligament.[42] Division of the transverse retinacular ligament may relieve the deformity, along with arthrolysis and postoperative splinting. In the authors' experience, surgical management of the PIPJ contracture often sufficiently resolves the Boutonniere deformity without the need for further surgery involving the DIPJ. Recalcitrant DIPJ hyperextension can be managed with terminal tenotomy distal to the triangular ligament.

SWAN NECK DEFORMITY IN DUPUYTREN DISEASE

Swan neck deformity in Dupuytren disease can be iatrogenic, via either overly aggressive excision of the volar plate or release of the collateral ligaments to correct a PIPJ flexion contracture. An oblique cord parallel to the oblique retinacular ligament has also been described to cause a swan neck deformity by tethering the central slip.[43] Although therapy or digital braces may be sufficient for some deformities, swan neck deformities associated with worsening Dupuytren contracture are

likely to be indicated for surgery. In these cases, arthrodesis may offer the most predictable means of preventing deformity.

COMPLICATIONS: COMPLEX REGIONAL PAIN SYNDROME

Complex regional pain syndrome (CRPS) has been reported in 0.3% to 5% of Dupuytren fasciectomy cases.[38,44] Although previous literature reported an increased risk of CRPS in Dupuytren's fasciectomy with concurrent carpal tunnel release, subsequent literature has not supported this association.[45,46]

ADJUVANT THERAPY

Adjuvant therapy may be an attractive alternative either for patients who are not ideal candidates for surgery or for younger patients with a higher recurrence risk. This increased risk is due both to increased disease "aggression" seen in younger patients and patients with Dupuytren diathesis, and due to a longer window of opportunity for recurrence.

Radiation may be an ideal adjunct treatment of young patients with aggressive disease but has been poorly studied to date.[47] The only prospective randomized trial, performed in 2001, involved 2 groups treated with different doses of radiation, without a control group.[48] The authors describe regression of cords, nodules, and skin changes at 3 and 12 months, with minimum follow-up of 1 year. The only long-term study, published in 2010, describes at that after 13 years of follow-up, 59% of patients were "stable," 10% improved, and 31% progressed, with 32% of patients experiencing late skin changes.[49] Radiation therapy of up to 30 Gy is generally well tolerated, with side effects including early skin erythema and late skin atrophy or desquamation.[48–50] Fibrosis or malignancies are potential long-term side effects of radiation that have not been described in therapy for Dupuytren disease.[47] Given the lack of a control group and minimal long-term follow-up, radiation therapy is considered "unproven" for Dupuytren disease at this time.

Radiation may also prove useful in the patient with recalcitrant disease who has undergone a desired "final" surgery and is not a good candidate for further surgery. In these settings, radiation may help to prevent recurrence.

Pharmacotherapy, such as anti-inflammatory, antimitotic, or hormonal therapy agents may prove to be a useful adjunct.[47] For example, the injection of a drug-blocking tumor necrosis factor (TNF), a regulator of myofibroblast activity in early

Dupuytren disease, may help to prevent progression of nodules to contractures.[51,52] To date, minimal evidence supports pharmacotherapy for Dupuytren disease.[47] Future randomized studies may shed light on whether anti-TNF injections, or other administration of other drugs, such as tamoxifen, will help to prevent the disease progression.[52,53]

SUMMARY

Management of recurrent Dupuytren disease can be both challenging and rewarding. Recognizing possible pitfalls to complex contractures will help the surgeon to be prepared for possible adjunct treatment. Skin grafting and careful attention to anatomy are still critical elements of treating recurrent disease. Progressive extension with external fixators may help to prevent the recurrence of PIPJ flexion contractures. Adjuvant treatment may offer further potential for patients with Dupuytren's diathesis.

CLINICS CARE POINTS

- Although dermatofasciectomy has not been proven to reduce the recurrence of Dupuytren disease, skin grafting remains an important element of management of severe, recurrent contracture.

- Patients should understand the risk of recurrence of PIPJ contractures. Volar plate release, postoperative therapy and splinting, and external fixators may help to reduce the risk of recurrence.

- Adjuvant treatment including radiation and pharmacotherapy may have a role in preventing the progression of Dupuytren disease.

DISCLOSURE

Dr J. Putnam has nothing to disclose.

REFERENCES

1. Black EM, Blazar PE. Dupuytren disease: an evolving understanding of an age-old disease. J Am Acad Orthop Surg 2011;19(12):746–57.
2. Hu FZ, Nystrom A, Ahmed A, et al. Mapping of an autosomal dominant gene for Dupuytren's contracture to chromosome 16q in a Swedish family. Clin Genet 2005;68(5):424–9.
3. Shih B, Wijeratne D, Armstrong DJ, et al. Identification of biomarkers in Dupuytren's disease by comparative analysis of fibroblasts versus tissue biopsies in disease-specific phenotypes. J Hand Surg 2009;34(1):124–36.
4. Satish L, LaFramboise WA, O'Gorman DB, et al. Identification of differentially expressed genes in fibroblasts derived from patients with Dupuytren's Contracture. BMC Med Genomics 2008;1:10.
5. Reilly RM, Stern PJ, Goldfarb CA. A retrospective review of the management of Dupuytren's nodules. J Hand Surg 2005;30(5):1014–8.
6. Lanting R, van den Heuvel ER, Westerink B, et al. Prevalence of Dupuytren disease in The Netherlands. Plast Reconstr Surg 2013;132(2):394–403.
7. Anthony SG, Lozano-Calderon SA, Simmons BP, et al. Gender ratio of Dupuytren's disease in the modern U.S. population. Hand N Y N 2008;3(2):87–90.
8. Burke FD, Proud G, Lawson IJ, et al. An assessment of the effects of exposure to vibration, smoking, alcohol and diabetes on the prevalence of Dupuytren's disease in 97,537 miners. J Hand Surg Eur 2007;32(4):400–6.
9. Hindocha S, Stanley JK, Watson S, et al. Dupuytren's diathesis revisited: Evaluation of prognostic indicators for risk of disease recurrence. J Hand Surg 2006;31(10):1626–34.
10. Dias JJ, Braybrooke J. Dupuytren's contracture: an audit of the outcomes of surgery. J Hand Surg Edinb Scotl 2006;31(5):514–21.
11. Stewart BD, Nascimento AF. Palmar and plantar fibromatosis: a review. J Pathol Transl Med 2021;55(4):265–70.
12. Ketchum LD, Donahue TK. The injection of nodules of Dupuytren's disease with triamcinolone acetonide. J Hand Surg 2000;25(6):1157–62.
13. Yin CY, Yu HHM, Wang JP, et al. Long-term follow-up of Dupuytren disease after injection of triamcinolone acetonide in Chinese patients in Taiwan. J Hand Surg Eur 2017;42(7):678–82.
14. Hueston JT. Table top test. Med J Aust 1976;2(5):189–90.
15. Diaz R, Curtin C. Needle aponeurotomy for the treatment of Dupuytren's disease. Hand Clin 2014;30(1):33–8.
16. Strömberg J, Ibsen Sörensen A, Fridén J. Percutaneous Needle Fasciotomy Versus Collagenase Treatment for Dupuytren Contracture: A Randomized Controlled Trial with a Two-Year Follow-up. J Bone Joint Surg Am 2018;100(13):1079–86.
17. van Rijssen AL, Ter Linden H, Werker PMN. Five-year results of a randomized clinical trial on treatment in Dupuytren's disease: percutaneous needle fasciotomy versus limited fasciectomy. Plast Reconstr Surg 2012;129(2):469–77.

18. Leafblad ND, Wagner E, Wanderman NR, et al. Outcomes and Direct Costs of Needle Aponeurotomy, Collagenase Injection, and Fasciectomy in the Treatment of Dupuytren Contracture. J Hand Surg 2019; 44(11):919–27.

19. Herrera FA, Mitchell S, Elzik M, et al. Modified percutaneous needle aponeurotomy for the treatment of dupuytren's contracture: early results and complications. Hand N Y N 2015;10(3):433–7.

20. Krefter C, Marks M, Hensler S, et al. Complications after treating Dupuytren's disease. A systematic literature review. Hand Surg Rehabil 2017;36(5):322–9.

21. Badalamente MA, Hurst LC, Benhaim P, et al. Efficacy and safety of collagenase clostridium histolyticum in the treatment of proximal interphalangeal joints in dupuytren contracture: combined analysis of 4 phase 3 clinical trials. J Hand Surg 2015; 40(5):975–83.

22. Peimer CA, Blazar P, Coleman S, et al. Dupuytren Contracture Recurrence Following Treatment With Collagenase Clostridium histolyticum (CORDLESS [Collagenase Option for Reduction of Dupuytren Long-Term Evaluation of Safety Study]): 5-Year Data. J Hand Surg 2015;40(8):1597–605.

23. David M, Smith G, Pinder R, et al. Outcomes and Early Recurrence Following Enzymatic (Collagenase) Treatment of Moderate and Severe Dupuytren Contractures. J Hand Surg 2020;45(12):1187.e1-11.

24. Skov ST, Bisgaard T, Søndergaard P, et al. Injectable Collagenase Versus Percutaneous Needle Fasciotomy for Dupuytren Contracture in Proximal Interphalangeal Joints: A Randomized Controlled Trial. J Hand Surg 2017;42(5):321–8.e3.

25. Scherman P, Jenmalm P, Dahlin LB. Three-year recurrence of Dupuytren's contracture after needle fasciotomy and collagenase injection: a two-centre randomized controlled trial. J Hand Surg Eur 2018; 43(8):836–40.

26. Citron ND, Nunez V. Recurrence after surgery for Dupuytren's disease: a randomized trial of two skin incisions. J Hand Surg Edinb Scotl 2005;30(6): 563–6.

27. Lesiak AC, Jarrett NJ, Imbriglia JE. Modified McCash Technique for Management of Dupuytren Contracture. J Hand Surg Am 2017;42(5):395.e1–5.

28. Hozack BA, Rayan GM. Surgical Treatment for Recurrent Dupuytren Disease. Hand N Y N 2021. 15589447211060448.

29. Ullah AS, Dias JJ, Bhowal B. Does a "firebreak" full-thickness skin graft prevent recurrence after surgery for Dupuytren's contracture?: a prospective, randomised trial. J Bone Joint Surg Br 2009;91(3):374–8.

30. McCann BG, Logan A, Belcher H, et al. The presence of myofibroblasts in the dermis of patients with Dupuytren's contracture. A possible source for recurrence. J Hand Surg Edinb Scotl 1993;18(5): 656–61.

31. Hay DC, Louie DL, Earp BE, et al. Surgical findings in the treatment of Dupuytren's disease after initial treatment with clostridial collagenase (Xiaflex). J Hand Surg Eur 2014;39(5):463–5.

32. Misra S, Wilkens SC, Chen NC, et al. Patients Transferred for Upper Extremity Amputation: Participation of Regional Trauma Centers. J Hand Surg 2017; 42(12):987–95.

33. Murphy A, Lalonde DH, Eaton C, et al. Minimally invasive options in Dupuytren's contracture: aponeurotomy, enzymes, stretching, and fat grafting. Plast Reconstr Surg 2014;134(5):822e–9e.

34. Craft RO, Smith AA, Coakley B, et al. Preliminary soft-tissue distraction versus checkrein ligament release after fasciectomy in the treatment of dupuytren proximal interphalangeal joint contractures. Plast Reconstr Surg 2011;128(5):1107–13.

35. Agee JM, Goss BC. The use of skeletal extension torque in reversing Dupuytren contractures of the proximal interphalangeal joint. J Hand Surg 2012; 37(7):1467–74.

36. Watson HK, Lovallo JL. Salvage of severe recurrent Dupuytren's contracture of the ring and small fingers. J Hand Surg 1987;12(2):287–9.

37. Pillukat T, Walle L, Stüber R, et al. [Treatment of recurrent Dupuytren's disease]. Orthopä 2017; 46(4):342–52.

38. Denkler K. Surgical complications associated with fasciectomy for dupuytren's disease: a 20-year review of the English literature. Eplasty 2010;10:e15.

39. Noland SS, Paul AW, Pflibsen LR, et al. The Effect of Anticoagulation on the Treatment of Dupuytren Contracture with Collagenase. Plast Reconstr Surg 2022;149(5):914e–20e.

40. Foucher G, Cornil C, Lenoble E. ["Open palm" technique in Dupuytren's disease. Postoperative complications and results after more than 5 years]. Chir Memoires Acad Chir 1992;118(4):189–94 [discussion: 195-196].

41. Cheung K, Walley KC, Rozental TD. Management of complications of Dupuytren contracture. Hand Clin 2015;31(2):345–54.

42. Kuhlmann JN, Boabighi A, Guero S, et al. Boutonniere deformity in Dupuytren's disease. J Hand Surg Edinb Scotl 1988;13(4):379–82.

43. Boyce DE, Tonkin MA. Dorsal Dupuytren's disease causing a swan-neck deformity. J Hand Surg Edinb Scotl 2004;29(6):636–7.

44. Rochlin DH, Sheckter CC, Satteson ES, et al. Separating Fact From Fiction: A Nationwide Longitudinal Examination of Complex Regional Pain Syndrome Following Treatment of Dupuytren Contracture. Hand N Y N 2020. https://doi.org/10.1177/1558944720963915. 1558944720963915.

45. Nissenbaum M, Kleinert HE. Treatment considerations in carpal tunnel syndrome with coexistent Dupuytren's disease. J Hand Surg 1980;5(6):544–7.

Advanced Dupuytren Contracture

46. Lilly SI, Stern PJ. Simultaneous carpal tunnel release and Dupuytren's fasciectomy. J Hand Surg 2010; 35(5):754–9.
47. Werker PMN, Degreef I. Alternative and Adjunctive Treatments for Dupuytren Disease. Hand Clin 2018;34(3):367–75.
48. Seegenschmiedt MH, Olschewski T, Guntrum F. Radiotherapy optimization in early-stage Dupuytren's contracture: first results of a randomized clinical study. Int J Radiat Oncol Biol Phys 2001;49(3): 785–98.
49. Betz N, Ott OJ, Adamietz B, et al. Radiotherapy in early-stage Dupuytren's contracture. Long-term results after 13 years. Strahlenther Onkol Organ Dtsch Rontgengesellschaft Al 2010;186(2):82–90.
50. Kadhum M, Smock E, Khan A, et al. Radiotherapy in Dupuytren's disease: a systematic review of the evidence. J Hand Surg Eur 2017;42(7):689–92.
51. Verjee LS, Verhoekx JSN, Chan JKK, et al. Unraveling the signaling pathways promoting fibrosis in Dupuytren's disease reveals TNF as a therapeutic target. Proc Natl Acad Sci U S A 2013;110(10): E928–37.
52. Png ME, Dritsaki M, Gray A, et al. Economic evaluation plan of a randomised controlled trial of intranodular injection of anti-TNF and placebo among patients with early Dupuytren's disease: Repurposing Anti-TNF for Treating Dupuytren's Disease (RIDD). Wellcome Open Res 2018;3:156.
53. Degreef I, Tejpar S, Sciot R, et al. High-dosage tamoxifen as neoadjuvant treatment in minimally invasive surgery for Dupuytren disease in patients with a strong predisposition toward fibrosis: a randomized controlled trial. J Bone Joint Surg Am 2014;96(8):655–62.

Infection Management for the Hand Surgeon

Victor King, MD[a], Nisha Crouser, MD[b], Amy Speeckaert, MD[b], Reena Bhatt, MD[c],*

KEYWORDS

- Hand infection • Flexor tenosynovitis • Septic arthritis • Osteomyelitis • Atypical pathogens

KEY POINTS

- It is important to consider underlying osteomyelitis in soft-tissue infections that are not responding to antibiotic management.
- Necrotizing infections of the extremity are most commonly secondary to polymicrobial infections (aerobic and anaerobic bacteria) or monomicrobial infections (Group A B-hemolytic *Streptococcus*, atypical bacteria such as *Vibrio vulnificus*).
- Atypical hand infections can be caused by various fungi, mycobacteria, and viruses that may not respond to standard treatments.
- Patients with immunocompromise secondary to immunosuppressive treatment, diabetes, or human immunodeficiency virus are more susceptible to common and atypical hand infections and have increased morbidity and mortality.

INTRODUCTION

Hand surgeons are frequently asked to manage complex infections caused by a number of insults, including trauma, adjacent spread, surgery, and systemic bacteremia. Once the acute infection is cleared, the transient and at times permanent sequelae can be equally challenging to manage. These include pain, numbness, stiffness, need for amputation, and loss of function. Critical in the treatment of hand infections is early diagnosis, timely surgical debridement, foreign body and necrotic tissue removal, and appropriate antibiotic coverage. Patients with a history of intravenous drug abuse, chronic diseases such as diabetes and chronic kidney disease, and immunocompromised state lend additional complexity for infection management.

DISCUSSION
Pyogenic Flexor Tenosynovitis

Pyogenic flexor tenosynovitis (PFT) is an infection within the flexor tendon sheath of the fingers or thumb. The most frequent etiology is traumatic inoculation of bacteria into the closed sheath. The relatively avascular and closed environment of the sheath allows the infection to spread while going unrecognized by the host's immune system. Proximally the flexor tendon sheaths communicate with the radial, ulnar, and palmar bursa, which, in turn, communicate with Parona's space. This communication allows for rapid progression of the infection throughout the hand and wrist.[1] Prompt diagnosis, therefore, remains imperative to prevent worsening infection both locally and systemically.

Although *Staphylococcus aureus* accounts for 80% of organisms cultured from PFT, it is important to recognize that broad-spectrum antibiotic coverage may be required until final cultures result. For example, the incidence of methicillin-resistant *Staphylococcus aureus* in PFT is increasing in recent years, and immunocompromised patients are at risk of atypical infections from organisms such as *Streptococcus mitis*, a strain of *Streptococcus*

a Division of Plastic Surgery, Warren Alpert Medical School fo Brown University, Coop Suite 500, 2 Dudley Street, Providence, RI 02905; b Hand & Upper Extremity Center, Wexner Medical Center, The Ohio State University, 915 Olentangy River Road, Suite 3200, Columbus, OH 43212, USA; c Division of Plastic Surgery, Warren Alpert Medical School fo Brown University, 235 Plain Street, Suite 203, Providence, RI 02905
* Corresponding author.
E-mail address: reena.bhatt.md@gmail.com

Hand Clin 39 (2023) 465–473
https://doi.org/10.1016/j.hcl.2023.04.003
0749-0712/23/Published by Elsevier Inc.

viridans.[2,3] Wounds sustained in the marine environment place patients at risk of infections from *Mycobacterium marinum* and *Shewanella algae.*[4,5]

Although antibiotics may successfully treat some early PFT, surgical management remains the mainstay of treatment.[6] Although there are many techniques described, they all result in opening and irrigating the flexor retinaculum. If there is any suspicion of associated septic arthritis, capsulotomies of the involved joints should be performed, and the joints should be irrigated. In addition, if there is any concern for proximal spread, the palm and or Parona's space should be opened and thoroughly irrigated and debrided. Due to the challenging nature of PFT, some recommend postoperative continuous irrigation of the sheath.[7]

Even when PFT is recognized and treated in a timely manner, it has a complication rate of 38%. These complications include stiffness, persistent infection, and amputation.[8] Pang and colleagues[9] reported a 17% amputation rate in patients presenting with PFT. Persistent infection can be due to a number of issues: persistent soft-tissue infection (locally or proximally) or involvement of a nearby bone or joint. Persistent infection warrants a thorough physical examination to evaluate the bones, joints, and soft tissues. Repeat surgical debridement is indicated if any suspicion of deep infection remains. Advanced imaging, such as a computed tomography scan or magnetic resonance imaging with and without contrast may aid in the diagnosis of deep space infection or osteomyelitis.

Pang and colleagues identified risk factors associated with poor outcomes in patients diagnosed with PFT.[9] They found the following to be associated with a poor outcome: age greater than 43 years; the presence of diabetes mellitus (DM), peripheral vascular disease, or renal failure; the presence of subcutaneous purulence; digital ischemia; and polymicrobial infection.[9] Although all patients with PFT should be treated promptly, patients who have these characteristics and/or comorbidities should also be warned of their elevated risk of poor outcome, including amputation.

Deep Hand Space Infections

Deep hand space infections spread throughout and between defined potential spaces of the hand: the thenar, midpalmar, hypothenar, interdigital subfascial web, dorsal subaponeurotic, and Parona's space. Deep space infections may develop as the result of direct inoculation from penetrating trauma to the defined space or from extension of an adjacent structure infection (such as an index flexor sheath infection). The closed

nature of these spaces leads to deep abscess formation that require urgent surgical decompression and debridement.

Thenar infections can occur secondary to spread of thumb, index, or long finger flexor sheath infections or via direct inoculation, while midpalmar infections can occur secondary to spread from long, ring, or small flexor sheath infections or direct inoculation. The hypothenar space does not communicate with the flexor sheaths.

The thenar space is separated ulnarly from the midpalmar space by the midpalmar septum extending from the long metacarpal volar diaphysis to the palmar fascia. The thenar space is bordered dorsally by the adductor pollicis muscle, index, and long metacarpals; palmarly by the index finger flexor tendon and palmar fascia; radially by the adductor insertion and thenar muscle fascia. On examination, a thenar space abscess presents with swelling, an abducted thumb, tenderness over the thenar eminence and first webspace, and pain elicited with passive adduction of the thumb. Drainage approaches may require both volar and dorsal incisions.[10]

The midpalmar space is bordered dorsally by the long, ring, and small metacarpals and second and third palmar interossei and volarly by the long, ring, small flexor tendons and lumbricals. The midpalmar oblique septum is the radial border; the hypothenar septum is the ulnar border. A midpalmar space infection can develop through a direct penetrating injury or from spread of a long/ring/small-finger flexor sheath infection. Patients will present with swelling both volarly and dorsally, while the long through small fingers are often in a flexed position with pain on passive extension of the same digits (**Fig. 1**).[10]

The hypothenar space is bordered radially by the hypothenar septum extending from the small metacarpal, bordered dorsally by the fifth metacarpal and hypothenar muscle fascia, and the volar borders are the superficial hypothenar muscle fascia and palmar fascia. These are not common infections, and the flexor tendons are not involved. Patients usually have swelling and pain elicited at the hypothenar region.[10]

Parona's space is the potential space in the volar wrist located deep to the digital flexors and superficial to the pronator quadratus. Infections of Parona's space can occur with an infection that has spread proximally from the radial or ulnar bursa or, less commonly, from direct inoculation. The radial bursa is contiguous with the flexor pollicis longus tendon sheath starting at the level of the metacarpophalangeal joint extending to the carpal tunnel. The ulnar bursa commences at the proximal aspect of the flexor tendon sheath of

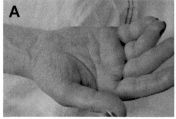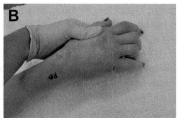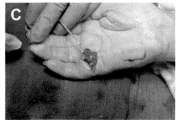

Fig. 1. A 59-year-old female with catbite infection with flexor tenosynovitis of the small finger with hypothenar involvement with subsequent spread to the midpalmar deep space. (*A-B*) Initial presentation. (*C*) After small finger washout with midpalmar and hypothenar involvement.

the small finger, continuing to the carpal tunnel. Infection can propagate from either bursa by rupture into Parona's space. Communication between the two bursae can occur within Parona's space, when the infection spreads and ascends along the bursa on the opposite side is called a horseshoe abscess. Patients traditionally present with signs of flexor tenosynovitis of the thumb or small finger with associated swelling and tenderness in the volar wrist. There may be numbness and tingling in the median nerve distribution as well.[11]

The dorsal subaponeurotic space is deep to the extensor tendons and superficial to the fascia of the interosseous muscles and periosteum of the metacarpals. Penetrating trauma to this space often is the culprit for inoculation. Patients traditionally present with dorsal hand swelling and erythema and difficulty with finger extension. Dorsal subcutaneous space infections have similar appearance and causes.[10]

Collar button abscesses are hourglass-shaped infections within the distal palm and webspaces. Often a result of inoculation through a fissure or callus, the infection tracts dorsally, away from the strong glabrous skin of the palm and underlying palmar fascia, tracking distal to the bifurcation of the common digital neurovascular bundles and intermetacarpal ligament. Patients present with redness, edema, induration at the webspace, and the adjacent fingers often sit in abduction.[11]

Bone and Joint Infections

Septic arthritis of the hand and wrist is a surgical emergency. Infection typically occurs as the result of hematogenous spread, direct trauma, or spread from adjacent tissue (such as postoperative infections). Infection within the joint can cause chondrolysis as early as 8 hours after infection with the potential for long-term joint damage.[12] In certain scenarios with a known contaminant, such as a fight bite injury (*Eikenella* inoculation), the concern for underlying infection is heightened

(**Fig. 2**). Meanwhile, in many cases, patients may present with atraumatic joint inflammation, wherein crystalline arthropathy and rheumatologic disease remain high on the differential diagnosis. Early joint aspiration is imperative in diagnosis, yet this becomes difficult in the hand where aspiration is technically challenging and may not yield significant fluid for analysis. If fluid is limited, cell count has been found to have the highest diagnostic yield with >50,000 white blood cells and greater than 75% polymorphonuclear leukocytes being diagnostic.[13] Surgical drainage is the mainstay of treatment, preferably within 16 hours of

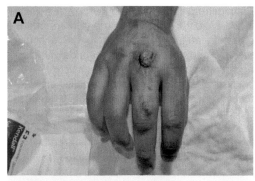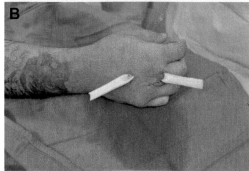

Fig. 2. Fight bite injury to the middle finger metacarpophalangeal joint with subsequent septic arthritis. (*A*) Clinical photograph of wound with associated soft-tissue swelling. (*B*) Status after irrigation and debridement with placement of penrose drain.

diagnosis. Both open and arthroscopic debridement are reasonable options with arthroscopic treatment having comparable results to open treatment for the wrist.[12,14]

Osteomyelitis of the hand is relatively uncommon, yet it is associated with significant morbidity. Amputation rates have been cited as high as 40%, with increased rates in patients with delayed presentation. Infection occurs generally from direct inoculation (trauma, surgery, or open fracture) or spread from adjacent tissue (such as from an abscess, septic arthritis, or tenosynovitis). Given the close proximity of the subcutaneous tissue to the bone throughout the hand, there is potential for chronic or untreated superficial infections to result in osteomyelitis. For example, felons in the acute or chronic setting can cause osteomyelitis of the distal phalanx.[13] The most common location for osteomyelitis in the hand is the distal phalanx (approximately 38% of all cases) (**Fig. 3**) followed by the proximal phalanx and metacarpal.[15] It is important to consider underlying osteomyelitis in soft-tissue infections that are not responding to antibiotic management. For example, chronic paronychia or nonhealing wounds in the hand can be a sign of underlying osteomyelitis. The mainstay of treatment for osteomyelitis is a combination of antibiotic and surgical management. Pathogen-specific antibiotic therapy for 4-6 weeks is the typical treatment. Surgery is important for obtaining culture specimens to guide antibiotic therapy and to adequately debride infected or necrotic tissue.[16]

Surgical site infections, specifically hardware infections, pose yet another challenge. Given the formation of biofilms on hardware, the potential for eradication of infection without removal of retained hardware is low. Yet the decision to remove hardware in the case of fracture fixation or surgical reconstruction is not always straight forward and requires a close evaluation of overall fracture stability. Studies have shown fracture union rates as high as 70%, with retention of implants in the setting of deep infection. Therefore, the argument can be made to treat deep infections with suppressive antibiotics while maintaining hardware until the fracture has healed. Once the fracture has healed, the hardware should be removed given the high probability of retained biofilm.[13,15]

Necrotizing Soft-tissue Infection

Necrotizing soft-tissue infection (NSTI) is a spectrum of diseases ranging from severe and rapidly spreading cutaneous and subcutaneous necrosis to necrosis of the underlying fascia and muscle with signs of septic shock. It is associated with a 50% misdiagnosis rate, high morbidity, and mortality of up to 30%.[17] Sequelae of NSTI in the upper extremity includes major disability and an amputation rate of 25%–37.5%.[18] It is principally a clinical diagnosis with symptoms of pain out of proportion and signs of edema, erythema, bullae, necrosis, tenderness (which often extends beyond the region where local signs are present), crepitus, and systemic signs. Necrotizing infections of the extremity are most commonly secondary to polymicrobial infections (aerobic and anaerobic bacteria) or monomicrobial infections (Group A B-hemolytic *Streptococcus*, atypical bacteria such as *Vibrio vulnificus*).

The Laboratory Risk Indicator for Necrotizing infection score (**Table 1**) was developed to predict the presence of NSTI, but a low score should not be used to rule out NSTI because of poor diagnostic accuracy, especially for *Vibrio* infections. Imaging may reveal subcutaneous emphysema, stranding, fluid collections, and thickened fascia but should never delay intervention. Invasive diagnosis includes fascial biopsy and the finger test, with fascial biopsy limited in practice due to practicality. The finger test may be performed under local anesthetic with a small incision, where minimal resistance to finger dissection at the level of the superficial fascia represents a positive test. Other findings such as "dishwater fluid," absence of bleeding, and tissue necrosis all suggest presence of NSTI.[17] Early suspicion and diagnosis followed by emergent surgical debridement and broad-spectrum antibiotic treatment are imperative to prevent rapid spread.

All NSTIs require a prompt surgical intervention, including incision and debridement of all necrotic and nonviable tissue. Initial empiric antibiotic therapy should be broad spectrum to cover gram-positive, gram-negative, and anaerobic organisms as it is impossible to exclude polymicrobial infections. Antibiotics should be administered within 1 hour of initial presentation. Cultures and tissue samples should be taken to assist with identification of the causative pathogen and tailoring of antimicrobial therapy. Mortality is significantly decreased in patients receiving surgical treatment within 6 hours of presentation versus more than 6 hours after presentation, with early surgical debridement being the most important determinant of outcomes.[17] Re-exploration and additional debridement should be performed 12-24 hours after the initial debridement and continued until the wound bed is healthy and without signs of pathologic progression (**Fig. 4**). Recent data suggest the strongest risk factors for infection persistence may be related to the tissues involved. Infections involving deeper tissues such as fascia, tendon,

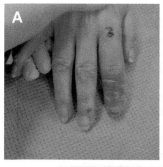
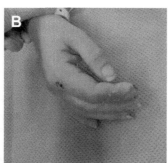
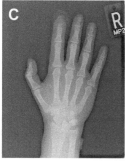
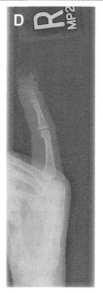

Fig. 3. Osteomyelitis of the index finger distal phalanx. (*A*) and (*B*) Clinical photographs of erythema and swelling of distal phalanx with associated skin changes. (*C*) Anteroposterior and (*D*) lateral radiographs of bony erosion of the distal phalanx associated with osteomyelitis.

bone, and joints are more likely to persist and require additional debridement for source control, with involvement of the fascia being the strongest predictor.[19] Wound management after source control includes dressing changes, negative pressure wound therapy, and reconstructive techniques from all rungs on the reconstructive ladder.

Atypical Pathogens

Atypical infections of the hand are rare and often pose a diagnostic challenge given their indolent, nonspecific presentation and need for special testing, which can lead to delays in treatment. Fungi, mycobacteria, and viruses can have various presentations ranging from cutaneous to deep infections in the hand.[20] Atypical pathogens should be considered when presumed typical hand infections are not responding to treatment.

The most common fungal infections affecting the hand are cutaneous and subcutaneous infections. Chronic paronychia is typically seen in patients that soak their hands often. The primary cause is *Candida albicans* (70–80%), although

secondary infection with *Pseudomonas aeruginosa* can occur which causes a green discoloration of the nail plate. Initial treatment involves application of topical clotrimazole, and oral antifungals can be used as well, although with limited success (approximately 40% resolution). Surgical treatment involves marsupialization of the affected nail fold.[21] *Sporotrichosis*, another fungal infection, is associated with agricultural activities and typically presents as an infected wound followed by lymphocutaneous spread. Although rare, deep infections are also possible with involvement of the wrist, hand, bursa, and tenosynovium. Superficial *Sporotrichosis* infections are treated with itraconazole, while deep infections often require surgical debridement in addition to antifungal therapy.[20,21]

Deep fungal infections are rare; however, it is important to be aware of the various etiologies given their need for multidisciplinary treatment. These infections are typically seen in immunocompromised hosts and, therefore, have a poor prognosis. Histoplasmosis, invasive aspergillosis, coccidiomycosis, mucormycosis, and deep

Table 1
Laboratory Risk Indicator for Necrotizing Fasciitis (LRINEC) score

Variable	Score
C-reactive protein (mg L)	
<150	0
150 or more	4
Total white cell count (per mm³)	
<15	0
15–25	1
>25	2
Hemoglobin (g/dL)	
>13.5	0
11–13.5	1
<11	2
Sodium (mmol/L)	
135 or more	0
<135	2
Creatinine (μmol/L)	
141 or less	0
> 41	2
Glucose (mmol/L)	
10 or less	0
>10	1

The maximum score is 13. A score of ≥6 should raise the suspicion of necrotizing fasciitis, and a score of ≥8 is strongly predictive of this disease.

From Wong CH, Wang YS. The diagnosis of necrotizing fasciitis. Curr Opin Infect Dis. 2005;18(2):101-106; with permission.

candidiasis are all causative agents of deep space hand infections. Often multiple surgical debridements or amputation are necessary to eradicate these deep fungal infections.[22]

Mycobacteria are gram-positive bacilli with a hydrophilic cell wall that pose a challenge to antibiotic treatment. *Mycobacterium marinum* is the most common cause of mycobacterial hand infections accounting for 40-80% of cases. Patients typically have a history of exposure to contaminated water or fish and may present with cutaneous lesions with granulomatous inflammation or deeper involvement with tenosynovitis. Culture is the gold standard; however, there is poor sensitivity, thus immunohistochemistry and polymerase chain reaction are recommended. Superficial infections can be treated with antibiotics while consideration for surgical debridement for deep infections may allow for better antimicrobial penetration and improved outcomes.[23] *Mycobacterium avium* complex is the second most common cause of mycobacteria hand infections. It typically presents

in immunocompromised patients with pulmonary manifestations but can also lead to soft-tissue infection of the hands.[20]

Mycobacterium tuberculosis (TB) of the hand, unlike systemic tuberculosis, may present with isolated hand involvement. It can cause a very wide range of presentations including cutaneous infections, tenosynovitis, osteomyelitis, bursitis, and septic arthritis, acting as a great mimicker of other common etiologies. Tenosynovitis is the most common presentation. Rice bodies, which are live bacteria found within the synovium, are the characteristic intraoperative finding. TB can be a diagnostic challenge, and advanced imaging and surgical biopsy are often needed for diagnosis. Acid fast staining is required for diagnosis, and pathologic specimens will demonstrate caseating granulomas. Tzanck smears can be diagnostic but often take 3-6 months to become positive. Treatment with multidrug therapy and surgical debridement is the gold standard.[23] It should be noted that steroids can cause exacerbation of disease progression in the setting of TB.[20]

Viral infections of the hand are typically self-limited and less severe. Herpetic whitlow caused by the Herpes simplex virus 1 or 2 is characterized by clear vesicular lesions that develop on a single digit after minor trauma. The lesions may coalesce and appear similar to a felon or paronychia; however, unlike a felon, they do not cause swelling of the digital pulp. The lesions usually self-resolve over 3 weeks. It is important to avoid surgical

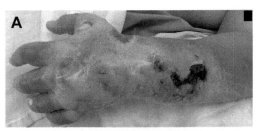
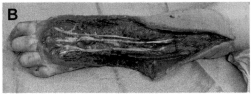

Fig. 4. Rapidly progressing necrotizing soft-tissue infection in 47-year-old male sustaining a dorsal hand abrasion 5 days before presentation. Despite immediate operative intervention and no cutaneous or clinical signs above the elbow on presentation, circumferential involvement of the hand, forearm, and upper arm necessitated subsequent transhumeral amputation (*A* initial, *B* after debridement).

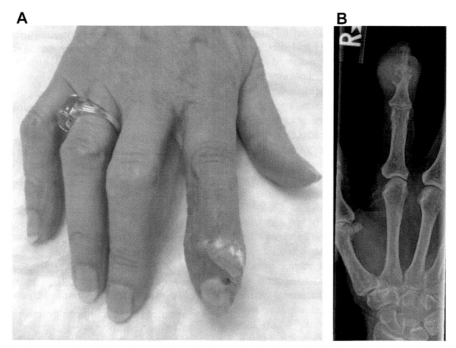

Fig. 5. Clinical examination (*A*) and x-ray (*B*) evaluation of articular gouty destruction in the right index finger.

drainage of the lesions given the risk of secondary bacterial infection.[20]

Complicating Factors

Not all dolor, calor, and rubor equates infection. One must approach these symptoms and signs keeping in mind other differential diagnoses that may mimic infection. The usual presentation of acute monoarticular arthritis, and more rarely tenosynovitis associated with gout and pseudogout, may be differentiated clinically by the absence of lymphangitis and microorganisms on aspiration. Gouty tophi may ulcerate and erupt through the skin with associated inflammation and drainage mimicking abscess (**Fig. 5**). The presence of crystals on microscopic examination remains the gold standard for diagnosis.[24] The constellation of polyarticular involvement, erosions on imaging, and

lack of more common signs of infection such as cellulitis and lymphangitis can aid in distinguishing crystalline arthropathy from infection.[24,25] Psoriatic arthritis can also mimic infection. Dactylitis, or the classic "sausage"-shaped finger, is seen in up to half of patients with psoriatic arthritis. Fusiform edema in multiple digits at baseline can make superimposed infection a challenge. Cutaneous psoriasis, oligoarticular disease, nail pitting, onycholysis, and pencil in cup deformity on plain films are also helpful in clinching the diagnosis of psoriatic arthritis rather than acute infection.[25]

Many comorbid conditions add complexity to management of hand and upper-extremity infections. Immunocompromised patients are more susceptible to infection and carry an increased morbidity and mortality when compared with immunocompetent hosts. Human immunodeficiency

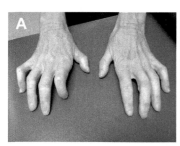
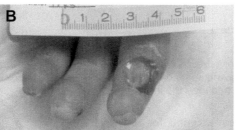
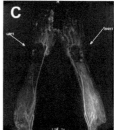

Fig. 6. Patient with scleroderma and sclerodactyly (*A*) and deep ulceration of soft-tissue in the index finger (*B*). Magnetic resonance imaging (*C*) demonstrates ulnar artery occlusion bilaterally at the level of the forearms.

virus (HIV) leads to a decreased immunocompetency from viral destruction of CD4 cells. Patients with HIV are at an increased risk of hand infections, as well as need for surgical intervention and longer hospital stays.[26] The increased susceptibility of patients suffering from DM is multifactorial, including hypoglycemic neutrophil dysfunction, associated vascular disease, and peripheral neuropathy. This increased susceptibility in DM patients also comes with an increased risk of osteomyelitis, septic arthritis, NSTI, need for repeat drainage, persistent infection, and amputation.[19,27] Patients on immunosuppressive therapy, such as transplant recipients, and patients with rheumatologic conditions, such as scleroderma, are at increased risk of soft-tissue infections in the upper extremity.[26] The complex interplay of immune system dysfunction, sclerotic skin, and vasculopathy in patients with scleroderma or systemic sclerosis (SSc) can lead to ulcerations and arterial occlusions and poor peripheral vascularity. For example, ulnar artery occlusion can lead to finger ischemia and ulcerations, which can become infected and require amputation (**Fig. 6**). One study found that infection was present in 37.8% of SSc patients with digital ulcerations, with the prevalence of osteomyelitis reported as 7.7%.[28]

SUMMARY

nfections of the upper extremity can be challenging to diagnose and treat because of the complex anatomy and range of offending pathogens. Early recognition of infections that require emergent surgical intervention, such as necrotizing fasciitis and septic joints, is imperative for good clinical outcomes. In addition, prompt diagnosis and intervention for deep closed space infections, such as deep abscesses or flexor tenosynovitis, is necessary to avoid chronic pain and dysfunction. Complicating factors such as underlying osteomyelitis, atypical pathogens, and immunocompromised states of patients should always be considered when treating upper-extremity infections.

CLINICS CARE POINTS

- For pyogenic flexor sheath tenosynovitis (PFT), the relatively avascular and closed environment of the sheath allows the infection to spread
- *Staphylococcus aureus* accounts for 80% of organisms cultured from PFT; however, broad-spectrum antibiotics should be used until cultures available.

- Deep hand space infections spread throughout and between defined potential spaces of the hand: thenar, midpalmar, hypothenar, interdigital subfascial web, dorsal subaponeurotic, and Parona's space.
- Infection within the joint can cause chondrolysis as early as 8 hours after infection with the potential for long-term joint damage.
- It is important to consider underlying osteomyelitis in soft-tissue infections that are not responding to antibiotic management.
- Necrotizing infections of the extremity are most commonly secondary to polymicrobial infections (aerobic and anaerobic bacteria) or monomicrobial infections (Group A *B*-hemolytic *Streptococcus*, atypical bacteria such as *Vibrio vulnificus*).
- Atypical hand infections can be caused by various fungi, mycobacteria, and viruses that may not respond to standard treatments.
- Patients with immunocompromise secondary to immunosuppressive treatment, diabetes, or human immunodeficiency virus are more susceptible to common and atypical hand infections and have increased morbidity and mortality.

DISCLOSURE

The authors have no financial disclosures.

REFERENCES

1. Doyle JR. Anatomy of the finger flexor tendon sheath and pulley system. J Hand Surg 1988;13(4):473–84.
2. O'Malley M, Fowler J, Ilyas AM. Community-acquired methicillin-resistant staphylococcus aureus infections of the hand: prevalence and timeliness of treatment. J Hand Surg 2009;34(3):504–8.
3. Bingol UA, Ulucay C, Ozler T. An unusual cause of flexor tenosynovitis: streptococcus mitis. Plast Reconstr Surg Glob Open 2014;2(12):e263.
4. Lopez CA, Magee CA, Belyea CC, Gumboc LR. Finger flexor tenosynovitis from stonefish envenomation injury. JAAOS Global Research & Reviews 2019;3(5):e024.
5. Fluke EC, Carayannopoulos NL, Lindsey RW. Pyogenic flexor tenosynovitis caused by shewanella algae. J Hand Surg 2016;41(7):e203–6.
6. Bolton LE, Bainbridge C. Current opinions regarding the management of pyogenic flexor tenosynovitis: a survey of Pulvertaft Hand Trauma Symposium attendees. Infection 2019;47(2):225–31.
7. Neviaser RJ. Closed tendon sheath irrigation for pyogenic flexor tenosynovitis. J Hand Surg 1978; 3(5):462–6.

8. Stern PJ, Staneck JL, McDonough JJ, et al. Established hand infections: a controlled, prospective study. J Hand Surg 1983;8(5, Part 1):553–9.

9. Pang H-N, Teoh L-C, Yam A, et al. Factors affecting the prognosis of pyogenic flexor tenosynovitis. J Bone Jt Surg 2007;89(8):1742–8.

10. Rekant MS, Tarr R. Hand abscesses: volar and dorsal. Hand Clin 2020;36(3):307–12.

11. Stevanovic M, Sharpe F. Acute infections of the hand. In: Wolfe SW, Pederson WC, Kozin SH, et al, editors. Green's operative hand surgery, 2, Eighth Edition. Chicago, IL: Elsevier; 2022. p. 17–62.

12. Jennings JD, Ilyas AM. Septic arthritis of the wrist. J Am Acad Orthop Surg 2018;26(4):109–15.

13. Koshy JC, Bell B. Hand Infections. J Hand Surg Am 2019;44(1):46–54.

14. Chow EMW, Lau JKY, Liyeung LLC, et al. Functional outcome for arthroscopic treatment of septic arthritis of the wrist. J Wrist Surg 2020;9(3):190–6.

15. Pinder R, Barlow G. Osteomyelitis of the hand. J Hand Surg Eur 2016;41(4):431–40.

16. Honda H, McDonald JR. Current recommendations in the management of osteomyelitis of the hand and wrist. J Hand Surg Am 2009 Jul-Aug;34(6):1135–6.

17. Sartelli M, Coccolini F, Kluger Y, et al. WSES/GAIS/WSIS/SIS-E/AAST global clinical pathways for patients with skin and soft tissue infections. World J Emerg Surg. BioMed Central 2022;17(1):3–23.

18. La Padula S, Pensato R, Zaffiro A, et al. Necrotizing fasciitis of the upper limb: optimizing management to reduce complications. J Clin Med. Multidisciplinary Digital Publishing Institute 2022;11(8):2182.

19. Sharma K, Mull A, Friedman J, et al. Development and validation of a prognostic, risk-adjusted scoring system for operative upper-extremity infections. J Hand Surg Am 2020;45(1):9–19.

20. Chan E, Bagg M. Atypical hand infections. Orthop Clin North Am 2017;48(2):229–40.

21. Fox MP, Jacoby SM. Fungal infections of the hand. Hand Clin 2020;36(3):355–60.

22. Al-Qattan MM, Helmi AA. Chronic hand infections. J Hand Surg Am 2014;39(8):1636–45.

23. Bachoura A, Zelouf DS. Mycobacterial infections in the hand and wrist. Hand Clin 2020;36(3):387–96.

24. Perez-Ruiz F, Castillo E, Chinchilla SP, et al. Clinical manifestations and diagnosis of gout. Rheum Dis Clin North Am 2014;40(2):193–206.

25. Rida MA, Chandran V. Challenges in the clinical diagnosis of psoriatic arthritis. Clin Immunol 2020;214:108390.

26. Schmidt G, Piponov H, Chuang D, et al. Hand Infections in the immunocompromised patient: an update. J Hand Surg Am 2019;44(2):144–9.

27. Sharma K, Pan D, Friedman J, et al. Quantifying the effect of diabetes on surgical hand and forearm infections. J Hand Surg Am 2018;43(2):105–14.

28. Giuggioli D, Manfredi A, Colaci M, et al. Osteomyelitis complicating scleroderma digital ulcers. Clin Rheumatol. Springer-Verlag 2013;32(5):623.

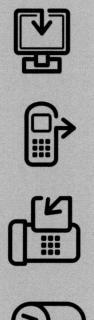